Crisis intervention
Theory and methodology

Crisis intervention
Theory and methodology

Donna C. Aguilera, Ph.D., F.A.A.N.
Consultant and Private Practice
Beverly Hills, California

and

Janice M. Messick, M.S., F.A.A.N.
Consultant
Laguna Hills, California

FIFTH EDITION

with **21** illustrations

The C. V. Mosby Company

ST. LOUIS • TORONTO • PRINCETON 1986

Editor: Nancy L. Mullins
Assistant editor: Maureen Slaten
Manuscript editor: Barbara D. Terrell
Book designer: Nancy Steinmeyer
Cover designer: John Rokusek
Production: Susan Trail

FIFTH EDITION ·

Previous editions copyrighted 1970, 1974, 1978, 1982

Printed in the United States of America

The C.V. Mosby Company
11830 Westline Industrial Drive, St. Louis, Missouri 63146

Library of Congress Cataloging in Publication Data

Aguilera, Donna C.
  Crisis intervention, theory and methodology.

  Includes index.
  1. Crisis intervention (Psychiatry) I. Messick,
Janice M. II. Title.
RC480.6.A38 1986   616.89′025   85-10612
ISBN 0-8016-0102-9

F/VH/VH 9 8 7 6 5 4 3 2   03/B/320

To
All from whom we have learned
and
all who will yet forever teach us

Foreword

In 1942 one of my close friends and colleagues lost several members of his family in the Boston holocaust known as the *Cocoanut Grove disaster*. Apart from the incredible loss and suffering of the family, that event also wrote an indelible page upon the history of American psychiatry, for it spurred Dr. Erik Lindemann of Massachusetts General Hospital to study in great detail the mourning reactions of the bereaved and to elaborate his early theories of crisis intervention. Later, his concepts were assiduously followed up and developed by our mutual friend and colleague, Dr. Gerald Caplan.

The idea of dealing immediately and vigorously with patients' acute reactions to overwhelming life situations to restore them to functional equilibrium as soon as possible began to compete with the notion of prolonged hospital care and with analytic doctrines demanding that therapists effect a thoroughgoing reorganization of personality before releasing clients to the stressful world outside the institution. Consistent with this concept, in the 1950s at Massachusetts Mental Health Center we established a "Community Extension Service," whose goals were to work with patients and their families as soon as they appeared on the waiting list; to relieve damaging feelings of anticipation, tension, and panic; and to forestall hospitalization wherever feasible. That project indeed prevented the hospitalization of a large percentage of clients who formerly would have languished on the waiting list, usually to be hospitalized and treated "as soon as the staff could get to them." Because use of the day hospital and of the halfway house as temporary way-stations enabled us to provide immediate care for all in need, eventually we were able to abolish the waiting list altogether.

At about the same time, at Boston State Hospital, Drs. Walter E. Barton and James Mann inaugurated their "Home Treatment Service," patterned after the Emergency Service developed by the pioneer Arie Querido for the city of Amsterdam. The motivating concepts of the Home Treatment Service were that it was best to treat the patient's disorder in his or her home as soon as symptoms became manifest in order not to disrupt the patient's family or community ties and to mobilize the family and all available community supports. This strategy was intended to help patients negotiate acute crises, forestall hospitalization, and prevent recurrences. But if, unfortunately, patients *had* to be hospitalized, at least they would have met the therapeutic personnel on their own turf, not in the strange hospital ward, and during home treatment they could have been oriented to the nature of the hospital's treatment program and to how they were expected to participate in it.

The times were favorable for the success of this program, the first of its kind in America. Not only was there a rising interest in crisis intervention and crisis theory, but also there existed a growing acceptance of family therapy, a great desire to find alternatives to hospitalization, an increased governmental concern with broad social issues—such as poverty, poor housing, lack of education, and racial discrimination—and a new awareness of the role of community in the genesis and treatment of mental illness. Such concerns also were apparent in reports of the first Joint Commission on Mental Illness and Health and in President John F. Kennedy's call for a "bold new approach" to the solution of the nation's problems. Interest in these social problems spawned a veritable revolution in the care and treatment of mentally ill and retarded persons.

Since the early 1960s, therefore, a whole new view of the task of psychiatry has been asserted. Psychiatrists must now think in terms of quickly restoring disabled individuals to social competence by using a public health orientation to treat defined populations; must mobilize community resources and networks on behalf of the patient; must attend to the underserved and poorly served, to minority groups, and to the poor; and also must become much more understanding of the beliefs, customs, and life-styles of hitherto more or less alienated subpopulations.

In the hundreds of community mental health centers created as a result of this movement to serve the public, we find a great proliferation of nonpsychiatric professionals and caregivers. Clearly, the task of providing mental health services has become too great to be carried out by psychiatrists alone. Furthermore, it is apparent that in many centers and clinics across the nation, allied professionals are doing a highly commendable job of providing direct personal care and treatment to clients. The role of the psychiatrist in such centers is gradually being defined as a *coordinator* of treatment plans in which a variety of professionals contribute; as a *consultant,* especially in cases complicated by medical and/or neurological disease; and as a *monitor* of medical and psychopharmacological aspects of therapy. At the same time, the role of ancillary professionals has been elevated, and their mastery of brief forms of therapy, such as strategies of crisis intervention, has continued to grow.

Crisis intervention, brief therapy, rapid resolution of emotional disequilibria, family therapy, and community support networks will, in all probability, be even more popular in the future. Professionals who today receive training and experience in these areas will become the valued teachers of tomorrow. This volume is an admirable and authoritative review of history, theory, and practice of crisis intervention, written in a most interesting and readable style. We recommend it to all those interested in modern methods of treatment of the mentally ill.

Milton Greenblatt, M.D.

Preface

We developed this textbook because we recognized the need for a comprehensive overview as well as an introduction and guide to crisis intervention from its historical development to its present utilization. Although the techniques and skills of a therapist must be learned and practiced under professional supervision, we believe that an awareness of the basic theory and principles of crisis intervention will be of value to all who are involved in the helping professions. The book should be of particular value as a guideline to those in the mental health field who are in constant proximity to persons in stressful situations who seek help because they are unable to cope alone.

Since it was not our intent in the previous editions of this textbook to imply that crisis intervention was limited only to one profession, we have revised and added selected sections in response to our readers' requests.

Chapter 1 deals with the historical development of crisis intervention methodology. Its intent is to create awareness of the broad base of knowledge incorporated into present practice, the fundamental procedures of brief psychotherapy, its implementation in community psychiatry, and an overview of the current trends in utilization of manpower resources in community mental health centers.

Chapter 2 explores the differences between the psychotherapeutic techniques of psychoanalysis and psychoanalytic psychotherapy and between brief psychotherapy and crisis intervention methodology in the major areas of their goals, foci, activities of the therapists, indications for treatment, and the average lengths of treatment.

Chapter 3 presents an overview of therapeutic groups and group therapy to show the bases from which crisis groups evolve. Two studies on crisis groups are presented to show their implementation, advantages, and disadvantages, and a case study is included to demonstrate the use of crisis intervention techniques in a group therapy session.

Chapter 4 presents some of the sociocultural factors that can act as barriers in the psychotherapeutic process. The purpose of this chapter is to discuss certain key areas that are usually considered to be problems and to make the reader aware of the nature of these difficulties.

Chapter 5 focuses on the problem-solving process and introduces the reader to basic terminology used in this method of treatment. We have devised a paradigm of intervention for the purpose of clarifying the sequential steps of crisis development and crisis resolution and have included a brief case study to illustrate its application as a guide to case studies in subsequent chapters.

Chapter 6 deals with stressful events that could precipitate a crisis in individuals regardless of socioeconomic or sociocultural status. These events include prematurity, child abuse, status and role change, rape, physical illness, Alzheimer's disease, chronic mental illness, wife abuse, divorce, cocaine abuse, suicide, and death and the grief process. Hypothetical case studies based on factual experience are presented to illustrate the techniques used by therapists in crisis resolution. Theoretical material preceding each case study is presented as an overview relevant to the crisis situation.

Chapter 7 is devoted to those changes that occur during concomitant biological and social role transitions, such as birth, puberty, young adulthood, marriage, illness or death of a family member, the climacteric, and old age. Maturational crises have been described as normal processes of growth and development and differ from situational crises in that they usually evolve over an extended period of time and frequently require more characterological changes of the individual. Case studies are included with appropriate theoretical material.

Chapter 8 focuses on the burn-out syndrome that occurs so frequently in high-stress work situations. A case study is also presented.

We are indebted to many people who have been of direct and indirect assistance in writing this book. Specifically we wish to thank several persons for their roles in bringing the manuscript to fruition. We want to acknowledge our gratitude to Dr. G.F. Jacobson, Dr. W.E. Morley, and the Research Committee of the Los Angeles Psychiatric Service—Benjamin Rush Centers for their encouragement and advice. We are especially grateful to Judy and Ken, without whose valuable and expert assistance the manuscript could not have been prepared in its final form. To our families, who were our kindest critics and strongest supporters, we owe a very special kind of debt.

Donna C. Aguilera
Janice M. Messick

Contents

chapter 1

Historical development of crisis intervention methodology

The Chinese characters that represent the word "crisis" mean both danger and opportunity. Crisis is a *danger* because it threatens to overwhelm the individual or his family, and it may result in suicide or a psychotic break. It is also an *opportunity* because during times of crisis individuals are more receptive to therapeutic influence. Prompt and skillful intervention may not only prevent the development of a serious long-term disability but may also allow new coping patterns to emerge that can help the individual function at a higher level of equilibrium than before the crisis.

A person in crisis is at a turning point. He* faces a problem that he cannot readily solve by using the coping mechanisms that have worked before. As a result, his tension and anxiety increase, and he becomes less able to find a solution. A person in this situation feels helpless—he is caught in a state of great emotional upset and feels unable to take action *on his own* to solve the problem.

Crisis intervention can offer the immediate help that a person in crisis needs to reestablish equilibrium. This is an inexpensive, short-term therapy that focuses on solving the immediate problem. Increasing awareness of sociocultural factors that could precipitate crisis situations has led to the rapid evolution of crisis intervention methodology. Therefore these factors will be discussed first in order to understand their social and cultural implications better.

Everywhere today we hear talk of the changes in our lives that have been made by "urbanization" and "technology." A closer study of these changes will add to our understanding of what they have meant to families and to individuals.

Before the revolution in technology and industrialization, most people lived on farms or in small rural communities. They were chiefly self-employed, either on their farms or in small, associated businesses. When sons and daughters married, they were likely to remain near their parents, working in the same occupations,

---

*Male and female pronouns have been used interchangeably throughout this book.

1

and, in this way, trades and occupations were a link between generations. Families therefore tended to be large, and because family members lived and worked together and relied chiefly on each other for social interaction, they developed strong loyalties and a sense of responsibility for one another.

Contemporary urban life, however, does not encourage or allow this kind of sheltered, close-knit family relationship. People who live in cities are likely to be employed by a company and paid a wage. They work with business associates and live within a neighborhood rather than with just their immediate family. Because of housing conditions and the necessity of living on a wage, families in cities usually consist of parents and unmarried children.

These differences between rural and urban life have important repercussions to individual security and stability. The large, extended rural family offered a large and relatively constant group of associates. Family size and the varying strength of blood ties meant that there was always someone to talk to, even about a problem involving two family members. But urban life is highly mobile. There is often a rapid turnover in business associates and neighbors, and there is no certainty that these relative strangers will share the same values, beliefs, and interests. All these factors make it difficult for people to develop real trust and interdependence outside the small immediate family. In addition, urban life requires that people meet each other only superficially, in specific roles, and in limited relationships rather than as total personalities.

All of these factors taken together mean that people in cities are more isolated than ever before from the emotional support provided by the family and close and familiar peers. As a result, there are no role models to follow—the demands of urban life are constantly changing, and coping behavior that was appropriate and successful several years before may be hopelessly ineffective today.

This creates a favorable environment for the development of crises. As defined by Caplan (1961), crisis may occur when the individual faces a problem that he cannot solve, which causes a rise in inner tension and signs of anxiety and inability to function in extended periods of emotional upset.

Historical development

The crisis approach to therapeutic intervention has been developed only within the past few decades and is based on a broad range of theories of human behavior, including those of Freud, Hartmann, Rado, Erikson, Lindemann, and Caplan. Its current acceptance as a recognized form of treatment cannot be directly related to any single theory of behavior; all have contributed to some degree.

Our intent in presenting an overview of historical development is to create awareness of the broad base of knowledge incorporated into present practice. Although not all theories of human behavior necessarily depend on Freudian concepts, and only a selected few are presented here, we chose to begin with the psychoanalytic theories of Freud because these are a major basis for further investigation of normal and abnormal human behavior. The fundamental procedures of brief psychotherapy are derived from hypotheses based on studies of the reasons for normal as well as abnormal human behavior.

Sigmund Freud was the first to demonstrate and apply the principle of causality as it relates to psychic determinism (Bellak and Small, 1965). Simply put, this principle states that every act of human behavior has its cause, or source, in the history and experience of the individual. It follows that causality is operative, whether or not the individual is aware of the reason for her behavior. Psychic determinism is the theoretical foundation of psychotherapy and psychoanalysis. The technique of free association, dream interpretation, and the assignment of meaning to symbols are all based on the assumption that causal connections operate unconsciously.

A particularly important outcome of Freud's deterministic position was his construction of a developmental or "genetic" psychology (Ford and Urban, 1963). Present behavior is understandable in terms of the life history or experience of the individual, and the crucial foundations for all future behavior are laid down in infancy and early childhood. The most significant determinants of present behavior are the "residues" of past experiences (learned responses), particularly those developed during the earliest years to reduce biological tensions.

Freud assumed that a reservoir of energy that exists in the individual initiates all behavior. Events function as guiding influences, but they do not initiate behavior; they only serve to help mold it in certain directions.

Since the end of the nineteenth century, the concept of determinism, as well as the scientific bases from which Freud formulated his ideas, have undergone many changes.

Although the ego-analytic theorists have tended to subscribe to much in the Freudian position, they differ in several respects. These seem to be extensions of Freudian theory rather than direct contradictions. As a group, they conclude that Freud has neglected the direct study of normal or healthy behavior.

Heinz Hartmann was an early ego analyst who was profoundly versed in Freud's theoretical contributions (Loewenstein, 1966). He postulated that the psychoanalytic theories of Freud could prove valid for normal as well as for pathological behavior. Hartmann began with the study of ego functions and distinguished between two groups: those that develop from conflict, and those that are "conflict free," such as memory, thinking, and language, which he labeled "primary autonomous functions of the ego." He considered these important in the adaptation of the individual to the environment. Hartmann emphasized that a person's adaptation in early childhood as well as her ability to maintain her adaptation to the environment in later life had to be considered. Hartmann's conception of the ego as an organ of adaptation required further study of the concept of reality.

He also described the search for an environment as another form of adaptation—the fitting together of the individual and society. He believed that although the behavior of the individual is strongly influenced by culture, a part of the personality remains relatively free of this influence.

Sandor Rado developed the concept of adaptational psychodynamics, providing a new approach to the unconscious as well as new goals and techniques of therapy (Salzman, 1962). Rado saw human behavior as being based on the dynamic principle of motivation and adaptation. An organism achieves adaptation through interaction with culture. Behavior is viewed in terms of its effect on the welfare of the individual, not just in terms of cause and effect. The organism's patterns of interaction improve through adaptation, with the goal being the increase of possibilities for survival. Freud's classical psychoanalytic technique emphasized the developmental past and the uncovering of unconscious memories, and little if any importance was attached to the reality of the present. Rado's adaptational psychotherapy, however, emphasizes the immediate present without neglecting the influence of the developmental past. Primary concern is with failures in adaptation "today," what caused them, and what the patient must do to learn to overcome them. Interpretations always begin and end with the present; preoccupation with the past is discouraged. As quickly as insight is achieved, it is used as a beginning to encourage the patient to enter into her present, real-life situation repeatedly. Through practice the patient automatizes new patterns of healthy behavior. According to Rado, it is this automatization factor that is ultimately the curative process, not insight. He believes that it takes place not passively, in the doctor's office, but actively, in the reality of daily living (Ovesy and Jameson, 1956).

Erik H. Erikson further developed the theories of ego psychology, which complement those of Freud, Hartmann, and Rado, by focusing on the epigenesis of the ego and on the theory of reality relationships (Rappaport, 1959). Epigenetic development is characterized by an orderly sequence of development at particular stages, each depending on the other for successful completion. Erikson perceived eight stages of psychosocial development, spanning the entire life cycle of the individual and involving specific developmental tasks that must be solved in each phase. The solution that is achieved in each previous phase is applied in subsequent phases. Erikson's theory is important in that it offers an explanation of the individual's social development as a result of encounters with the social environment. Another significant feature is his elaboration on the normal rather than the pathological development of social interactions. He dealt in particular with the problems of adolescence and saw this period in life as a "normative crisis," that is, a normal maturational phase of increased conflicts, with apparent fluctuations in ego strength (Pumpian-Mindlin, 1966). Erikson integrated the biological, cultural, and self-deterministic points of view in his eight stages of human development and broadened the scope of traditional psychotherapy with his theoretical formulations concerning identity and identity crises. His theories have provided a basis for the work of others who further developed the concept of maturational crises and began serious consideration of situational crises and individual adaptation to the current environmental dilemma.

Lindemann's (1956) initial concern was in developing approaches that might contribute to the maintenance of good mental health and the prevention of emotional disorganization on a community-wide level. He chose to study bereavement reactions in his search for social events or situations that predictably would be followed by emotional disturbances in a considerable portion of the population. In his study of bereavement reactions among the survivors of those killed in the Coconut Grove nightclub fire, he described both brief and abnormally prolonged reactions occurring in different individuals as a result of a loss of a significant person in their lives.

In his experiences in working with grief reactions Lindemann concluded that it might be profitable for investigation and useful for the development of preventive efforts if a conceptual frame of reference were to be constructed around the concept of an emotional crisis, as exemplified by bereavement reactions. Certain inevitable events in the course of the life cycle of every individual can be described as hazardous situations, for example, bereavement, the birth of a child, and marriage. He postulated that in each of these situations emotional strain would be generated, stress would be experienced, and a series of adaptive mechanisms would occur that could lead either to mastery of the new situation or to failure with more or less lasting impairment to function. Although such situations create stress for all people who are exposed to them, they become crises for those individuals who by personality, previous experience, or other factors in the present situation are especially vulnerable to this stress and whose emotional resources are taxed beyond their usual adaptive resources.

Lindemann's theoretical frame of reference led to the development of crisis intervention techniques, and in 1946 he and Caplan established a community-wide program of mental health in the Harvard area, called the Wellesley Project.

According to Caplan (1961), the most important aspects of mental health are the state of the ego, the stage of its maturity, and the quality of its structure. Assessment of its state is based on three main areas: (1) the capacity of the person to withstand stress and anxiety and to maintain ego equilibrium, (2) the degree of reality recognized and faced in solving problems, and (3) the repertoire of effective coping mechanisms employable by the person in maintaining a balance in his biopsychosocial field.

Caplan believes that all the elements that compose the total emotional milieu of the person must be assessed in an approach to preventive mental health. The material, physical, and social demands of reality, as well as the needs, instincts, and impulses of the individual, must all be considered as important behavioral determinants.

As a result of his work in Israel (1948) and his later experiences in Massachusetts with Lindemann and with the Community Mental Health Program at Harvard University, he evolved the concept of the importance of *crisis* periods in individual and group development (Caplan, 1951).

Crisis is defined as occurring "when a person faces an obstacle to important life goals that is, for a time, insurmountable through the utilization of customary methods of problem solving. A period of disorganization ensues, a period of upset, during which many abortive attempts at solution are made" (Caplan, 1961:18).

In essence, the individual is viewed as living in a state of emotional equilibrium, with the goal always to return to or to maintain that state. When customary problem-solving techniques cannot be used to meet the daily problems of living, the balance or equilibrium is upset. The individual must either solve the problem or adapt to nonsolution. In either case a new state of equilibrium will develop, sometimes better and sometimes worse insofar as positive mental health is concerned. There is a rise in inner tension, there are signs of anxiety, and there is disorganization of function, resulting in a protracted period of emotional upset. This he refers to as "crisis." The outcome is governed by the kind of interaction that takes place during that period between the individual and the key figures in his emotional milieu.

Evolution of community psychiatry

Community psychiatry has emerged as a new field. New concepts and new biopsychosocial problems arise continually in rapidly changing cultures so that it is a broad, fluid field. A difference is now perceived between long-term, psychoanalytic therapy of the individual and short-term, reality-oriented psychotherapy as practiced in community psychiatry.

In the middle 1960s the term *crisis intervention* was not yet included in psychiatric dictionaries. In 1970 the fourth edition of Hinsie and Campbell's *Psychiatric Dictionary* listed crisis intervention as one of several modes of community psychiatry: "In the crisis-intervention model, the focus is on transitional-situational demands for novel adaptational responses. Because minimal intervention at such times tends to achieve maximal and optimal effects, such a model is more readily applicable to population groups than the medical model" (Hinsie and Campbell, 1970:606).

According to Bellak (1964), community psychiatry evolved from multiple disciplines and is intrinsically bound to the development of psychoanalytic theory. The social and behavioral sciences that advanced during the first half of the century were predicated on psychodynamic hypotheses. At the same time, concepts of public health and epidemiology were advancing in community health programs.

After World War II the general public's increasing awareness and acceptance of the high incidence of psychiatric problems created changes in attitudes and demands for community action.

The discovery and use of psychotropic drugs were important steps forward, which resulted in opportunities for open wards and rehabilitation of the hospitalized patient in his home milieu.

It would be incorrect to assume that all of these factors merged spontaneously, creating a successful, structured cure for mental illness. Rather, this was a slow process of trial and error. Widely different programs, each striving to meet problems involving different cultures, interests, knowledge, and skills, communicated and related to other programs similarly initiated. Disciplines once separated in goals became cognizant of their interdependence in attaining mutually recognized goals. New, allied disciplines developed; roles changed and expanded. Tasks were diffused and lines between disciplines became more flexible.

The origin of day hospitals for the care of psychiatric patients grew out of a shortage of hospital beds (Ross, 1964), which forced premature discharges of patients to their homes, rather than as a treatment innovation. The first reported day hospital was associated with the First Psychiatric Hospital in Moscow in 1933. As Dzhagarov (1937) states: "The need to continue treatment and for special observation in a setting similar to that of a hospital suggested a practical solution in the form of admission to the preventive section of the hospital. In a short time a transformation took place, the day hospital was created, proving to be adequately prepared to meet the new needs." In referring to this day hospital in Moscow, Kramer, as quoted by Ross (1964:190) says: "While this day center is little known and probably had little effect on later developments in the Western world, it is accurate to say that this was the first organized Day Hospital for individuals with severe mental illness."

In the late 1930s Bierer (1964) began the Marlborough Experiment in England. Patients, as members of a "therapeutic social club," lived outside the hospital and were treated at day hospitals or part-time facilities. According to Bierer, the primary goal of the program was to change the patient's role concept from that of a passive object of treatment to one of an active participant-collaborator. At the same time, the psychiatrist and staff had to reconceptualize the patient as a human being accessible to reason, emphasizing his assets rather than concentrating on his psychopathology and conflicts. The reality of here and now was the focus of attention.

These innovations in attitude gave rise to the concept of "therapeutic community." The patient became a partner and collaborator with the staff and was granted equal rights, opportunities, and facilities. The medical staff and their assistants functioned as advisors.

The patient group assumed responsibility for the behavior of its members, as well as planning for activities, planning their futures, and offering support to each other. Group and social methods that encouraged the constant interaction of the members were used.

Other complementary projects developed in the Marlborough Program were the Day Hospital, the Night Hospital, the Aftercare Rehabilitation Center, the Self-Governed Community Hosel, Neurotics Nomine, and the Weekend Hospital.

Linn (1964) describes Cameron's first day hospital in Montreal (1946), in which he and others were responsible for defining and giving formal structure to the program as a treatment innovation.

With this frame of reference it was only natural that the general hospital should add to the various roles in which it serves the community—that of becoming a focal point of preventive medicine and public health functions in psychiatry.

In 1958 a "Trouble Shooting Clinic" was initiated by Bellak (1960) as part of City Hospital of Elmhurst, New York, a general hospital with 1000 beds. The clinic was designed to offer first aid for emotional problems and was not limited to urgent crises. It combined two aspects of service on a walk-in basis around the clock: major emergencies as well as minor problems involving guidance, legal problems, and marital relations.

After the passage of the California Community Mental Health Act (1958) the California Department of Mental Hygiene established the first state agency in the country (1961) to undertake the training of specialists in community psychiatry.

It was recognized that clinics were needed to accommodate those individuals in the community who were unfamiliar with established forms of psychiatric treatment. A cause for these individuals' exclusion from treatment conceivably could have been the divergency in social-cultural background, lack of communication, and lack of recognition of the need for services by both the population and the existing agencies.

In January 1962 the Benjamin Rush Center for Problems of Living, a division of the Los Angeles Psychiatric Service, was opened as a no-waiting, unrestricted intake, walk-in crisis intervention center. The center is currently under the aegis of the Didi Hirsch Community Mental Health Center. After nearly 25 years of operation, the Benjamin Rush Center has accumulated considerable evidence that persons who come to the center are often those who would not typically seek treatment in a traditional clinic. The approach has been to bring forth persons who, while judged to be genuinely in need of psychiatric treatment, would not have sought traditional treatment because of reluctance to consider themselves "sick," to assume the patient role, or to accept the stigma of psychiatric treatment.

In 1967 crisis intervention replaced emergency detention at the San Francisco General Hospital. On each of the psychiatric units interdisciplinary teams were established whose primary goals were to reestablish independent functioning of the clients as soon as possible. In a follow-up study in 1972 Decker and Stubblebine (1972) concluded that the crisis intervention program achieved the anticipated reduction in psychiatric inpatient-treatment.

In the early 1970s the Bronx Mental Health Center (Centro de Hygiene Mental del Bronx) (Morales, 1971) was created for crisis intervention for the low socioeconomic Spanish-speaking people and was staffed by Spanish-speaking psychiatrists.

At about the same time, suburban churches in Montreal, Canada, offered brief crisis-intervention services on an experimental basis (Lecker, 1971). The goal of the program was to reach families undergoing a variety of stress through a roving walk-in clinic. The clinics served to facilitate delivery of these services to a latent population at risk, not reached by other means and at a point early in the evolution of a life crisis.

The first hot line was started at Children's Hospital in Los Angeles in 1968. Hot lines and youth crisis centers have been created in recognition of the failure of traditional approaches to make contacts among adolescents. Twenty-four–hour crisis telephones, free counseling with a minimum of red tape, walk-in contacts, crash pads, and young people serving as volunteer staff in such services continue to be increasingly attractive to the youth who have emerged as the locus of a counter-culture.

Trends such as these are being repeated around the country as all community mental health programs recognize the value of providing services in primary and secondary prevention unique to the needs of their particular clients. Increasing recognition is also being given to the need to provide more services for those clients whose needs are for continuing support in rehabilitation after resolution of the immediate crisis.

A major concern confronting community mental health centers is no longer that of discerning just what services are appropriate to the needs of potential clients. It is not even that of recruiting clients for the services provided. The centers are being faced with the problem of obtaining an adequate supply of human resources to meet demands for their services. Professionals and nonprofessionals alike have been recruited and trained to fill the gap between supply and demand for their services. This has led to the deprofessionalization of many mental health functions previously considered to be solely within the scope of the professional's skills. Role boundaries have undergone increasing diffusion as the needs of the individual client and his community have become the determining factors in establishing the appropriateness of services.

It is not our purpose to define the levels of educational preparation and experience of the various disciplines now practicing crisis intervention. Our intent is, however, to provide an overview of the continuing trends being reported in the utilization of available human resources.

Paraprofessionals

Increasing numbers of paraprofessionals are being provided with additional education and training to function as consultants or "therapists" in mental health centers. Rusk (1972) reported an increased trend toward the use of paraprofessionals in functions once considered to be only within the domain of the highly skilled professional. Leaders in community mental health were keenly aware of the many dangers inherent in random, unplanned deprofessionalization of major mental health functions. Increasing concern is being voiced about the lack of definitive criteria established for the different levels of educational preparation and experience required of those who conduct the various "therapies."

As new roles and careers are created, some are being formed within well-structured, formal educational and training programs. Others, however, have tended to evolve gradually and informally, often in response to specific needs of innovative programs.

Interest in developing more innovative uses for the relatively untrained nonprofessional worker is leading to a wide variety of training programs being offered in community colleges around the country. Currently wide differences in admission criteria and program content exist.

Lincoln Hospital Mental Health Services in New York City established a prototype for careers in mental health in which indigenous people were trained to serve as mental health aides in neighborhood service centers. Rather than functioning as an ancillary extension of the professional, these individuals served as liaison between the social and experiential gap separating the middle-class professionals and the lower-class clients.

Christmas, Wallace, and Edwards (1970) expressed concern that the inappropriate use of the paraprofessional in community programs could lead to perpetuating the past patterns of providing second-class services for the poor and minorities. This reflected a predominant theme of concern being expressed that the same patterns of care reported by Hollingshead and Redlich (1958) might be perpetuated in the new community programs.

All emphasized that the functions for which paraprofessional staff members are utilized must not be determined by the scope of preparation alone. They must also be determined by the amount of professional supervision and consultation that will be made available to them. The public has become increasingly sophisticated in its understanding of its human rights to equal care and treatment.

Non-mental health professionals

Other resources for manpower that have been recruited into liaison activities with community programs are the non-mental health professionals. These are the professional individuals who serve as the official caretakers within their communities. Common to all is their traditional role of helping people who are in trouble.

Included in this group are the medical professionals, teachers, lawyers, clergy, police officers, firefighters, social and welfare workers, and so on. In the course of their daily work activities these highly skilled individuals can be found functioning in what could be called the front lines of preventive mental health care. They are frequently in contact with both individuals and groups who are in potential crisis situations because of a loss or the threat of a loss in their lives. Most often these professional community caretakers become the initial contact made by a person in crisis.

The contributions that this group is making to positive mental health education and practices have not gone unrecognized. Many new programs have been developed to include them as active participants on the treatment teams. How little or how much each can do is highly dependent on the availability and willingness of the mental health professionals to provide them with training and consultation services.

Nonprofessional volunteers

Nonprofessional volunteers are another human resource being recruited by mental health centers. Not only do they fill the traditional volunteer roles, but they are also seeking training to develop skills to meet their human needs to be creative, to help others, to be recognized, to learn new skills, and to become meaningful members of the treatment teams.

Crisis hot lines, initially established by professionals and community leaders, rely heavily upon the nonprofessional volunteer for their 24-hour, 7-day services. According to Clark and Jaffe (1972), these hot lines seem to have originated in both the traditional and counterculture models of crisis intervention. Nonprofessionals are carefully selected, intensively trained, and closely supervised in these psychiatric emergency centers.

Torop and Torop (1972), in their report on the use of volunteers in a crisis hot line program, called attention to the potential dangers for clients when unskilled volunteers are not provided with consistent and skillful professional supervision. In particular they pointed out the need to recognize and intervene when a volunteer may be responding to personal intuition and bias.

Later developments in crisis intervention history were the organization of free clinics and similar community help centers. These are predominantly staffed by volunteers from the counterculture communities to whom they provide services.

Team approach to crisis

Another development has been the increasing use of the team approach to crisis intervention. Crisis team members are selected on the basis of their expertise to meet the specific needs of each patient in crisis. Members will vary with the structure and requirements of the individual mental health centers, as well as with the geographical and socioeconomic needs of the community. The unique skills of each member are utilized from the time of initial contact until the crisis is resolved and follow-up support is no longer believed to be necessary.

Team membership is open ended, expanding and contracting within highly flexible boundaries. Leadership of each team depends upon who has the skills and expertise most appropriate to help the individual resolve his crisis. This is not to say, however, that ultimate professional responsibility is removed from the physician. Rather, there is a greater scope in delegation of authority to make decisions in treatment planning.

Informal and at times unrecognized members of the community mental health team are the nonprofessional community caretakers. These individuals in the course of their usual daily activities have many contacts with fellow members of the community or are sought out for help and advice. They act as a source of information and are an integral part of the communication channels within the social systems of the community. In their formal roles, such as cab drivers, bartenders, grocers, barbers, beauticians, and neighbors, they provide a sympathetic ear and situational support to those in trouble and looking for help. If informed and aware of the purpose and services provided by the center, they can be a reliable and direct referral source for those in need of crisis intervention.

The non–mental health professional caretaker's function is a more formal role relationship with members of the community. These caretakers receive their communications within the system from a nonprofessional caretaker or directly from the individual who needs help. They are incorporated into the community mental health team as consultants or as persons who make direct referrals to the center for treatment.

Selected nonprofessional volunteers are used in liaison within the community as interpreters with foreign language population groups and as sources of referral. With appropriate training in crisis intervention techniques they are utilized as "therapists" under the supervision of mental health professionals at some centers.

Paraprofessionals function as members of the team in accord with their basic training and educational preparation. In their roles at the center they focus on initial assessments and observations of behavioral changes in the clients. If a client were retained for 24 to 72 hours on a crisis ward, members of this group are prepared to participate in various adjunctive therapies under professional guidance and supervision. Their realm of functioning is within the immediate environs of the center.

The mental health professionals function on the crisis team much as they function on any mental health team. The psychiatrist, psychologist, psychiatric nurse, and psychiatric social worker conduct individual, family, or group therapy as needed by the clients. The diversity of local demands and problems underscores ability and accomplishment of individual team members more than professional background alone. Generalization, frequently required on the part of the staff, is one factor accounting for the less strict division of roles and responsibilities among the professional personnel in a community mental health center.

The administrator's task is to create a climate in which each team member is free enough and challenged enough to actively participate in the care needed by the clients seeking help to resolve their crises.

References

Bellak, L.: A general hospital as a focus of community psychiatry, J.A.M.A. **174:**2214, 1960.

Bellak, L., editor: Handbook of community psychiatry and community mental health, New York, 1964, Grune & Stratton, Inc.

Bellak, L., and Small, L.: Emergency psychotherapy and brief psychotherapy, New York, 1965, Grune & Stratton, Inc.

Bierer, J.: The Marlborough experiment. In Bellak, L., editor: Handbook of community psychiatry and community mental health, New York, 1964, Grune & Stratton, Inc.

Caplan, G.: A public health approach to child psychiatry, Ment. Health **35:**235, 1951.

Caplan, G.: An approach to community mental health, New York, 1961, Grune & Stratton, Inc.

Caplan, G., Principles of preventive psychiatry, New York, 1964, Basic Books, Inc., Publishers.

Christmas, J.J., Wallace, H., and Edwards, J.: New careers and new mental health services: fantasy or future? Am. J. Psychiatry **126:**1480, April 1970.

Clark, T., and Jaffe, D.T.: Change within youth crisis centers, Am. J. Orthopsychiatry **42:**675, July 1972.

Collins, J.A., and Cavanaugh, M.: The paraprofessional. II. Brief mental health training for the community health worker, Hosp. Community Psychiatry **22:**367, Dec. 1971.

Decker, J.B., and Stubblebine, J.M.: Crisis intervention and prevention of psychiatric disability; a follow-up study, Am. J. Psychiatry **129:**101, Dec. 1972.

Dzhagarov, M.A.: Experience in organizing a day hospital for mental patients, Neurapathologia Psikhiatria **6:**147, 1937. (Translated by G. Wachbrit.)

Eastman, K., Coates, D., and Allodi, F.: The concepts of crisis: an expository review, Can. Psychiatr. Assoc. J. **15:**463, 1970.

Ford, D., and Urban, H.: Systems of psychotherapy, New York, 1963, John Wiley & Sons, Inc.

Golan, N.: When is a client in crisis? Soc. Casework **50:**389, July 1969.

Hinsie, L.E., and Campbell, R.J.: Psychiatric dictionary, ed. 4, New York, 1970, Oxford University Press, Inc.

Hollingshead, A.B., and Redlich, F.C.: Social class and mental illness, New York, 1958, John Wiley & Sons, Inc.

Janis, L.: Psychological stress, New York, 1958, John Wiley & Sons, Inc.

Lecker, S., and others: Brief interventions: a pilot walk-in clinic in suburban churches, Can. Psychiatr. Assoc. J. **16**(2):141, 1971.

Lindemann, E.: The meaning of crisis in individual and family, Teachers Coll. Rec. **57:**310, 1956.

Linn, L.: Psychiatric program in a general hospital. In Bellak, L., editor: Handbook of community psychiatry and community mental health, New York, Grune & Stratton, Inc., 1964.

Loewenstein, R.M.: Psychology of the ego. In Alexander, F., Eisenstein, S., and Grotjahn, M., editors: Psychoanalytic pioneers, New York, 1966, Basic Books, Inc., Publishers.

Morales, H.M.: Bronx Mental Health Center, N.Y. State Division Bronx Bull. **13**(8):6, 1971.

Ovesy, L., and Jameson, J.: Adaptational techniques of psychodynamic therapy. In Rado, S., and Daniels, G., editors: Changing concepts of psychoanalytic medicine, New York, 1956, Grune & Stratton, Inc.

Pumpian-Mindlin, E.: Contributions to the theory and practice of psychoanalysis and psychotherapy. In Alexander, F., Eisenstein, S., and Grotjahn, M., editors: Psychoanalytic pioneers, New York, 1966, Basic Books, Inc., Publishers.

Rapoport, L.: The state of crisis: some theoretical considerations, Soc. Service Rev. **36:**211, June 1962.

Rappaport, D.: A historical survey of psychoanalytic ego psychology. In Klein, G.S., editor: Psychological issues, New York, 1959, International Universities Press.

Reiff, R.: Mental health manpower and community change, Am. Psychologist 21:540, 1966.

Ross, M.: Extramural treatment techniques. In Bellak, L., editor: Handbook of community psychiatry and community mental health, New York, 1964, Grune & Stratton, Inc.

Rusk, T.: Future changes in mental health care, Hosp. Community Psychiatry 22:7, Jan. 1972.

Salzman, L.: Developments in psychoanalysis, New York, 1962, Grune & Stratton, Inc.

Sifneos, P.E.: A concept of emotional crisis, Ment. Hyg. 44:169, 1960.

Torop, P., and Torop, K.: Hotlines and youth culture values, Am. J. Psychiatry 129:106, Dec. 1972.

United States House of Representatives: A bill to provide for the assistance in the construction and initial operation of community mental health centers and for other purposes, No. 3688, Eighty-eighth Congress, first session, 1963.

Additional readings

The antidote to ivory-tower psychiatry? Lancet No. 8162, p. 241, 1980.

Baldwin, B.A.: Training in crisis intervention for students in the mental health professions, Prof. Psychol. 10(2):161, 1979.

Barzilay, R.: Towards tomorrow's world. Five families in precrisis: the key people, Nurs. Times 80(15):50, 1984.

Barzilay, R.: Towards tomorrow's world. Six families in precrisis: a case study, Nurs. Times 80(16):47, 1984.

Bell, C.C.: The role of psychiatric emergency services in aiding community alternatives to hospitalization in an inner-city population, J. Nat. Med. Assoc., 70:931, 1978.

Bowen, A.: Some mental health premises, Milbank Mem. Fund Q. 57(4):533, 1979.

Britton, J.: The crisis home program, Minn. Nurs. Accent 55(4):45, 1983.

Burgess, A.W., and Baldwin, B.A.: Crisis intervention theory and practice: a clinical handbook, Englewood Cliffs, N.J., 1981, Prentice-Hall, Inc.

Butcher, J.N., and Maudel, G.R.: Crisis intervention. In Weiner, I., editor: Clinical methods in psychology, New York, 1976, John Wiley & Sons, Inc.

Cobb, C.W.: Community mental health services and the lower socioeconomic classes: a summary of research literature on outpatient treatment (1963–1969), Am. J. Orthopsychiatry 42:404, April 1972.

Cohen, D.: Psychiatry at home, New Society (London) 43:486, 1978.

Cormier, W.H., and Cormier, L.S.: Interviewing strategies for helpers: a guide to assessment, treatment, and evaluation, Monterey Park, Calif., 1979, Brooks/Cole Publishing Co.

Cowen, E.L., and Gesten, L.: Community approaches to intervention. In Woodwonan, B., editor: Handbook of treatment of mental disorders in childhood, Englewood Cliffs, N.J., 1978, Prentice-Hall, Inc.

Dayle, W.W., and others: Effects of supervision in the training of nonprofessional crisis-intervention counselors, J. Couns. Psychol. 24(1):72, 1977.

Delfin, P.E., and Hartsough, D.M.: Increasing informational competence in crisis workers through programmed instruction, Am. J. Community Psychol. 7:111, Jan. 1979.

de Smit, N.W.: The crisis center in community psychiatry: an Amsterdam experiment. In Masserman, J.H., editor: Current psychiatric therapies, vol. 2, New York, 1971, Grune & Stratton, Inc.

de Smit, N.W.: Crisis intervention and crisis centers: their possible relevance for community psychiatry and mental health care, Psychiatr. Neurol. Neurochir. 75:299, 1973.

Dixon, S.L.: Working with people in crisis: theory and practice, St. Louis, 1979, The C.V. Mosby Co.

Donovan, C.M.: Problems of psychiatric practice in community mental health centers, Am. J. Psychiatry 139(4):456, 1982.

Elias, P.: The state of crisis: implications for practice, Hong Kong J. Soc. Work 8(2):17, 1974.

Ewing, C.P.: Crisis intervention as psychotherapy, New York, 1978, Oxford University Press.

Fadda, S.: Psychiatric hospital as a crisis intervention center, Rev. Med. Suisse Romande 104(2):163, 1984.

Farberow, N.: The crisis is chronic, Am. Psychol. **28**(5):388, 1973.

Galatzer, A., and others: Crisis intervention program in newly diagnosed diabetic children, Diabetes Care **5**(4):414, 1982.

Gordon, J.S.: The runaway center as a community mental health center, Am. J. Psychiatry **135**(8):932, 1978.

Gordon, J.S.: Alternative mental health services and psychiatry, Am. J. Psychiatry **193**(5):653, 1982.

Hafner, H., and Helmchen, H.: Psychiatric emergency and psychiatric crisis—conceptual issues, Nervenarzt (Berlin) **49**:82, 1978.

Hobbs, M.: Crisis intervention in theory and practice: a selective review, Br. J. Med. Psychol. **57**(Pt 1):23, 1984.

Hodovanic, B.H., and others: Family crisis intervention program in the medical intensive care unit, Heart Lung **13**(3):243, 1984.

Hoffman, J.A., and Forssmann-Falck, R.: Emergency psychiatry training: the new old problem, Gen. Hosp. Psychiatry **6**(2):143, 1984.

Hose, M.A., and Hirschman, R.: Psychological training of emergency medical technicians: an evaluation, Am. J. Community Psychol. **12**(L):127, 1984.

Huessy, H.R.: Rural models. In Barten, H.H., and Bellak, L., editors: Progress in community mental health, vol. 2, New York, 1972, Grune & Stratton, Inc., pp. 199–220.

Jacobson, G.F.: Crisis oriented therapy, Psychiatr. Clin. North Am. Symp. Brief Psychother. **2**(1):39, 1979.

Kaforey, E.C.: Crisis intervention and the new unemployed, Occup. Health Nurs. **32**(3):154, 1984.

Klerman, G.L.: National trends in hospitalization, Hosp. Community Psychiatry **30**:110, 1979.

Kresky-Wolff, M., and others: Crossing Place: a residential model for crisis intervention, Hosp. Community Psychiatry **35**(1):72, 1984.

Larsen, K.S.: A black community health program —perspectives on training, Aust. Psychologist **14**:29, Jan. 1979.

Lindeman, E.: Beyond grief: studies in crisis intervention, New York, 1979, Jason Aronson, Inc.

Linn, L.: Crisis intervention in private medical practice, N.Y. State J. Med. **80**(2):209, 1980.

McGee, R.K.: Crisis intervention in the community, Baltimore, 1974, University Park Press.

McGowen, R., and King, G.D.: Expectations about effectiveness of telephone crisis intervention, Psychol. Rep. **46**(2):640, 1980.

Messick, J.M.: Crisis intervention concepts: implications for nursing practices, J. Psychiatr. Nurs. Ment. Health Services **10**(5):3, 1972.

Parad, H.J., Resnick, H.L.P., and Parad, L., (editors): Emergency and disaster management, Bowie, Md., 1976, Charles Press.

Pascoe, E.A., and Thoreson, R.W.: The employee assistance program: a systems intervention model for health care settings, Professional Psychol. **11**(2):169, 1980.

Perlmutter, F.D.: Primary prevention in mental health services: the U.S.A. experience, Israel Ann. Psychiatry Related Disciplines **17**:45, Jan. 1979.

Rabin, P.L., and Hussain, G.: Crisis intervention in an emergency setting, Ann. Emerg. Med. **12**(5):300, 1983.

Ratna, L.: Crisis intervention in psychogeriatrics: a two-year follow-up study, Br. J. Psychiatry **141**:296, 1982.

Sands, R.G.: Crisis intervention and social work practice in hospitals, Health Soc. Work **8**(4): 253, 1983.

Schinke, S.P., and others: Crisis intervention training with paraprofessionals, J. Community Psychol. **7**(4):343, 1979.

Seligman, M.E.P.: Abnormal psychology, New York, 1982, W.W. Norton & Co., Inc.

Skodol, A.E., and others: Crisis in psychotherapy: principles of emergency consultation and intervention, Am. J. Orthopsychiatry **49**(4): 585, 1979.

Slaikew, K.A., and Duffy, M.: Mental health consultation with campus ministers: a pilot program, Professional Psychol. **10**(3):338, 1979.

Smith, L.L.: Crisis intervention theory and practice: a source book, Washington, D.C., 1976, University Press of America, Inc.

Stein, D.M., and Lambert, M.J.: Telephone counseling and crisis intervention: a review, Am. J. Community Psychol. **12**(1):101, 1984.

Sterling, M.: Visiting aides training program, Health Soc. Work **3**:155, Mar. 1978.

Sundel, M., and others: The impact of a psychiatric hospital crisis unit on admissions and use of community resources, Hosp. Community Psychiatry **19:**569, Sept. 1978.

Tierney, K.J., and Baisden, B.: Crisis intervention programs for disaster victims: a source book and manual for smaller communities, Washington, D.C., DHEW Pub. No. (ADM)79-65, 1979, U.S. Government Printing Office.

Torre, J.: Brief encounters: general and technical psychoanalytic considerations, Psychiatry, Journal of the Study of Interpersonal Process **41:**184, 1978.

Weal, E.: Indigenous workers trained to reach out, Innovations **6**(2):19, 1979.

Wicks, R.J.: Counseling strategies and intervention techniques for the human services, Philadelphia, 1977, J.B. Lippincott Co.

chapter 2

Differentiation between psychotherapeutic techniques

Psychotherapy as a form of treatment has had many definitions, some conflicting and others concurring. Areas of divergence are generally those of methodology, therapeutic goals, length of therapy, and indications for treatment. All apparently agree that psychotherapy is a set of procedures for changing behaviors based primarily on the establishment of a relationship between two (or more) people.

Psychoanalysis and psychoanalytic psychotherapy

The original theories of Sigmund Freud, the founder of psychoanalysis, passed through several phases as he subjected changing hypotheses to the tests of experience and observation, all directed toward the goal of making the unconscious available to the conscious.

In collaboration with Breuer, Freud first developed the psychotherapeutic technique of "cathartic hypnosis." Recognizing that ego control of the unconscious was released under the influence of hypnosis, Freud used hypnotism to induce the patient to answer direct questions in an effort to uncover the unconscious causes of his symptomatology and to allow free expression of pent-up feelings.

Freud observed, however, that to obtain therapeutic results, the procedure had to be repeated. He recognized that material brought to consciousness during hypnosis returned to the unconscious as the awakening patient regained control over his emotions. The therapeutic task of making the conscious patient recall and face repressed emotions in order to gain insight and increased ego strength was only transiently achieved by this technique.

Freud then experimented with what he referred to as "waking suggestion." Laying his hand on the patient's forehead, he would strongly suggest that the patient could recall the past if he tried. He soon learned that a person could not be forced to recall repressed, conflictual emotional events through this approach.

He next devised an indirect method of freeing unconsciously repressed material for confrontation by the conscious. Using the process of "free association," the patient was expected to verbalize whatever thoughts came into his mind, freely associating events from his whole life span of experiences, feelings, fantasies, and dreams without concern for logic or continuity. Freud concentrated on gaining an intellectual understanding of the patient's psychogenic past. He insisted on the "basic rule" that the patient tell the therapist everything that came into his mind during each interview. Nothing, no matter how inconsequential the patient might think it was, could be withheld from the analyst. In this process of a search for repressed memories he found that repressed emotions were gradually discharged as they emerged, although not as dramatically as in cathartic hypnosis.

One of the most important discoveries by Freud is considered to be "transference phenomena." He deemed transference to be a valuable therapeutic tool in overcoming the patient's defenses in resisting the release of unconscious, repressed emotional experiences. He thought of transference as an emotional reaction of the patient to the therapist in which the patient would relive her conflicts and emotions as they emerged from the past, from her unconscious. She would transfer to the therapist emotions she felt toward authority figures in her childhood.

Freud referred to this reliving of the neurotic past in a present relationship with the therapist as transference neurosis. The principal factor in this process was that the patient expressed her aggressions against the therapist without any fears of the reprisal or censure that she may have been subjected to by the authority figure in her childhood. Through the therapist's nonjudgmental acceptance the patient was encouraged to face new material released from her own unconscious with reduced fear and anxiety. As these new experiences were assimilated into the conscious ego, coping skills increased. This in turn facilitated further release of repressed material. Alexander (1956) refers to this process as a "corrective emotional experience."

Psychoanalysis is concerned with theory as well as techniques. Alexander and French (1946) also state that the traditional approach in psychoanalytic therapy has been nondirective. The therapist is a passive observer who would follow the lead of the patient's verbal expressions as they unfolded. Tarachow (1963) indicates that psychoanalytic therapy is for those whose personalities and ego strengths are relatively intact, despite neurotic symptoms or mild to moderately severe characterological disturbances due to unconscious conflicts.

Stone (1951) lists eight factors in the situation and technique of psychoanalysis from which technical variations have derived: "(1) Practically exclusive reliance during the hour on the patient's free associations for communications; (2) regularity of the time, frequency and duration of appointments and clearly defined financial agreement; (3) three to five appointments a week (originally six), with daily appointments the dominant tendency; (4) recumbent position, in most instances with some impediment against seeing the analyst directly; (5) confinement of the analyst's activity essentially to interpretation or other purely informative interventions such as reality testing, or an occasional question; (6) the analyst's emotional passivity and neutrality (benevolent objectivity), specifically abstention from gratifying the analysand's transference wishes; (7) abstention from advice or any other direct intervention or participation in the patient's daily life; (8) no immediate emphasis on curing symptoms, the procedure being guided largely by the patient's free associations from day to day. In a sense the analyst regards the whole scope of the patient's psychic life as his field of observation.''

In psychoanalytic psychotherapy the therapist is more active than in psychoanalysis. The therapist interacts more with the patient and does not interpret the transference attitudes as completely as in analysis. The most helpful attitude is one of calmness, continued interest, and sympathetic, understanding helpfulness. This differs from the neutral attitude of the analyst in psychoanalysis. Contention is that this calm, helpful, interested attitude of the therapist in psychotherapy provides support for the patient in dealing with tensions, sustains contact with reality, and provides gratifications and rewards in the therapeutic relationship. These, in turn, provide incentives for the patient to continue to deal with emerging unconscious material.

Freud (1924) expressed the opinion that any digression from classical psychoanalysis that still recognizes the two basic facts of transference and resistance and takes them as the starting point of its work may call itself psychoanalysis, even though it arrives at results other than his own.

Alexander (1956) has noted that in procedures that deviate from the classical psychoanalysis of Freud, one or another of the basic phenomena is emphasized from the standpoint of therapeutic significance and is often being dealt with in isolation from others. For example, Rank centered on life situation, believing that insight into infantile history had no therapeutic significance. Feranczi placed emphasis on the emotional experience in transference (abreaction factor). Reich concentrated on the analysis of the resistances in order to allow, by their removal, the discharge of highly charged emotional experiences. He emphasized the importance of hidden forms of resistance and the understanding of the patient's behavior apart from his verbal communication.

Psychoanalytic psychotherapy procedures have customarily been divided into two functional categories based on methodology; these are frequently referred to as supportive (suppressive) and uncovering (exploratory or expressive) procedures.

According to Alexander (1956), the aim of the uncovering procedure is to intensify the ego's ability to handle repressed emotional conflict situations that are unconscious. Through the use of transference the patient relives her early interpersonal conflicts in relation to the therapist. Supportive and uncovering procedures overlap, but it is not difficult to differentiate between them. Primarily, supportive methods of treatment are indicated when functional impairment of the ego is temporary in nature and caused by acute emotional distress. Alexander designated therapeutic tasks in supportive methodology as follows: (1) gratifying dependency needs of the patient during stress situations, thereby reducing anxiety; (2) reducing stress by giving the patient an opportunity for abreaction; (3) giving intellectual guidance by objectively reviewing with the patient her acute stress situation and assisting the patient in making judgments, thereby enabling her to gain proper perspective of the total situation; (4) supporting the patient's neurotic defenses until the ego can handle the emotional discharges; and (5) actively participating in manipulation of the life situation when this might be the only hopeful approach in the given circumstances.

Psychoanalysis and psychoanalytic psychotherapy require many years of intensive training on the part of the therapist; this in itself has limited the number of therapists available. Both methods may require that the individual remain in therapy over an extended period of time, often for years. The obligation of time as well as expense for such extensive treatment also limits its availability for many.

Brief psychotherapy

Brief psychotherapy as a treatment form developed as the result of the increased demand for mental health services and the lack of personnel trained to meet this demand. Initially, much of it was conducted by psychiatric residents as part of their training. Later, psychiatric social workers and psychologists became involved in this form of treatment.

Brief psychotherapy has its roots in psychoanalytic theory but differs from psychoanalysis in terms of goals and other factors. It is limited to removing or alleviating specific symptoms when possible. Intervention may lead to some reconstruction of personality, although it is not considered as the primary goal. As in more traditional forms of psychotherapy, the therapy must be guided by an orderly series of concepts directed toward beneficial change in the patient. It is concerned with the degree of abatement of the symptoms presented and the return to or maintenance of the individual's ability to function adequately. To attain this goal the individual may choose to get involved in a longer form of therapy. Another goal is assistance in preventing the development of deeper neurotic or psychotic symptoms after catastrophies or emergencies in life situations.

Free association, interpretation, and the analysis of transference are also used successfully in a modified manner. According to Bellak and Small (1965), free association is not a basic tool in short-term therapy. It may arise in response to a stimulus from the therapist. Interpretation is modified by the time limit and the immediacy of the problem. Although it may occur in brief psychotherapy, it is commonly used with medical or environmental types of intervention.

Bellak also believes that positive transference should be encouraged. It is crucial in brief therapy that the patient sees the therapist as being likeable, reliable, and understanding. The patient *must* believe that the therapist will be able to help. This type of relationship is necessary if treatment goals are to be accomplished in a short period of time. This does not mean that negative transference feelings are to be ignored, but it does mean that these feelings are not analyzed in terms of defenses.

The therapist assumes a more active role than in the traditional methods. Trends not directly related to the presenting problem are avoided. The positive is accentuated, and the therapist acts as an interested, helpful person. The difficulties faced by the patient are circumscribed. The environmental position in which the patient finds himself is used by the therapist to help the patient evaluate the reality of his situation in an attempt to modify and change it. Productive behavior is encouraged.

Diagnostic evaluation is extremely important in short-term therapy. Its aim is to understand the symptoms and the patient dynamically and to formulate hypotheses that can be validated by the historical data. The result of the diagnosis will enable the therapist to decide which factors are most susceptible to change and to select the appropriate method of intervention. Part of the evaluation should be the degree of discrepancy or accord between the patient's fantasies and reality. The patient's probable ability to tolerate past and future frustrations should also be considered; the adequacy of his past and present relationships is also pertinent. The question ''Why do you come now?'' must be asked and means not only ''What is it that is going on in your life that distresses you?'' but ''What is it that you expect in the way of help?'' It is reasonable to assume that a request for help is motivated by emotional necessities, both external and internal, which are meaningful to the patient. Short-term goals can be beneficial for *all* patients.

After determining the causes of the symptoms, the therapist elects the appropriate intervention. Interpretation in order to achieve insight is used with care. Direct confrontation is used sparingly. An attempt is made to strengthen the ego by increasing the patient's self-esteem. One facet of this approach is to help the patient feel on a level with the therapist and no less worthwhile. Nor are his problems more unusual than those of others. This technique not only relieves the patient's anxiety but also facilitates communication between the patient and the therapist. Other basic procedures used include the following: catharsis, drive repression and restraint, reality testing, intellectualization, reassurance and support, counseling and guidance to move the patient along a line of behavior, and conjoint counseling (Bellak and Small, 1965).

The ending of treatment is an important phase in brief therapy. The patient must be left with a positive transference and the feeling that she may return if the need arises. The learning that has taken place during therapy must be reinforced in order to encourage the patient to realize that she has begun to understand and solve her own problems. This has a preventive effect that will help the patient to recognize possible future problems.

As an adjunct, drug therapy may be used in selected cases. This is in contrast to pure psychoanalysis, where drugs are seldom used. Environmental manipulation is considered when it is necessary to remove or modify an element causing disruption in the patient's life pattern. Included might be close scrutiny of family and friends, job and job training, education, and plans for travel (Bellak and Small, 1965).

Brief psychotherapy is indicated in cases of acutely disruptive emotional pain, in cases of severely destructive circumstances, and in situations endangering the life of the patient or others. Another indication involves the life circumstances of the in-dividual. If the person cannot participate in the long-term therapeutic situation, which implies a stable residence, job, and so forth, brief therapy is advocated to alleviate disruptive symptoms.

It is imperative that the patient feel relief as rapidly as possible, even during the first therapeutic session. The span of treatment can be any reasonable, limited number of sessions but usually is more than six. Most clinics expect the number of visits to be under twenty. Treatment goals can be attained in this short period of time if the patient is seen quickly and intensively after requesting help. Circum-stances associated with disrupted functioning are more easily accessible if they are recent. Only active conflicts are amenable to therapeutic intervention. Disequili-brated states are more easily resolved *before* they have crystallized, acquired second-ary gain features, or developed into highly maladaptive behavior patterns.

Crisis intervention

Crisis intervention extends logically from brief psychotherapy. The minimum therapeutic goal of crisis intervention is psychological resolution of the individual's immediate crisis and restoration to at least the level of functioning that existed be-fore the crisis period. A maximum goal is improvement in functioning above the precrisis level.

Caplan emphasizes that crisis is characteristically self-limiting and lasts from 4 to 6 weeks. This constitutes a transitional period, representing both the danger of in-creased psychological vulnerability and an opportunity for personality growth. In any particular situation the outcome may depend to a significant degree on the ready availability of appropriate help. On this basis the length of time for interven-tion is from 4 to 6 weeks, with the median being 4 weeks (Jacobson, 1965).

Since time is at a premium, a therapeutic climate is generated that commands the concentrated attention of both therapist and patient. A goal-oriented sense of commitment develops in sharp contrast to the more modest pace of traditional treatment modes.

Methodology

Jacobson and associates (1968, 1980) state that crisis intervention may be divided into two major categories, which may be designated as generic and individual. These two approaches are complementary.

Generic approach

A leading proposition of the generic approach is that there are certain recognized patterns of behavior in most crises. Many studies have substantiated this thesis. For example, Lindemann's (1944) studies of bereavement found that there is a well-defined process that a person goes through in adjusting to the death of a relative. He refers to these sequential phases as "grief work" and found that failure of a person to grieve appropriately or to complete the process of bereavement could potentially lead to future emotional illness.

Subsequent studies of generic patterns of response to stressful situations have been reported. Kaplan and Mason (1960)* and Caplan (1964)* studied the effect on the mother of the birth of a premature baby and identified four phases or tasks that she must work through to ensure healthy adaptation to the experience. Janis (1958) suggests several hypotheses concerning the psychological stress of impending surgery and the patterns of emotional response that follow a diagnosis of chronic illness. Rapoport (1963)* defines three subphases of marriage, during which unusual stress could precipitate crises. These are only a few of the broad research studies being done in this field.

The generic approach focuses on the characteristic course of the *particular kind of crisis* rather than on the psychodynamics of each individual in crisis. A treatment plan is directed toward an adaptive resolution of the crisis. Specific intervention measures are designed to be effective for all members of a given group rather than for the unique differences of one individual. Recognition of these behavioral patterns is an important aspect of preventive mental health.

Tyhurst (1957) has suggested that knowledge of patterned behaviors in transitional states occurring during intense or sudden change from one life situation to another might provide an empirical basis for the management of these states and the prevention of subsequent mental illness. He cites as examples the studies of individual responses to community disaster, migration, and retirement of pensioners.

Jacobson and associates (1968) state that generic approaches to crisis intervention include "direct encouragement of adaptive behavior, general support, environmental manipulation and anticipatory guidance. . . . In brief, the generic approach emphasizes (1) specific situational and maturational events occurring to significant population groups, (2) intervention oriented to crisis related to these specific events, and (3) intervention carried out by non-mental health professionals."

---

*These studies are also discussed in Chapters 6 and 7 of this text.

This approach has been found to be a feasible mode of intervention that can be learned and implemented by nonpsychiatric physicians, nurses, social workers, and so forth. It does not require a mastery of knowledge of the intrapsychic and interpersonal processes of an individual in crisis.

Individual approach

The individual approach differs from the generic in its emphasis on assessment, by a professional, of the interpersonal and intrapsychic processes of the person in crisis. It is used in selected cases, usually those not responding to the generic approach. Intervention is planned to meet the unique needs of the individual in crisis and to reach a solution for the particular situation and circumstances that precipitated the crisis. This differs from the generic approach, which focuses on the characteristic course of a particular kind of crisis.

Unlike extended psychotherapy, this approach deals relatively little with the developmental past of the individual. Information from this source is seen as relevant only for the clues that may result in a better understanding of the present crisis situation. Emphasis is placed on the immediate causes for disturbed equilibrium and on the processes necessary for regaining a precrisis or higher level of functioning. Jacobson cites the inclusion of family members or other important persons in the process of the individual's crisis resolution as another area of differentiation from most individual psychotherapy.

In comparison with the generic approach he views the individual approach as emphasizing the need for greater depth of understanding of the biopsychosocial process, intervention oriented to the individual's unique situation and carried out only by mental health professionals.

Morley and associates (1967) recommend several attitudes that are important adjuncts to the specific techniques. In essence these comprise the general philosophical orientation necessary for the full effectiveness of the therapist.

1. It is essential that the therapist view the work being done not as a "second-best" approach but as the treatment of choice with persons in crisis.
2. Accurate assessment of the presenting problem, *not* a thorough diagnostic evaluation, is essential to an effective intervention.
3. Both the therapist and the individual should keep in mind throughout the contacts that the treatment is sharply time limited and should persistently direct their energies toward resolution of the presenting problem.
4. Dealing with material not directly related to the crisis has no place as an intervention of this kind.
5. The therapist must be willing to take an active and sometimes directive role in the intervention. The relatively slow-paced approach of more traditional treatment is inappropriate in this type of therapy.

6. Maximum flexibility of approach is encouraged. Such diverse techniques as serving as a resource person or information giver and taking an active role in established liaison with other helping resources are often appropriate in particular situations.

7. The goal toward which the therapist is striving is explicit. Energy is directed entirely toward returning the individual to at least his precrisis level of functioning.

Steps in crisis intervention

There are certain specific steps involved in the technique of crisis intervention (Morley and associates, 1967). Although each cannot be placed in a clearly defined category, typical intervention would pass through the following sequence of phases:

1. The first phase is the assessment of the individual and his problem. This requires the use of active focusing techniques on the part of the therapist to obtain an accurate assessment of the precipitating event and the resulting crisis that brought the individual to seek professional help. The therapist may have to judge whether the help-seeking person presents a high suicidal or homicidal risk. If the patient is thought to be a high level of danger to himself or to others, referral is made to a psychiatrist for consideration of hospitalization. If hospitalization is not deemed necessary, the intervention proceeds.

The initial hour may be spent entirely on assessing the circumstances directly relating to the immediate crisis situation.

2. Planning of therapeutic intervention: After accurate assessment is made of the precipitating event(s) and the crisis, intervention is planned. This is not designed to bring about major changes in the personality structure but to restore the person to at least the precrisis level of equilibrium. In this phase, determination is made of the length of time since onset of the crisis. The precipitating event usually occurs from 1 to 2 weeks before the individual seeks help. Frequently it may have occurred within the past 24 hours. It is important to know how much the crisis has disrupted the person's life and the effects of this disruption on others in his environment. Information is also sought to determine what strengths he has, what coping skills he may have used successfully in the past and is not using presently, and what other people in his life might be used as supports. Search is made for alternative methods of coping that for some reason are not presently being used.

3. Intervention: The nature of intervention techniques is highly dependent on the preexisting skills, creativity, and flexibility of the therapist. Morley suggests some of the following, which have been found useful:

    a. *Helping the individual to gain an intellectual understanding of his crisis.* Often the individual sees no relationship between a hazardous situation occurring in life and the extreme discomfort of disequilibrium that he is experiencing. The therapist could use a direct approach, describing to the patient the relationship between crisis and the event in his life.

b. *Helping the individual bring into the open his present feelings to which he may not have access.* Frequently the person may have suppressed some very real feelings, such as anger or other inadmissible emotions toward someone he "should love or honor." It may also be denial of grief, feelings of guilt, or failure to complete of the mourning process following bereavement. An immediate goal of intervention is the reduction of tension by providing means for the individual to recognize these feelings and bring them into the open. It is sometimes necessary to produce emotional catharsis and reduce immobilizing tension.

c. *Exploration of coping mechanisms.* This approach requires assisting the person to examine alternate ways of coping. If for some reason the behaviors used in the past for successfully reducing anxiety have not been tried, the possibility of their use in the present situation is explored. New coping methods are sought, and frequently the person devises some highly original methods that he has never tried before.

d. *Reopening the social world.* If the crisis has been precipitated by loss of someone significant to the person's life, the possibility of introducing new people to fill the void can be highly effective. It is particularly effective if supports and gratifications provided by the "lost" person in the past can be achieved to a similar degree from new relationships.

4. The last phase is the resolution of the crisis and anticipatory planning. The therapist reinforces those adaptive coping mechanisms that the individual has used successfully to reduce tension and anxiety. As coping abilities increase and positive changes occur, they may be summarized to allow the person to reexperience and reconfirm the progress made. Assistance is given as needed in making realistic plans for the future, and there is discussion of ways in which the present experience may help in coping with future crises.

Summary

A differentiation between psychoanalysis, brief psychotherapy, and crisis intervention methodology has been explored. No attempt has been made to state that one type of therapy is superior to another. In Table 1 we have provided the reader with a succinct profile of some of their major differences.

In psychoanalysis the goal of therapy is that of restructuring the personality, the focus of treatment is on the genetic past and the freeing of the unconscious. Psychoanalytic psychotherapeutic procedures are usually divided into two functional categories: the supportive (suppressive) and uncovering (exploratory or expressive)

Table 1

Major differences between psychoanalysis, brief psychotherapy, and crisis intervention methodology

	Psychoanalysis	Brief psychotherapy	Crisis intervention
Goals of therapy	Restructuring the personality	Removal of specific symptoms	Resolution of immediate crisis
Focus of treatment	1. Genetic past	1. Genetic past as it relates to present situation	1. Genetic present
	2. Freeing the unconscious	2. Repression of unconscious and restraining of drives	2. Restoration to level of functioning prior to crisis
Usual activity of therapist	1. Exploratory	1. Suppressive	1. Suppressive
	2. Passive observer	2. Participant observer	2. Active participant
	3. Nondirective	3. Indirect	3. Direct
Indications	Neurotic personality patterns	Acutely disruptive emotional pain and severely disruptive circumstances	Sudden loss of ability to cope with a life situation
Average length of treatment	Indefinite	From one to twenty sessions	From one to six sessions

procedures. The therapist's role is nondirective, exploratory, and that of a passive observer. This type of therapy is indicated for those individuals with neurotic personality patterns. Lengths of the therapy is indefinite and depends on the individual and the therapist.

Brief psychotherapy has as its goal removing specific symptoms and aiding in the prevention of developing deeper neurotic or psychotic symptoms. Its focus is on the genetic past as it relates to the present situation, repression of the unconscious, and restraining of drives. The role of the therapist is indirect, suppressive, and that of a participant observer. Basic tools used are psychodynamic intervention coupled with medical or environmental types of intervention. Indications for brief psychotherapy are acutely disruptive emotional pain, severely disruptive circumstances, and situations endangering the life of the individual or others. It is also indicated for those who have problems that do not require psychoanalytic intervention. The average length of treatment is from one to twenty sessions.

The goal of crisis intervention is the resolution of an immediate crisis. Its focus is on the genetic present, with the restoration of the individual to her precrisis level of functioning or possibly to a higher level of functioning. The therapist's role is direct, suppressive, and that of an active participant. Techniques are varied and limited only by the flexibility and creativity of the therapist. Some of these techniques include helping the individual gain an intellectual understanding of the crisis, assisting the individual in bringing her feelings into the open, exploring past and present coping mechanisms, finding and using situational supports, and anticipatory planning with the individual to reduce the possibility of future crises. This type of therapy is indicated when a person (or family) suddenly loses her ability to cope with a life situation. The average length of treatment is from one to six sessions.

References

Alexander, F.: Psychoanalysis and psychotherapy, New York, 1956, W.W. Norton & Co., Inc.

Alexander F., and French, T.M.: Psychoanalytic therapy, New York, 1946, The Ronald Press Co.

Bellak, L., and Small, L.: Emergency psychotherapy and brief psychotherapy, New York, 1965, Grune & Stratton, Inc.

Caplan, G.: Principles of preventive psychiatry, New York, 1964, Basic Books, Inc., Publishers.

Freud, S.: Collected papers, vol. 1, translated by Joan Riviere, Alex Strachey, and James Strachey, London, 1924, The Hogarth Press, Ltd.

Jacobson, G.: Crisis theory and treatment strategy: some sociocultural and psychodynamic considerations, J. Nerv. Ment. Dis. **141:**209, 1965.

Jacobson, G.: Crisis theory, New Directions for Mental Health Services **6:**1, 1980.

Jacobson, G., Strickler, M., and Morley, W.E.: Generic and individual approaches to crisis intervention, Am. J. Public Health **58:**339, 1968.

Janis, I.L.: Psychological stress, psychoanalytical and behavioral studies of surgical patients, New York, 1958, John Wiley & Sons, Inc.

Kaplan, D.M., and Mason, E.A.: Maternal reactions to premature birth viewed as an acute emotional disorder, Am. J. Orthopsychiatry **30:**539, 1960.

Lindemann, E.: Symptomatology and management of acute grief, Am. J. Psychiatry **101:**101, Sept. 1944.

Mason, E.A.: Method of predicting crisis outcome for mothers of premature babies, Public Health Rep. **78:**1031, 1963.

Morley, W.E., Messick, J.M., and Aguilera, D.C.: Crisis: paradigms of intervention, J. Psychiatr. Nurs. **5:**537, 1967.

Rapoport, R.: Normal crises, family structure, and mental health, Fam. Process **2:**68, 1963.

Stone, L.: Psychoanalysis and brief psychotherapy, Psychoanal. Q. **20:**217, 1951.

Tarachow, S.: An introduction to psychotherapy, New York, 1963, International Universities Press.

Tyhurst, J.A.: Role of transition states—including disasters—in mental illness, Symposium on Preventive and Social Psychiatry sponsored by Walter Reed Institute of Research, Walter Reed Medical Center, and National Research Council, April 15-17, Washington, D.C., 1957, U.S. Government Printing Office.

Additional readings

Baldwin, B.A.: A paradigm for the classification of emotional crises, implications for crisis intervention, Am. J. Orthopsychiatry **48:**538, 1978.

Baldwin, B.A.: Crisis intervention: an overview of theory and practice, Counseling Psychologist **8:**43, Feb. 1979.

Beck, A.T., and others: Cognitive therapy, New York, 1979, The Guilford Press.

Beers, T.M., Jr., and Foreman, M.E.: Intervention patterns in crisis interviews, J. Counsult. Clin. Psychol. **3**(2):87, 1976.

Bernstein, A.E., and Warner, G.M.: An introduction to contemporary psychoanalysis, New York, 1981, Jason Aronson, Inc.

Bloom, B.L.: Social and community interventions, Ann. Rev. Psychol. **31:**111, 1980.

Budman, S.H.: Forms of brief therapy, New York, 1981, The Guilford Press.

Caplan, G.: Emotional crisis. In Deutsch, A., and Fishbein, H., editors: The encyclopedia of mental health, vol. 2, New York, 1963, Franklin Watts, Inc.

Caplan, G., and Grunebaum, H.: Perspectives on primary prevention, Arch. Gen. Psychiatry **17:**331, Sept. 1967.

Connally, J.: Therapy options in psychiatry, Turnbridge Welk, England, 1978, Pitman Medical.

Corsini, R.J.: Current psychotherapies, ed. 2, Itasca, Ill., 1979, F.E. Peacock Publishers, Inc.

Dixon, S.L.: Working with people in crisis, St. Louis, 1979, The C.V. Mosby Co.

Flegenheimer, W.V.: The patient-therapist relationship in crisis intervention, J. Clin. Psychiatry **39**:348, April 1978.

Frank, J.: Thirty years of group therapy: a personal perspective, Int. J. Group Psychother. **29**:439, 1979.

Fromm-Reichmann, F.: Psychoanalysis and psychotherapy, Chicago, 1959, University of Chicago Press.

Garfield, S.L.: Psychotherapy: an eclectic approach, New York, 1980, John Wiley & Sons, Inc.

Ivey, A.E., and Simek-Downing, L.: Counselling and psychotherapy: skills, theory, and practice, Englewood Cliffs, N.J., 1980, Prentice-Hall, Inc.

Jacobson, G.F.: Crisis-oriented therapy, Psychiatr. Clin. North Am. **2**:39, 1979.

Karasu, T.B.: Psychotherapies: an overview, Am. J. Psychiatry **134**:851, 1977.

Kardener, S.H.: A methodological approach to crisis theory, Am. J. Psychother. **29**:4, 1975.

Langsley, D.G., and Kaplan, D.M.: The treatment of families in crisis, New York, 1968, Grune & Stratton, Inc.

Lazare, A., editor: Outpatient psychiatry: diagnosis and treatment, Baltimore, 1979, The William & Wilkins Co.

London, P., and Klerman, G.L.: Evaluating psychotherapy, Am. J. Psychiatry 139:709, 1982.

Marguiles, A., and Havens, L.L.: The initial encounter: what to do first, Am. J. Psychiatry **138**:421, 1981.

Marmor, J.: Short-term dynamic psychotherapy, Am. J. Psychiatry **136**:149, Feb. 1979.

Podolnick, E.E., and others: A psychodynamic approach to brief therapy, College Health, **28**:109, 1979.

Rapoport, L.: The state of crisis: some theoretical considerations, Chicago, 1972, University of Chicago Press.

Rosenbaum, C.P., and Beebe, J.E.: Psychiatric treatment: crisis/clinic/consultation, New York, 1975, McGraw-Hill Book Co.

Silver, R.J., and others: The group psychotherapy literature: 1980, Int. J. Group Psychother. **31**(4):469, 1981.

Small, L.: The briefer psychotherapies, ed. 2, New York, 1979, Brunner/Mazel, Inc.

Smith, L.L.: A review of crisis intervention theory, Soc. Casework, 7:396, 1978.

Smith, L.L.: A review of crisis intervention theory, Soc. Casework 59:396, 1978.

Yalom, I.: The theory and practice of group psychotherapy, ed. 2, New York, 1975, Basic Books, Inc., Publishers.

Yalom, I.: Existential psychotherapy, New York, 1980, Basic Books, Inc., Publishers.

chapter 3

Group therapy concepts in crisis intervention

Group concepts

From birth on, the individual is a member of a group composed of himself and his parents. His life becomes a succession of group memberships, expanding from the basic family unit to peer groups, play groups, and groups in school, business, and church. An individual may remain in some groups permanently or temporarily, voluntarily or involuntarily, and in some directly or indirectly, but he will usually participate in some form of group activity until death.

A helpless infant depending on the actions of others for survival progresses through intellectual, emotional, and social development. Forms of behavior that communicate feelings, needs, and ideas develop through interactions with others. At the same time, perceptions and reactions toward the feelings, needs, and ideas of others develop.

It has been suggested that an individual's behavior can be controlled and influenced by the forces of groups of which she is a member and that she becomes what she is because of the roles, status, and functions that are taken or given in the groups (Asch, 1951; Merton, 1968). Interpersonal skills are neither inherited nor instinctive but are acquired through a continual learning process involving use of all the senses. Facial expressions, vocal tones, body movements, odors, touch, and so forth are all a part of the language of interpersonal communications. Since human beings communicate through nonverbal as well as verbal clues, deprivation of any one of the senses could lead to distorted perceptions of the actions and responses of others.

Experiences that bring feelings of comfort and satisfaction are usually tried again, whereas those that result in frustration and discomfort are avoided whenever possible so that progressive learning is based on past experiences. If a child's first important group, the immediate family, fails to provide gratifying, positive interpersonal learning experiences, his future psychosocial development could be impaired. For example, the child who has never learned how to obtain gratifying feelings of approval from his family may be less than secure in establishing relationships with authority figures in other groups later, such as a teacher-pupil relationship in school. He may also have added difficulties in early peer groups, where beginning competition and leadership skills are first learned.

In recent years practical and scientific knowledge has been synthesized to form new concepts about the manipulation of group structures and group processes to effect change, both on the group and on its individual members. In psychiatry emphasis has shifted from considering a person as a biological entity to considering him as a biopsychosocial entity. Movement has been increasingly away from an organism-centered to a social-centered conceptualization of personality dynamics. Other professions and social institutions have also been increasingly aware of the effects of group influences upon the individual.

During and immediately after World War II there was an increased recognition of the necessity to meet the special needs of groups of people for whom individual care was impossible. This contributed to a rapid rise in the development and acceptance of group therapy and other therapeutic groups in the military, veterans' hospitals, and state and private institutions and clinics. Since then, an increasing variety of therapy groups has been developed in community and institutional settings, not only for patients with psychiatric problems but also for people unable to cope with many situational and maturational problems and stresses in daily life.

Therapy groups

Any simple definition of the term *group therapy* would be difficult because of a wide variety of concepts, methods, and interpretations of its meaning. In reference to people a group means, primarily, more than one person. If combined with the word therapy, it could mean, simply, a treatment given simultaneously to more than one person. When the group goal of effecting a change is included, it becomes more complicated because consideration must then be given to the methods and processes of group action, of individual action, and of the wide differences in group accomplishments.

Corsini and Rosenberg (1955) proposed a classification of group therapies in terms of involvement of intellectual, emotional, or action factors. Luchins (1964) suggests classifications based on concrete activities. According to Hinckley and Hermann (1951), one approach to understanding the differences between the many types of therapy groups has been to focus on their purposes and results. They suggest two main categories: *social group work* and *group therapy*.

Social group work

In social group work the purpose is to achieve a common group goal with the aid of a leader. A project or an activity is used to unite the members, and the chief result is socialization. Examples of this are recreational groups, calling for teamwork and sportsmanship, or rhythm and games groups; another example is sociodrama, in which symptomatic behavior is indirectly touched on by participants through playacting. In this way discussions of feelings and behavior can be directed toward the *part* that is acted out, not toward the participant. Scouting and camping groups for children and adolescents are other means of fostering socialization and group-unifying activities.

In any of these social groups the leader serves as a director, discussant, or counselor. The leader must have skills in special areas, and her understanding of the dynamics of personality is secondary in importance to her understanding of group action and cultural patterns and mores. She is usually directive in leading group activities along a prescribed course.

Slavson's (1964) approach to classifying therapy groups is to focus on the concept of depth in therapy for differentiating between types of psychotherapies. He acknowledges the concept of depth in therapy to be a controversial one, and apparently no absolute criterion exists for determining the absolute values of any one method in relation to another. The absence of accurate measuring devices makes it difficult to measure quantitatively changes in the psyche, functions, or attitudes resulting from therapy, and comparisons between methods could be misleading.

If the choice of method and course of psychotherapy is determined by the nature and intensity of individual needs, Slavson suggests a differentiation of psychotherapies based on the level of a person's psyche that requires change. Using this concept he has differentiated psychotherapy into the main categories of counseling, guidance, and psychotherapy.

Counseling

Counseling is reality oriented and focuses on solving specific problems arising from situational or interpersonal difficulties. The counselor is not required to be a trained psychotherapist but should have a greater knowledge than the counselee of the factors affecting the situation. The role is to direct actively toward the finding and acceptance of a solution to an immediate difficulty while not intentionally exposing the counselee's feelings or attitudes for the purpose of changing them. It is assumed that once the solutions are made clear, the ego will be able to function adequately toward solving the problem. The length of time in interviews is comparatively brief, and the sessions terminate as soon as the immediate specific difficulty is resolved. This method is least effective in group use.

Guidance

Guidance is a reality-oriented approach that may be used when a person is incapable of coping with increased stresses because the emotional significance of a specific problem begins to affect simple ego functioning. The aims and techniques are toward holding or reducing anxiety to a tolerable level and preventing disorganization. The focus is on correcting feelings and requires a professionally trained person with a sound understanding of psychodynamics and experience in psychotherapy that will enable the professional to work at this deeper level. The therapist's role is to supply clarification and support through empathy, acceptance, and permissiveness, thus enabling a client to bring conflictual feelings about the specific problem into conscious awareness and to ventilate them without increasing anxiety, guilt, or fear.

This approach may require a much longer period of time and more sessions than the counseling approach because additional stress and discomfort need to be prevented, since the client is confronted with personal feelings and may be expected to change some perceptions, attitudes, and behaviors.

The use of groups appears to accelerate the guidance process, particularly when people with problems of a similar nature are brought together. There is mutual identification with the problem area, and interactions occur rapidly, members possibly providing each other with greater support of self-esteem through empathy, acceptance, and permissiveness than the therapist alone could provide. Negative feelings of being alone in needing help with a problem are alleviated.

Guidance has been found particularly effective in dealing with adolescents, persons with marital problems, families, parents of handicapped children, and so on. The therapist's role requires the ability to use skills necessary for psychotherapy, recognizing and avoiding threatening areas for each member while working with the group as a whole. Feelings and behaviors are explored only as they are significant to the reality of each member's life situation; unrestricted exploration of feelings is avoided.

Group psychotherapy

Group psychotherapy is intended to make fundamental personality changes and to investigate reasons for personal emotional problems (Hinckley and Hermann, 1951). Unlike counseling or guidance, it does not aim to solve a single specific situational problem; rather, it aims toward correction of intrapsychic processes that will make the person more capable of dealing with many problems.

The group approach is based on concepts of individual psychotherapy. Free association and unrestricted exploration of emotions are encouraged. Unlike social or guidance groups, the group approach has no one specific group goal, and each member has specific personal aims and expectations about what the group experience can offer. Cohesiveness of members develops from the stresses and pain they experience as they focus on emotional problems, traumatic memories, and uncovered feelings, and possibly from mutual identification with any specific reality problem area. Efforts to minimize these feelings by resorting to gamelike activities are not permitted. Rather than avoiding threatening areas, the therapist takes relatively few precautions and encourages ventilation or catharsis of feelings. General therapeutic goals for patients with functional illness are to relieve tensions and anxiety, help them to gain some insights into their problems, assist them to resolve some of their conflicts, and support them in replacing or changing maladaptive behaviors for adaptive ones.

Group therapy employs a variety of techniques to obtain its general aims, and therapists often differ in their leadership roles. Some actively direct, whereas others may deem it more therapeutic to take a passive, indirect role to a degree that the group appears to be self-directed.

Although there is a relationship between technique and theory, few present-day techniques have been derived *solely* from theory. The therapist will undoubtedly be testing out certain theories and hypotheses and psychodynamics and group dynamics; this is an intrinsic part of a professional-scientific role. At the same time, the therapist also has the role of "healer," assuming responsibilities to help individuals solve concrete problems encountered in their daily living.

Some therapists may focus on the psychodynamics of individual behavior; others may focus on group dynamics. Sometimes the focus will remain on the theoretical, intellectual level rather than on the specific individual behavioral responses taking place within the immediate interactions of the group; more often than not there is a combination of both going on, and no one method can be criticized as being better or worse than another.

A most important responsibility for the therapist is interpreting to patients the purpose for bringing the group together and the principles or rules under which they will operate. The patient's acceptance of this mode of therapy is determined in large part by whether he sees it as meeting his needs and whether he will be able to function under the principles of the group's operation. For example, the basic difficulties of a person may stem from early negative experiences in his primary family, and resultant avoidance reactions to group contacts could further increase his anxieties. Not only might this lead to increasing areas of conflict but the necessary positive transference phenomena would be unlikely. Selection criteria for members vary widely according to their needs, the availability and special areas of expertise of qualified therapists, and the purpose of the groups. These factors may also influence the size of membership, and there is no general agreement about the number of sessions needed to accomplish specific goals.

The group process provides more than one person with whom the individual may identify and test out reactions to past experiences. The therapist is most likely to be seen as the parental role figure. Also there are the sibling role figures of other members with whom interactions take place. In this way group psychotherapy provides on a small scale a situation in which a problem in interpersonal relationships can be exposed and a setting for action, reaction, and interaction within a therapeutic environment. Distorted perceptions of interpersonal experiences in the past can be revealed and examined. Varied interpersonal stimuli will be received from more than one source, and increasing opportunities for transference phenomena to take place and to be worked through will occur. Briefly, a transference phenomenon occurs when a person reacts to someone in the present as he did to someone in the past. This is because everyone has a tendency to carry over, into the present, attitudes and impressions gained from past interpersonal experiences. Although the present person may possess only one or two of the characteristics of the past person, a generalized distortion of the relationship can be triggered. The present person becomes the recipient of the emotional responses and reactive behaviors that, in reality, were learned in the past relationship.

One therapeutic goal is to modify and clarify feelings; feelings must be labeled and then verbalized in order for this to take place. The group provides an incentive in this area by open discussion during which patients are stimulated by the fact of emotions expressed by others and by the opportunity to relate their own problems to others in the group. Changed or new behavior responses can be tried out, observed in action, reflected back, and the dynamics explored for cause-and-effect reactions. Providing opportunities to increase coping capacities is important because this reflects the ability to resolve emotional issues and interpersonal problems that create conflicts.

For the individual, group experience is primarily an emotional one, and through interactions with other members he is confronted by relationships that may be supportive, critical, or a combination of both. Members are encouraged to both criticize and support each other, support occurring most often through mutual acceptance and empathic responses from other members. The presence of others is perceived as a protection against being the only object of the therapist's attention. Acceptance by a peer group rather than by just one person, the therapist, is reassuring, and feelings of being different and isolated are counteracted by the discovery that these same feelings and problems may be shared by others. It seems generally agreed that intergroup support is essential to the growth of a therapy group. Group interaction should assist the members to achieve insight into past behavior and to gain self-awareness in learning to adapt to more positive and satisfying interpersonal experiences in the future.

Crisis groups

Since the term *group therapy* may mean any two individuals who are in therapy together with a therapist, certain terms that may be unfamiliar to those who have not been involved in conducting therapy will be clarified. When *individual* crisis intervention therapy is mentioned, it means that an individual is in therapy on a one-to-one relationship with the therapist (Case study: Status and role change, p. 99). *Conjoint* therapy refers to therapy that is conducted with a husband and wife who are seen by the therapist together (Case study: Prematurity, p. 79). *Family* therapy includes those members of the family who are involved or affected by the crisis situation (Case study: Prepuberty, p. 195). *Collateral* therapy could include almost any combination of two individuals who are involved in the crisis: mother-son, father-son, mother-daughter, father-daughter, boyfriend-girlfriend, boyfriend-boyfriend, roommates, and so forth (Case study: Young adulthood, p. 207). The term *crisis group* refers to a collection of individuals who are unknown and unrelated to each other who meet as a group with a therapist to work together toward resolution of their individual crises through group interaction (Case study: Mrs. L., p. 41).

Treatment goals

The goal of a crisis group is that of returning the individual members of the group to at least their precrisis level of functioning and possibly to a higher level with an increased ability in problem solving. The focus of treatment (like that of crisis intervention individual therapy) is oriented to the present and to the problem that is of concern at the time the individuals request help. It deals with the stresses and balancing factors that are either absent or ineffective in the present crisis situations and is directed toward assisting the members to achieve resolution of their crises. With the therapist the members explore the crisis-precipitating events, the crises, past coping skills (what they usually do when they cannot handle anxiety, tension, and so on), situational supports (whom they usually turn to for help), and what is going on at the present time that is preventing them from solving their problems. The group members quickly become a cohesive group, actively involved in helping other members develop new coping skills and find situational supports. The therapist keeps them aware that the number of sessions is limited to six, using such methods as reminding them that a certain member has only two more sessions left.

Selection of participants

The determination of whether individuals requesting help in a crisis situation would benefit more from group therapy sessions than from individual therapy sessions is initially left to the discretion of the intake worker who sees the patient first. It might be that a group is being formed or that an ongoing group is oriented toward problems similar to the one in which the individual is involved. For example, there may be groups of married couples experiencing marital discord, parents with problems that involve their children, a group whose members are trying to break the drug habit, and adolescents with problems (family, drugs, juvenile authority, and so forth). Another consideration is whether another member can be added to the group. The crisis group is open ended—its members enter and leave at different times; some will be beginning in the group, others will be halfway through, and others will be terminating. Five to eight members is usually considered the best size for a crisis group; it can fluctuate weekly as some members are absent or are terminated and new members are added. The therapist who conducts the group can control this by limiting the number of intake interviews scheduled each week.

Other crisis groups have differing rather than common problems as their focus. The purpose of including individuals in one of these groups would be because the interviewer believes that the individual would benefit more by interaction in a group than in a one-to-one relationship. It may be decided that part of the problem is the result of inadequate interpersonal relations. The individual may be a social isolate by choice or by necessity, and her problem may be that she has never been able to establish satisfactory relationships with others because of low self-esteem, poor self-concept, or a real or imagined handicap; or she may be new to the area, functioning in a new job or school and having difficulty meeting and making friends and would benefit from a group experience. This also could be true with individuals who, although they might resist accepting the "advice of experts," would be more agreeable to changing faulty coping skills through group pressure.

If it is thought that a person would benefit from group therapy, she is told the time and day the group meets and is asked to participate. If she agrees, she is given an appointment for a pregroup interview with the therapist who will be conducting the group. In this interview the therapist assesses the individual and makes the final decision of recommending group or individual therapy. Determinations are made of the stressful event(s) that precipitated the crisis, the symptoms that are present, and the degree of disruption that the crisis is creating in the individual's life. If group therapy is the treatment of choice, the therapist discusses the format of the sessions. Explanations are made of the time element (6 weekly sessions that last for 1½ to 2 hours), the necessity for focus on immediate problems, and the fact that some members will be new to the group and others will be terminating. If the group comprises members with a common problem area, a brief explanation may be made of who is in the group—for example, Mr. and Mrs. X. have been married for 4 years and are having problems in their marriage similar to those of other members. This technique assists those seeking help to relax and assures them that their problem is not unique, that they are not alone, and that they can expect other members of the group to understand and help them reach a solution to their problem.

Format of sessions

The format of sessions is highly individual, depending on the therapist and the physical environment or setting where the group sessions meet. Members may be asked to wait in a reception room until the scheduled hour before they are brought into the office (or room) that has been assigned. Or a room may be set aside, the members going directly to the room and, in some cases, "starting" the session informally before the therapist arrives.

In the first part of the group session the therapist very briefly introduces new members and asks them to tell the reason why they came for help. The other members then tell the reason why they are there and will usually add at what stage they are in therapy and what they believe is being accomplished in the group.

Role of therapist

The role of the therapist is active and direct. The therapist functions as a participant leader in the group sessions, assisting the members to focus on the problem areas under discussion by restricting and diverting general social conversation and lengthy discussions of past occurrences that have no relevance to the present crisis of the individuals in the group. The therapist also acts as group facilitator and must be alert to the quiet, passive members and encourage their participation. Conversely, highly verbal and dominant members must be controlled and directed without completely silencing them as participants. Therapists must be skillful in understanding and acting on nonverbal clues from the members of the group. An example of this is the silent wife who appeared to the group to be calm and unruffled while her verbal, aggressive husband, in an angry tirade, told the rest of the group about the problems he was having with their son, who never talked to him, refused to mind, was never home, and so on. The therapist, observing the wife's nonverbal behavior (tense posture, hands folding her handkerchief over and over, lips tightly compressed—as if she did not dare to speak), interrupted the husband politely but firmly and asked the wife directly if this was the way their son acted toward his father. The wife looked at the rest of the group; they encouraged her, saying that she should know her son better than his father because she was with him more. Thus encouraged by the therapist and the group, she replied that their son did act this way toward his father and she believed that he had every reason to because he had no respect for him. Turning to her husband she said, "Why should he? Every time he sees you, you are either drunk or mad and you are always fighting with him."

Studies of crisis groups

Relatively little has been written about the effectiveness or ineffectiveness of crisis group therapy. Strickler and Allgeyer's (1967) pilot study at the Benjamin Rush Center in Los Angeles was one of the first to test the feasibility of conducting group therapy using the crisis intervention model. In this study consideration was given to the unique role of the therapist, the dynamics of the group process, and the group instrument that was structured to lend itself to the characteristic phases of crisis resolution.

Selection of members and structure of the group were in most respects similar to the general admission procedures for individual crisis intervention. No one was eliminated from group therapy because of severe pathological illness. After the initiation of the pilot group, it was found necessary to eliminate the following two groups of individuals: (1) those whom the therapist believed were seriously suicidal or homicidal and in need of more concentrated and individualized attention; and (2) those who were unable to relate to others because of a psychotic state or who, because of a language barrier, were unable to communicate in English. In the intake interview people were allowed the opportunity to choose individual therapy over group therapy if they so desired.

The study, which was conducted over a six-month period, served thirty patients and had an average weekly attendance of four to five sessions for each member. The size of the group in each session varied from four to eight members; a group of five to six members each session was considered to be the optimum for treatment purposes.

The crisis group at the Benjamin Rush Center was structured to correspond to the three sequential phases of crisis resolution. The first phase involved the formulation of the crisis situation for the patient, which was accomplished in the pre-group interview. The second phase constituted the utilization of the group to help the patient attempt to solve his problem. In the third phase the group reinforced and helped sustain the patient's confidence in new ways of coping.

A study by Morley and Brown (1968) explored the disadvantages and advantages of crisis intervention groups. Their study was carried out at the Venice branch of the Benjamin Rush Center. This clinic serves people who are usually underrepresented in most mental health facilities: families with an annual income of less than $4000, blacks, those of Mexican or Spanish-American descent, or those whose main family wage earner is a blue-collar worker. The criteria for accepting individuals into the group were similar to those previously used by Strickler and Allgeyer.

Morley and Brown listed several advantages of crisis groups and individual crisis intervention not typically available in "traditional" group or individual psychotherapy. First, it brings help to a number of individuals in need of treatment who might be unwilling or unable to enter into traditional treatment. This would include individuals who are willing to accept help with a problem but who do not consider themselves in need of psychiatric treatment for a mental or emotional illness. Second, many individuals are unwilling to agree to long-term therapy but will accept help for a particular problem carried out over a short period of time. Third, the universality of crisis provides a common meeting ground between patient and therapist, and the terminology and concepts seem to be more understandable and more acceptable to many individuals.

It was concluded that there seemed to be some disadvantages that occurred in the crisis group approach when compared with a traditional group approach. First and primarily, the analysis of group process, which is a powerful tool in traditional group work, had to be sacrificed to a certain extent. The time-limited and problem-oriented crisis groups made it impossible to make as much use of process analysis as is possible with a longer-term group. The need to focus on each individual's presenting problem limited dealing with group interaction on any but a superficial level. Second, some spontaneity seemed to be lost. It was often necessary for the therapist to use the technique of "going around" to be certain that all members became active participants as soon as possible. Third, there was some loss of continuity and a greater need for repetition. The members were constantly changing, and new members needed to be brought up to date on the problem areas of the other members. Finally, transference interpretation was minimized. Negative transference interpretation was minimized because there was not a long-term relationship to give the individuals support if there was a sharp focus on strong negative feelings.

The study also compared crisis groups with individual crisis intervention. On the positive side, group support was apparent to a significant degree, and members of the group offered a considerable amount of help and assurance to particularly disturbed group members, both within and outside the group therapy session; significant social relationships often grew out of the group contacts, and group members were effective in suggesting alternate coping mechanisms to others in the group. The group provided an avenue for encouraging expression of feelings, and members who saw others in the group openly expressing their feelings were thus encouraged to express their own feelings.

On the negative side the primary problem was keeping each individual's crisis in sharp focus. With members presenting a wide variety of different crises, it was often difficult to keep each person dealing solely with the specific area necessary for successful resolution of the crisis. It was also difficult to identify the "correct crisis." In the second or third hour of therapy the original area identified as the crisis might be supplanted by another. In individual crisis therapy this could be reassessed and identified easier than in a group setting. Another problem area was that of destructive coping mechanisms offered by other members of the group. Because they did not understand the underlying dynamics operating within a particular individual, the suggestions they would make might be more maladaptive than adaptive. Morley and Brown believed that the group approach offered little or no saving of professional time. The pregroup interviews and cancellations seemed to have been of primary importance in producing this result.

One of the authors (Aguilera) also conducted crisis group therapy at this same center in Venice and concurs with the findings of Strickler and Allgeyer and those of Morley and Brown. The format of the sessions and admission to the group were essentially the same as those for the other studies cited, with one exception: the selection of members was made with a specific problem area in which to work. The problem area of the group was defined as those parents who were having problems with their young adolescents. These parents were seen in one group with the therapist, and their adolescent children were seen in another group with another therapist. The sessions usually lasted from 1 to 1½ hours and were scheduled concurrently for the same evening. There was close communication between therapists, usually immediately after each session. Occasionally the therapists decided that the parents and adolescents would benefit from a collateral session with both therapists present. This was usually scheduled either before or immediately following the group therapy session. These crises groups seemed extremely effective because of the specific focus on a problem area, and the interaction between the group members was exceptionally high. The members were able to support each other in decisions regarding their problems and to explore alternate ways of coping. During the intake interview and the pregroup interview the parent(s) and child were seen individually, and, if necessary, together, to determine their reasons for requesting help, their willingness to enter a group, and the appropriateness of their membership in the group.

As a brief overview of how group therapy functions using crisis-intervention techniques, a case study is presented depicting how the therapist and the group members interrelated in resolving their crises.

It was initially believed by the intake worker that Mrs. L. would benefit more from group therapy than from individual therapy. She was by choice a social isolate and in all probability would resist efforts to modify her behavior with her daughter because she strongly believed that she was "right" and a "good mother." Cindy, in turn, would benefit from group therapy with those of her own age group to gain their support or to have her actions invalidated by them. They were scheduled for their pregroup interview with the therapist.

Case study

Mrs. L., 42 years of age and a grandmotherly appearing woman, came to a crisis intervention center for her pregroup interview with the therapist, accompanied by her 14-year-old daughter, Cindy. Cindy and her mother had been referred to the center for therapy by juvenile authorities. Cindy had run away from home and had been picked up by the police while trying to hitchhike to a well-known commune in northern California. When Mrs. L. was notified that Cindy had been found and was at the police station, she refused to come down, stating to the officer, "You had better keep her; I can't do anything with her!" She was told to come to court the next morning.

Cindy was held overnight in a juvenile hall. This apparently had been a terrifying experience for her. She said that she had shared a room with two other girls but had been too frightened to sleep because they threatened to kill her if she "reported on their lesbian activities." She stated she would do anything to avoid going back to juvenile hall or a similar corrective institution.

Cindy was very attractive and mature socially as well as physically. She was soft spoken and poised, was of above-average intelligence with A and B grades in school, and enjoyed tennis and playing the piano. She was well liked by her teachers but had few friends in her peer group.

Cindy told the therapist that she thought her mother's standards were too rigid and that her mother tried to keep her isolated from her own age group. She refused to let Cindy participate in social activities or dating and would even wait for Cindy to get out of school and "walk" her home.

Mrs. L. said that Cindy had been a "good" girl until recently—very obedient and so forth—and she could not understand her present behavior. When questioned about Cindy's father, Mrs. L. became quite angry and defensive and said they had been divorced for 6 years. She implied that she had "married beneath her" and that he drank too much and had difficulty keeping jobs. A small amount of alimony and support for Cindy had forced them to move from their original "middle-class" neighborhood to their present low socioeconomic area. She was apparently attempting to isolate Cindy from the "undesirable elements and people" in the environment. She saw herself as a "good" mother who was trying to maintain middle-class morality while living among a lower class.

GROUP SESSION

Phase 1: Formulation of crisis situation. Mrs. L. was introduced to the other members of the group and asked by the therapist to state what problem she was having with Cindy. She repeated her previous remarks to the group about Cindy running away and what she had done and said to the officer. When asked what had preceded Cindy's running away (the precipitating event), she became quite verbal. She said Cindy had asked to go to a neighborhood teen social center where a dance was being held. Mrs. L. refused, feeling that "Cindy was too young . . . she would meet the 'wrong' kind of people . . . the events were not properly chaperoned, etc., etc." While Mrs. L. was watching television in the living room, Cindy sneaked out of the house, went to the dance, and got back without being found out. The next day a neighbor informed Mrs. L. that her daughter had seen Cindy at the dance.

Mrs. L. immediately went to school, had Cindy called out of class, and confronted Cindy with the information. Cindy admitted she had attended the dance and that she would sneak out again if she got the chance. Mrs. L. slapped her, and Cindy ran from the school crying. When Cindy failed to come home that evening, Mrs. L. reported her missing to the police. Cindy was picked up the next afternoon. Mrs. L.'s previous method of coping, by denying the reality of the situation and by trying to isolate herself and Cindy from their environment, was no longer effective: Cindy was growing up and demanding more freedom and independence.

Group response. Some of the members of the group responded to Mrs. L.'s comments by making superficial supportive statements such as, "It sure is difficult to raise kids these days!'' and, ''The kids must be acting this way because of the kind of world we live in.'' Others suggested that she was ''too rigid,'' and, ''You have to give the girl some freedom . . . she's not a baby anymore . . . you can't keep her a prisoner.'' Another offered alternate ways of coping: ''You don't have to give in all the way, but give her a chance; if it doesn't work, then try something else.'' One member reminded her that her present behavior had *caused* Cindy to run away. Others challenged her with, ''If you don't like the neighborhood, move; no one is keeping you there!'' and, ''If you don't have the money, go to work instead of staying home and playing the good mother.''

Mrs. L.'s response to group. At first Mrs. L. reacted with hostility toward the group suggestions and confrontations. She still maintained her rigidity and saw her actions and behavior as justified. She rationalized them by stating firmly that she ''couldn't care less what other people think,'' she knew she was right. Later, when the group members began making suggestions for different ways of maintaining discipline and still allowing Cindy some freedom, she responded with, ''I'll consider it.'' She reacted warmly to those members who made supportive statements or suggestions and directed most of her remarks toward them. To the members who made negative statements she responded in an aloof, superior, cold manner and avoided conversation with them if she could.

Phase II: Intervention. In subsequent sessions Mrs. L. became more comfortable with the group members and felt less threatened. She began to adopt some of their suggestions in coping with Cindy. When the suggestions ''worked,'' she always expressed her thanks to the member who had made the suggestion. She soon dropped her superior attitude toward group members and was able to express her feelings of guilt over slapping Cindy. She stated that she rarely had to punish Cindy because she was usually able to reason with her. She still maintained her ''good mother'' role in the group, and the group accepted her as an authority figure because she was very verbal and intelligent. They still challenged her rigidity and inconsistency about not wanting to work while Cindy was in school. She believed that she and her daughter were beginning to understand each other a little better.

The group members worked cohesively and sharply focused on specific problem areas. By the end of the third session they were interacting freely, testing new coping devices and reality testing within the group. Before the fourth group session the therapist had a pregroup interview with a Mr. G. His problems with his son appeared to be so similar to Mrs. L.'s that the therapist thought he would be a valuable addition to the group and would benefit from the group experience.

In the pregroup interview with the therapist Mr. G. expressed great concern over his son's changed behavior and appeared genuinely at a loss as to why he should now be presenting problems. He had also run away from home and had been picked up by authorities. Mr. G. said he had tried hard to be a ''good father'' since his wife had left him 5 years ago, and he stated repeatedly how much he loved his son and what a good boy the son had always been before running away. Mr. G. appeared to be a very mild-mannered man and was quiet almost to the point of shyness.

He entered the group at the fourth session. After being introduced he began talking about his son and his problems with him. Very matter-of-factly, with little emotional expression, he calmly stated: "I'm a good father, I love my son, I can't understand why he has changed. I've beaten the hell out of him since he was 5 years old, and with the buckle end of the belt half the time, and he still won't mind." The group members were shocked into silence. The therapist, recognizing this, remained silent to observe the responses of the individual members to this different attitude about disciplining a child.

Group response. The group recovered from their state of shock over Mr. G.'s announcement and immediately began to attack him verbally. Mrs. L. emerged as their "leader" in the attack. Their comments were personal and cutting. Mr. G. countered their attack by becoming hostile and just as verbally aggressive. It was obvious that the focus of the group was, at this time, shattered because the group had deviated from problem areas to attacking an individual's attitude and character. The therapist stopped the "debate" and confronted the group with their behavior. After a discussion period the group, at the insistence of the therapist, began to redirect the focus to problem areas of concern. Mrs. L., as the group leader, began to explain to Mr. G. how the group functioned and brought him up-to-date on the problems they had been working on together. Mr. G. remained mostly silent for the rest of the session, giving his opinion only if asked directly by a group member or the therapist.

(Therapist's note: Mr. G.'s attitude and statements in the pregroup interview were totally different from those displayed in the group. The therapist was caught completely unaware by his change in behavior. It was a very valuable learning experience for the group *and* the therapist!)

Phase III: Termination. By the sixth session Mrs. L. had apparently resolved her crisis with the help of group support. She and Cindy were getting along well together. (This information was verified by Cindy and her therapist.) She admitted that occasionally minor problems occurred but that she and Cindy were usually able to reach an agreeable compromise. She became quite friendly with several members of the group. They even visited at each other's homes. Thus Mrs. L. was able to overcome her illogical isolation of herself and Cindy from the low-income community. The most dramatic and encouraging change in behavior in Mrs. L. was apparent when she announced in the last session that through the encouragement and help of another member, she had gotten a part-time job as a secretary at a local junior college. She had worked three days and, as she stated it, "I love it! I've never been happier and Cindy is so proud of me!"

It was at this session that the therapist and the group reviewed the progress and work they had done in the previous sessions to help Mrs. L. resolve her problem. Mrs. L. expressed some reluctance over terminating with the group. She was reassured by the members that they would "keep in touch." In an attempt to overcome her feeling of loss, Mrs. L. invited the entire group to her house for cake and coffee after the session. Everyone accepted the invitation.

Summary

The behavior and personality of the individual may be changed by the forces of any group in which he is a member. Since World War II the increasing awareness of the need to treat large groups of people has contributed to the rapid advances in the development and acceptance of group therapy and other therapeutic groups. An overview of therapeutic groups and group therapy has been presented to show the basis from which crisis groups evolved.

Two representative studies have been discussed for the purpose of showing their implementation, advantages, and disadvantages. A case study has been presented to demonstrate the use of crisis intervention techniques in a group therapy session.

References

Asch, G.: Effects of group pressure upon the modification and distortion of judgment. In Guetzkow, H., editor: Groups, leadership and men, Pittsburgh, 1951, Carnegie Press.

Corsini, R.J., and Rosenberg, B.: Mechanisms of group psychotherapy, J. Abnorm. Soc. Psychol. **51**:406, 1955.

Hinckley, R.G., and Hermann, L.: Group treatment in psychotherapy, Minneapolis, 1951, University of Minnesota Press.

Luchins, A.S.: Group therapy: a guide, New York, 1964, Random House, Inc.

Merton, R.K.: Social theory and social structure, enlarged ed., New York, 1968, The Free Press.

Morley, W.E., and Brown, V.B.: The crisis-intervention group: a natural mating or a marriage of convenience? Psychother. Theory Res. Prac. **6**:30, Winter 1968.

Slavson, S.R.: A textbook in analytic group psychotherapy, New York, 1964, International Universities Press.

Strickler, M., and Allgeyer, J.: The crisis group: a new application of crisis theory, Soc. Work **12**:28, July 1967.

Additional readings

Allgeyer, J.: The crisis group: its unique usefulness to the disadvantaged, Int. J. Group Psychother. **20**:235, April 1970.

Bonham, H.E., and others: Group psychotherapy with deaf adolescents, Am. Ann. Deaf **126**(7): 806, 1981.

Brown, D., and Pedder, J.: Introduction of psychotherapy, London, 1979, Tavistock Publications.

Calhoun, L.G., and others: Dealing with crisis, Englewood Cliffs, N.J., 1976, Prentice-Hall, Inc.

Chen, M.E.: Applying Yalom's principles to crisis work: some intriguing results, J. Psychiatr. Nurs. **16**:15, 1978.

Democker, J.D., and Zimpfer, D.G.: Group approaches to psychosocial intervention in medical care: a synthesis, Int. J. Group Psychother. **31**(2):247, 1981.

Donovan, J.M., and others: The crisis group: an outcome study, Am. J. Psychiatry **136**(7):906, 1979.

Elizur, A., and others: The treatment of adolescents and their parents in group settings in a psychiatric hospital, Int. J. Soc. Psychiatry **27**(2):83, 1981.

Erickson, R.C.: Small-group psychotherapy with patients on a short-stay ward: an opportunity for innovation, Hosp. Community Psychiatry **32**(4):269, 1981.

Goldstein, S., and Giddings, J.: Multiple impact therapy: an approach to crisis intervention with families. In Specter, G.: Crisis intervention, New York, 1973, Behavioral Publications, No. 210, pp. 193–204.

Hatton, C.L., and Valente, S.M.: Bereavement group for parents who suffered a suicidal loss of a child, Suicide Life Threat Behav. **11**(3):141, 1981.

Herink, R., editor: The psychotherapy handbook, New York, 1980, New American Library.

Imber, S.D., and others: Uses and abuses of the brief intervention group, Int. J. Group Ther. **19**:39, Jan. 1979.

Moreno, J.L., and others, editors: The international handbook of group psychotherapy, New York, 1966, Philosophical Library, Inc.

Satir, V.M.: Conjoint family therapy, Palo Alto, Calif., 1964, Science & Behavior Books, Inc.

Small, L.: The briefer psychotherapies, New York, 1971, Brunner/Mazel, Inc.

Smith, L.L.: A review of crisis intervention theory, Soc. Casework **7**:396, 1978.

Specter, G.A., and Claiborn, W.L., editors: Crisis intervention, New York, 1973, Human Sciences Press.

Testa, J.A.: Group systematic desensitization and implosive therapy for death anxiety, Psychol. Rep. **48**(2): 376, 1981.

Thornton, J.F., and others: Schizophrenia: group support for relatives, Can. J. Psychiatry **26**(5): 341, 1981.

Tozman, S., and others: The rap group: a milieu treatment model for the chronically mentally ill in an outpatient setting, Int. J. Group Psychother. **31**(2):233, 1981.

chapter 4

Sociocultural factors affecting therapeutic intervention

In a discussion of some of the sociocultural factors that can act as barriers in the psychotherapeutic process two aspects should be considered. First, there are the professionals who are frustrated when they try to help someone from a different and unfamiliar sociocultural background; and second, there are those in need of help who are frustrated when they do not receive the kind of assistance they feel they need.

In this chapter we will not attempt to cover the gamut of specific ethnic and cultural factors present in today's society, but we will make an effort to discuss certain key areas that are usually considered to be problems and to help the reader become aware of the nature of these difficulties.

The inability to understand and accept the attitudes and values of those who are not in our same educational, economic, or ethnic group is a major barrier. Professionals are aware of this barrier, since they have difficulty and are uncomfortable when trying to communicate with those who do not share their same standards and ideas.

One reason for this is the sociocultural background of the professionals. The majority are from the middle-class culture and have no difficulty in understanding and working comfortably with members of their own class culture. They speak the same language, have the same values ethically and morally, and share essentially the same expectations from life. When confronted with someone from a different sociocultural background seeking help, the professionals are frustrated in their desire to help because they may not understand what is being asked of them. Language and terminology are a mutual problem because codes of conduct and behavioral expectations are not always understood. Mutual suspicion is aroused; the professional feels that the person does not really want help, and the person in need of help, not understanding what is expected of him, is uncomfortable and aggravates the problem of noncommunication.

Behavior and beliefs that are acceptable and highly valued in one cultural group may be unacceptable and devalued in another, or what is viewed as normal in one group could be abnormal in another.

Normal is the term society uses for social behaviors that are preferred, and *abnormal,* for those to which it objects (Benedict, 1934; Opler, 1956; Redlich, 1952). One of the big problems for social psychiatry is to determine just which feelings, thoughts, and actions are normal and which are abnormal. Who or what determines this? The term *normal* has several definitions. Statistically it can mean average, or the "norm." This is most likely to be seen in mathematical samples. When the term *adaptive* is used to mean normal behavior, it is more likely to be used psychiatrically. For example, normal behavior is the ability of the individual to adapt to ordinary environmental conditions without undue stress or anxiety. If an individual has more difficulty adapting to ordinary environmental conditions than the general group, his behavior could be labeled as being abnormal or maladaptive.

Benedict suggests that normality is culturally defined and cites as an example the behavior of the mystic who experiences trancelike states and catalepsy. In our general culture this could be considered abnormal behavior; in some cultures the greatest prestige is awarded to those who have trancelike experiences. They are considered blessed and are accorded the reverence due them as shaman in their communities. Their behavior is given cultural approval, and their roles as counselors and diviners are a necessary part of the social structure of their communities. It can be demonstrated in all cultures that honorable roles are assigned by society to those behaviors it needs and accepts, and devalued roles are assigned to those it no longer needs and rejects. From this frame of reference normality is defined by culture.

In the traditional Chinese culture the grandparents were revered by their descendants, bowed to, and given full obedience to their demands. Such expectations from grandparents in our culture would be considered abnormal. In some cultures suicide is considered to be a traditionally normal and honorable way to resolve problems. In Western culture it is generally considered abnormal to the degree that there are laws against it, religious as well as societal, and any attempts may be punishable as a crime against society. The same extremes of views among cultures may be held toward such actions as homicide, homosexuality, and polygamy.

Differing cultural values

Widely divergent cultural perceptions are also found between the values accorded family roles, child-rearing methods, and the roles and status given individuals relative to their age, sex, occupation, marital status, religion, education, and so forth. Changes vary with the conditions under which society must function. Constant problems face every culture in adapting to the environs and attempting to maintain cultural equilibrium. Most of their norms are directed toward their basic needs for survival (Opler, 1956).

It is important to avoid stereotyping if there is to be understanding and communication between members of different cultural classes. Preconceived ideas about who does what and why it is done are the strongest barriers to understanding behavior and effecting change.

An example of this is the traditional middle-class culture. It has been both attacked and supported in recent decades. Its values and ideals have been called the backbone of our society and the cause of our weaknesses. Both opinions probably hold elements of truth. Because of its pervasive influence on all facets of our society, it has been scrutinized, criticized, praised, and derogated. Today many think it an insult to be accused of "middle-class thinking." Values and ideals that were once considered to be inviolate are now being challenged.

Traditional middle-class culture

Before the depression years of the 1930s the traditional middle-class ideals and values were based on the Protestant ethic—the idea that hard work and self-control would lead to success. Traditions of social behavior were strongly adhered to, with emphasis on self-discipline, individualism, and clearly defined roles in the family and community (Haas, 1963; Seward, 1956). Social stability was the key word.

This was the culture in which proverbs were lived, not hung on the walls as pop art decorations. "Early to bed and early to rise makes a man healthy, wealthy, and wise" was a way of life. So also were "A stitch in time saves nine," "A rolling stone gathers no moss," "Virtue is its own reward," and the dozens of others that emphasized the goodness of industriousness, stability, and self-discipline and the evils of laziness, instability, and lack of self-control.

The father was expected by society to reign unchallenged in his role as patriarch and breadwinner in his family. His wife obeyed him, and her role was relegated to the family, kitchen, and church. The children were expected to be obedient to both parents. Impulsive actions and aggressive hostility were frowned on. Family roles were clearly defined and were reinforced by the social institutions of the times (Seward, 1956). Traditional education emphasized discipline, order, and authority. Christian morality still held the puritanical tenets of fear of God's judgment for any real or imagined sins against His teachings. Sex was only a three-letter word, not acceptable for use in mixed company or "polite" conversation.

This was the era of strong conscience and of fear of punishment and social disfavor if any deviance were discovered. Today it would be said that the middle-class culture of that era was ruled by overly severe superegos. Those were a tradition-bound, hardworking people who were, in many ways, the necessary source of stability in the rapidly changing society in the United States. As progressive changes occurred in the overall society, cultural changes took place.

New middle-class culture

The values and ideals of any culture reflect the attitudes and needs of its society. With technological advances the United States has become increasingly industrialized and urbanized. The core of the "old" middle class decreased in numbers. The predominating cultural values and needs of the rural independent farmers and the small-town entrepreneurs were supplanted by the changing needs of the urban middle class (Riessman and Miller, 1964). The children no longer were expected to be the tradition bearers of their rural home communities. They moved on to less stable urban areas, and the old ideals, attitudes, and values failed to meet their changing needs. Industriousness no longer was a guarantee of personal success. Too often a person was working for someone else, and self-employment was the exception rather than the rule. Authoritarianism and self-control were coming into conflict with the changing values of an increasingly technological society. Creativity, individual autonomy, and self-expression grew in cultural value.

Child-rearing and educational goals reflected these changing ideals, attitudes, and values. Permissiveness and self-expression gained in favor (Riessman and Miller, 1964). Individualism gave way to the concepts of group membership, cooperation, and teamwork. High value was placed on the individual's ability to interrelate with others. Cultural emphasis on these last factors was exemplified by the neverfailing request for evaluations of a person's interpersonal and communication skills in reference questionnaires sent out by employers.

Educational, business, and professional opportunities have been steadily opening to women. In 1948 only 13% of women with preschool children were employed outside of the home. By 1976 this number had risen to 37% (Kenniston, 1977). By 1978 approximately 6.5 million children younger than 6 years of age and 18 million children between 6 and 14 years of age had working mothers (Authier, 1979). Evolving patterns of labor force participation have affected both trends and practices in parenting.

The "new" middle-class culture shows the effects of the vast changes introduced into American society since World War II. Yet it retains the basic high valuation of thrift, industriousness, and self-control, which still permeate the structure of its institutions. Socioeconomic stratification of classes has diffused these values into other sociocultural classes.

Traditional treatment methods

Federal legislation made increased funding available for development of community programs and facilities. Professional disciplines refocused their activities to include consideration of sociocultural components of mental illness. Accumulation of data over the past decade suggests that several important factors are considered barriers to effective therapeutic intervention. Until ways are found to overcome these barriers, successful programs will be limited in the scope of their activities.

One of the main criticisms of the traditional psychiatric treatment methods has been that they have become self-limiting by the very nature of their origins. Theories and techniques have been developed by professionals who come predominantly from the middle class and identify with its cultural values and goals. For example, Freud's psychoanalytic theories were based on his observations made in a middle-class continental culture with a relatively stable environment (Seward, 1956). His norms were a reflection of the norms of his culture, and his therapy was focused toward adaptation to those norms. One of his basic assumptions was that a patient would have enough time and money to continue in a long course of private therapy sessions. A prevailing theme in literature has been the dominant middle-class character of the mental health movement (Haas, 1963; Riessman and Scribner, 1965; Yamamoto and Goin, 1965).

A number of studies (Heine and Trossman, 1960; McMahon, 1964; Myers, Bean, and Pepper, 1968) have attempted to identify the character traits of patients who might be most likely to "succeed" in psychodynamic-based therapies. The consensus describes them as persons who feel a strong need to relate to people, particularly when they have problems. They are psychologically oriented, have intellectual capacity to deal with abstracts, are sophisticated in the jargon of psychiatry, and have some idea of the values and goals of psychotherapy. All these factors make it easier for them to communicate their feelings to the therapist. A basis for mutual understanding is more readily established. They are introspective in nature and probably have a strong tendency to blame themselves, rather than others, for their problems. They are highly motivated to find out why they feel the way they do and how they can change their life-style to make things better for themselves. They place a high value on self-control and on their ability to accept delayed gratification of their needs, and they expect to have to put much of their own efforts into getting those needs met. For these reasons they accept the lengthy time that they may have to spend in therapy and have positive feelings that it will be worth their efforts. These characterological traits reflect many of the basic ones reported for the middle-class culture.

Until the early 1940s the main focus of treatment was derived from theories stressing the organic and psychological causes of mental illness. This was followed by a shift, which included the effects of interpersonal relationships on behavior and personality. Current emphasis on sociocultural factors influencing mental health has stimulated broad research in this area, particularly in the relatively new field of social psychiatry.

The basis of psychiatric treatment is the establishment of meaningful communication between the therapist and his patient. If unable to accomplish this, the therapist has few alternatives to offer. In order to establish a meaningful base of communication the therapist's responsibility is to have some awareness, if not a full understanding, of the needs, values, and goals of his patient.

Members of one socioeconomic class may not actually understand or be aware of the needs, values, and goals of another. As a result of the increasing number of mental health programs being maintained by state and local governments, more individuals from substandard sociocultural groups are having their first contacts with mental health professionals. At the same time, many of the mental health professionals are having *their* first contacts with these groups in their home environments. The appropriateness of treatment modalities is being questioned not only by the professionals but also by the public receiving them.

Class stratification systems

Since Hollingshead and Redlich (1958) completed their study of the relationships between social class and mental illness, further studies in the field have supported their findings (Albronda, Dean, and Starkweather, 1964; Brill and Storrow, 1960; Haas, 1963; Myers, Bean, and Pepper, 1968). Relationships have been found to exist between social class and the development, type, prevalence, and treatment of mental illness. It appears that the lower a person's location is on the socioeconomic class scale, the more restricted is the range of available therapies.

Defining social classes might be done through either of two main approaches. The first, the *statistical* approach, can be drawn from the socioeconomic levels of education, income, occupation, and place of residence. This is most frequently seen in industrial and government reports. Although this approach will convey a concrete differentiation between socioeconomic classes in the American class structure, it does not include any criteria for the sociocultural life-styles of different groups of people. If only the statistical method is used, there may be a strong tendency to stereotype people into classes using only the available economic information about them. Poverty level in one part of the country might well be a comfortable lower middle-class level in another.

The second method of defining social classes, *life-styles,* recognizes and accounts for the influences of the less well-defined, systematized behavior patterns, values, and life-styles of groups of people and their interrelated effects on the socioeconomic classifications. In their study of a selected population group that was receiving psychiatric treatment, Hollingshead and Redlich (1958) used a classification format that took into consideration the values the subjects placed upon their education, income, occupation, and place of residence. They also developed a two-factor index (occupation and education) to determine social position. Occupation presumably reflected the skill and power that individuals possessed in society; education reflected not only knowledge but also cultural tastes. By using statistical techniques with the proper combination of these two factors they were able to determine the approximate social position occupied by an individual in the structure of society.

In the collection and organization of their data they used a pattern of vertical divisions such as race, religion, and ethnic groupings. In addition, they classified subjects in horizontal divisions according to their commonly held values attached to places of residence, occupations, educational backgrounds, and associations. This meant that, regardless of race, religion, or ethnic grouping, an unskilled laborer with little formal education who lived in a poverty area of the community was ranked low in all of the vertical divisions' groupings.

Class I. This class consisted of the community's business and professional leaders. Its members lived in the best areas of the community; the men were college graduates, and their wives usually had completed from 1 to 4 years of college. Income was the highest of any class, and members of the core group were descendants of the pioneers who settled in New England. The core group family was stable, secure, and socially responsible for its members and the welfare of the community. These families dominated the private clubs, and play was a prominent part of this group's use of leisure time.

Class II. Most of the adults in this class had some formal education beyond high school. The men occupied managerial positions, and many were engaged in lesser-ranking professions. Its members lived in one-family houses in the better residential areas. The families were well-to-do, but there was no inherited or acquired wealth. The nuclear family was composed predominantly of married adults and their minor children. They belonged to neighborhood clique groups, local church organizations, political clubs, and so on. Family members of all ages were "joiners."

Class III. The typical Class III man or woman was a high school graduate. The men were employees in various salaried positions: clerical, semiprofessional, or technical. The women also worked in clerical, sales, or technical positions. They tended to live in the "good" sections of the residential areas. The family included father, mother, and minor children but no other relatives or nonrelatives. Most members belonged to community organizations of one kind or another: fraternal orders, church clubs, athletic clubs, lodges, or veterans' groups. More were dissatisfied with their present living conditions and less optimistic about the future than were those in Class II.

Class IV. The median years of school completed by the men was 9.4 years and by their wives, 10.5 years. The men were primarily semiskilled employees, skilled manual employees, or clerical and sales workers. Almost all of the women were working as semiskilled factory workers, clerical workers, or sales workers. The majority of the families lived in two-, three-, or multiple-family dwellings in the working-class sections of the city. The family income was spent, for the most part, as it was earned. The family constellation differed from that of Class III in four ways: (1) there were more broken homes, (2) more households had boarders and roomers, (3) the families were larger, and (4) there were more three-generation families living under one roof. Recreation consisted of "working around the place," watching television, listening to the radio, and family visiting. The husband belonged to the union but no other organization; the wife belonged to no formal organization but was a member of informal neighborhood women's groups.

Class V. This class had the poorest education in the population. The median years of school was 6 for the men and slightly less than 8 for the women. The men worked as semiskilled and unskilled workers, and some had never had a regular job. Jobs in this class were poorly paid, required long hours for 6 or 7 days a week, and were in industries that were not unionized. Over two thirds of Class V persons lived in crowded tenement areas, the tenements housing from ten to fifty families. Family ties were more brittle in this class. Five types of families existed: the nuclear family of father, mother, and children, the three- or four-generation family; the broken nuclear residual families consisting of widows, widowers, or elderly couples; mixed families of one parent, children, and roomers; and the common-law groups. Only a small number of family members belonged to organized community institutions. Their social life took place in the household, on the street, or in neighborhood social agencies. Adults were resentful of the way they were treated by employers, clergymen, teachers, physicians, police, and other representatives of organized society.

A person, for example, from Class IV or Class V cannot invest the money or the time for extensive psychotherapy. His education level limits his understanding of the psychotherapeutic goals and terminology. He is more concrete and direct in his thinking and not particularly introspective. If he seeks help, he wants it immediately, not 6 months from now. He is inclined to regard authorities with suspicion and dislike and will seek their help only as a last resort.

In the follow-up study by Myers, Bean, and Pepper (1968), individuals in Class V of the Hollingshead and Redlich study were the ones who had remained institutionalized and usually ended up dying there or had repeated admissions. This validates their suspicions that they should not ask for help unless absolutely forced to because the only help available to them is in institutions.

Lower sociocultural groups

Current literature puts various labels on the lower sociocultural groups. These are, for the most part, indications of the specific areas within the lower-class structure being studied. Designations have been made such as the "underprivileged," the "poor," the "culturally disadvantaged," the "culturally deprived," the "migratory worker," the "blue-collar worker," the "disenfranchised," ad infinitum. The one fact that they all seem to hold in agreement is that there are people who, for one reason or another, will always be found clustered at the lower level of any class-stratification system. A clear-cut criterion for just exactly "who" these people are has not been developed, and inconsistencies in results of studies of similar populations bear out this fact.

Many scales of class measurement exist, and a person does not necessarily fall into all lower categories at the same time. Just because an individual is the unemployed head of a household and living on the fringes of a poverty area is no reason to categorize that person as culturally deprived. If this were so, a large mass of college students would be eligible for cultural poverty programs! On the other hand, a blue-collar laborer making a good salary could feasibly be described as culturally deprived if there were a lack of cultural programs available to her.

Societies are usually structured around institutions that they have created to provide for the "normal" needs of their population. Judgments about their "abnormal" needs are most often made by the same group that has determined the norms for their culture. Only in the recent history of the United States has there been active recognition of the high variability of cultural norms and values, and values of the dominant sociocultural class are no longer being left unchallenged as being "good" or "bad" for all of the society's members.

Barriers to therapy

All of the groups (ethnic, racial, occupational, age, and so forth) who live in the culturally and economically lower margins of society have been categorized as "lower class." Much of the tone of literature about them tends to have a negative quality. In terms of socioeconomic programs there has always seemed to be more interest in what could be done *for* them rather than *with* them. This was particularly evident in programs to effect changes in their ways of life; little confidence was expressed in their ability to change. Only recently has there been emphasis on a new theme—that of recognizing their strenghts rather than just their weaknesses and of going into their communities and working in a cooperative effort with them to make the changes *they* feel are most necessary.

Mental health professionals are well aware that the attitudes of the general community toward mental illness are a keystone in the development of any treatment program and these attitudes should be recognized as determinants of the goals of the services offered. To be effective, a program should be meaningful and seen as needed by the community groups it is meant to reach.

Crisis intervention is by *no* means restricted to people at the lower sociocultural levels; however, because of certain inherent factors it is thought that its techniques are more effective for those at this level than are the techniques of other types of therapy.

Jacobson (1965) has stated that motivating forces have universal elements and precede cultural differences. Typically, people are wary of strangers, and time is needed to assess new situations and strangers in the environment. Under such circumstances they are usually guarded in their speech and controlled in their actions. In emergency situations such as fires, earthquakes, and other catastrophes, individuals work together freely, barriers to communication are lowered, and sociocultural levels are disregarded. This occurs similarly when a person is in a crisis and comes for help. The element of strangeness is quickly overcome as the person and the therapist concentrate on relieving the symptoms of stress even though they may be from different sociocultural backgrounds.

The time-limiting factor of crisis intervention is a distinct advantage with individuals in the lower sociocultural group, who are focused on the here and now and want relief of their symptoms as soon as possible. Crisis intervention is directed toward helping the individual solve a specific problem. Many characterological and behavioral changes are not expected, nor are they dwelt on in the therapy sessions. This lessens the threat because the individual does not have to expose a complete pattern of living, which may be different from that of the therapist.

A community mental health center conceivably serves individuals from different sociocultural levels. Psychotherapy for an extended period of time may be too expensive for an average middle-class family or person, and it may not be needed if a crisis situation exists. Those who may now be considered middle class may have originally come from a lower sociocultural background and may retain their views on the value of psychotherapy and their misconceptions about mental illness.

Referrals to a community mental health center come from multiple sources. Family physicians may decide that certain individuals need help with an emotional problem and make the referral; attorneys, juvenile authorities, clergymen, family service agencies, and others may also make referrals. The community itself is usually aware through publicity (radio, television, newspapers, word-of-mouth, and liaison personnel) of a community center's function and the services available. Because of this publicity and location in the community they may serve many who "walk-in" for help.

Conversely, referrals from a community mental health center are also diversified and are usually highly individualized. A person may be referred directly for hospitalization if dangerously suicidal or homicidal, for longer-term therapy after crisis intervention for chronic problems, to a family service agency if needed, or to a rehabilitation center.

The prevalent attitudes toward mental illness in our society continue to be less than favorable. An aura of fear and anxiety still surrounds overt mental disturbance. Much of this is the result of the distorted ideas about what happens when a person "goes crazy" or "insane," ideas which have been reinforced by the mass media (Tershakovek, 1964). Basic to many movies, television programs, or fiction that have been put out for the public are elements of fear, loss of control, and questionable "recovery"—believable yet grossly exaggerated for impact and saleability.

The lower sociocultural groups, in particular, fear mental illness (Myers, Bean, and Pepper, 1968; Myers and Roberts, 1959; Riessman and Scribner, 1965). Often they fail even to admit its presence until there is overt psychotic behavior present. Frequently, they ask for outside help only when a person becomes a threat and a danger to himself or others. And, just as frequently, the first "help" the people in these sociocultural groups receive is from the police, who are called in to protect the family and others from the mentally ill person. Too often the family still tries to keep the disturbed member at home until it is too late and he becomes unmanageable.

Many cultural reasons for this exist. Many still consider mental illness to be inherited and passed on from generation to generation. To admit it is "in the family" could destroy any pending marriages, business associations, and, most certainly, the family status in the community.

Realistically the lower classes fear mental illness for good reason. Hollingshead and Redlich's study (1958) shows that Class V individuals had the greatest percentage who were in state hospitals and receiving custodial care.

Class V individuals saw mental illness as craziness, not as being sick. For this they saw only institutionalization as the answer. Fearing this end, they avoided seeking any help, even when it was obviously needed.

Other factors have been recognized as pertinent, basic needs of the lower sociocultural groups that must be met in treatment programs (Bloch, 1968; Hartog, 1967; McMahon, 1964; Riessman and Scribner, 1965; Yamamoto and Goin, 1965). Generally, they are oriented to the here and now; they cannot afford to wait for tomorrow and later. Too often theirs is a day-to-day existence. They have no reason to save up for a rainy day because for them it may rain every day.

Long-term therapy is not for them if for no other reason than its cost. If a day laborer has to choose between keeping a clinical appointment and getting a few hours' work, she will have to have concrete proof that she will get help if she keeps the appointment and she will expect immediate feelings of relief for her symptoms.

The lower sociocultural families have had long experience with help from outsiders, and the past history of social intervention from outsiders has not done much to build their trust. Many have learned to mistrust the well-intentioned social welfare agencies that saw fit to move the aged or infirm away from their homes and into institutions "for their own good." They are familiar with situations in which children have been taken from "unfit" parents and placed in foster homes or similar child-care agencies. Too often their families have been measured against middle-class norms and found lacking in stability. Ineffective outside action has led only to further instability. How can they be expected to trust the mental health profession? Historically it has taken either adverse actions against them or neglected them completely.

Even more concretely, until they have active proof that conversation or "talking treatment" will help them, their basic needs for survival will outweigh any appeals to them to help identify their emotional needs. Not knowing what to expect or value from psychiatry, they cannot be expected to immediately feed back their needs.

The following case study illustrates how a therapist worked effectively in crisis intervention with a married couple whose sociocultural background was different from her own.

Case study

Tony and Marta, a young married couple with four small children, came to a crisis intervention center and requested help. They had originally gone to their parish priest for advice, and he had recommended that they seek professional help at a nearby community center. Tony was an unskilled laborer who worked for an airline as a maintenance man. He had finished the eighth grade in school; Marta had finished 9 years of school and had worked in a garment factory until right before the birth of their first child. They lived in a poor section of town in a house owned by Tony's mother. Their only recreation was watching television. Tony usually worked 6 to 7 days a week.

Tony was very angry and suspicious at the beginning of the session, whereas Marta appeared frightened and was reluctant to talk. When asked by the therapist "why they had come to the center," Tony replied that he thought his wife was crazy; he then began to explain her "crazy" behavior. The afternoon before, Marta had caught their oldest son (Joe, 9 years old) playing with matches behind the house. She flew into a rage, pulled him into the house, and burned his arm by holding it over the flame of the kitchen stove. Tony's mother had walked in while Joe was screaming. The grandmother learned what had happened, and she had grabbed Marta and forced her arm over the flame so she "could see how it felt." When the therapist asked Marta if this were "true," she nodded her head and began to cry. The therapist asked if she could see her arm. Together they removed the bandage from the rather large second-degree burn. Marta said she had put a patented burn medicine on it and a dressing. The therapist told Marta that she would like the doctor to see her arm to give her an antibiotic prescription and some medicine to help her control herself. A medical consultation was arranged and while Marta saw the physician, the therapist met with Tony.

(Therapist's note: This maneuver served two purposes: first, it showed Marta and Tony that she wanted to provide immediate help; and second, by her nonjudgmental attitude and acceptance of their behavior, she established a basis for rapport.)

When Tony was alone with the therapist, he dropped his defensive attitude and showed his true concern for Marta's irrational behavior. When questioned about Marta's usual manner of coping with problems, he stated that he really did not know—usually she just "blew up" at him, and since it did not bother him, he ignored it. He stated that he loved his wife and children and he believed that she loved him and the children, too. When asked what he and Marta usually did together and with the children for pleasure, he said, "Are you kidding? I work 6 or 7 days a week—hard! I come home and I'm tired; I have a few beers, eat, and usually fall asleep in front of T.V." When asked what Marta usually did, he stated that she "took care of the house and kids."

When Marta returned from the medical consultation, the therapist repeated what Tony had told her. Marta said, "That's true—that's *all* I do: take care of his mother's crummy house and the kids!" Tony jumped on this immediately and said, "You have never gotten along with my mother—you hate her!" Marta said that she did not hate her; she just did not like her "always butting into our business and you always taking her side against me and the kids! I've told you I don't like living in her house, where she can walk in and out anytime she wants to; I want a place I can call my own. We pay her rent; we can pay rent someplace else—and get a better house too!"

Tony said, "You never told me you didn't want to live in Mother's house." Marta said, "I have—but you never listen!"

When asked about the possibility of moving, since Marta was unhappy with the living arrangements, Tony said his mother would "not understand," but "Marta and the kids mean more to me than anything."

The therapist thought at this time she could refocus on the problem that had brought them into the center. She asked Marta about burning Joe's arm. Marta said, "I was tired and upset; all I ever hear are the kids yelling and Tony's mother butting in and telling me everything I'm doing wrong—with the kids and the house; and Tony never tries to help or even listen to me. I just felt like I was cracking up!"

Tony was asked if there were any way he could help Marta. It was explained that taking care of four small children every day without a few hours "off" can be very exhausting. The therapist went on to tell Tony that his work kept him in contact with people all day, whereas Marta had no contact with anyone except his mother (who was an added irritant) and the children. Marta said that if only she could look forward to talking with him when she was upset, or even if she could go over to a friend's house for a few hours once or twice a week, "anything to get away for a few hours!" she knew she would be all right.

Tony very reluctantly said that he would put the kids to bed one night for her so she could go to a friend's house. The therapist said that it sounded like a wonderful idea and that what would really be good for them both would be getting out for a few hours together to talk things over. Their reaction was a cautious silence.

When Tony and Marta came for their next session, it was very obvious that they had had a good week. They were talking together quite animatedly when the therapist came into the waiting room to get them for their appointment. She remarked how well they looked and how happy. Marta started talking about their week: Tony had put the kids to bed one night, as he had said he would, and she had gone to a friend's house to visit. She said it was really great to be out for a few hours. When Tony was asked how he had managed with the children, he looked embarrassed and said, "It was a mess! I don't know how she ever manages them all; no wonder she gets so tired!" It seemed that Tony could not get the children to go to sleep—or even stay in bed—without Marta there to control them. What he finally did was bring them all into the living room to watch television, and when they fell asleep, he carried them one by one to bed. The highlight of the week came when Tony told his mother not to come to the house and bother Marta. He had said that if she did, he and Marta would find another house and move. This made Marta feel so much better that she backed down a bit and told her mother-in-law that she could visit them but that she ought to call in advance to say that she was coming. The therapist told them how well they were doing in working toward solving their problem but cautioned them that there would be good weeks and bad weeks and if they began to talk *with* each other when problems arose rather than *at* each other, they could work out solutions more easily.

At the next session Marta had apparently stabilized, and Tony and she were relaxed and comfortable with each other and the therapist. Tony began by saying that they both really felt that they were capable of handling their problems now and did not want to return for more visits. He said that he could really understand Marta's feelings of being "hemmed in" and "trapped" when she was with the children constantly, all day and every day. He said a friend at work had invited them over for dinner the Saturday before, and instead of refusing as he usually did, he had accepted. He asked his mother to stay with the children, and he and Marta went to dinner. He said that as he watched Marta laughing and talking, he realized how much he had missed their being together, alone, "like before we were married. I watched her and realized how pretty and young she really is and how much I love her. I'm going to do everything I can to help her with the kids—I know we can make it now!" The therapist agreed and wished them luck and told them that if they needed help again to feel free to return to the center.

SUMMARY OF CASE STUDY

The therapist in this situation, even though from a middle-class background, was aware of the sociocultural background of her patients, and this knowledge was invaluable in the approach. Her attitude was nonjudgmental, concentrated on getting some immediate "help" (the medical consultation), and focused on assisting them with their problem. She made no attempt at characterological or insightful changes in their behavior, but worked on the "here and now" and was very directive. Although she offered suggestions, no attempt was made at major changes in behavior. The terminology was kept at a concrete level, so she was able to talk with them in language they could understand. She attempted to give them the feeling that she was there to help them and that she would be there in the future if necessary.

Summary

It is our contention that crisis intervention is a logical treatment modality that transcends sociocultural classes. It can fulfill needs for immediate problem solving, it is direct and short term, and the therapist's role in it is an active one. No attempt is made to produce drastic behavioral changes. Its object is to reduce the symptoms of disequilibrium and to restore the individual to a precrisis level of functioning, with improved abilities to solve problems and more effective coping skills.

Community mental health centers, rather than large, isolated institutions, are where the "people" are. If therapists are to work successfully with people from all sociocultural levels, they should understand and accept the possibility that those who seek their help may have different attitudes and values. It should be the therapists' commitment to learn how to communicate with and meet the needs of those who seek help. The burden should not be placed upon them to change their lifestyle and patterns of living in order to get the help they are seeking.

References

Albronda, H.F., Dean, R.L., and Starkweather, J.A.: Social class and psychotherapy, Arch. Gen. Psychiatry **10**:276, 1964.

Authier, K.: Defining the care in child care, Social Work **24**:500, 1979.

Benedict, R.: Anthropology and the abnormal, J. Gen. Psychol. **10**:59–82, 1934.

Bloch, H.S.: An open-ended crisis-oriented group for the poor who are sick, Arch. Gen. Psychiatry **18**:178, 1968.

Brill, N.Q., and Storrow, H.A.: Social class and psychiatric treatment, Arch. Gen. Psychiatry **3**:340, 1960.

Haas, K.: The middle-class professional and the lower-class patient, Ment. Hyg. **47**:408, 1963.

Hartog, J.: The mental health problems of poverty's youth, Ment. Hyg. **51**:85, 1967.

Heine, R.W., and Trossman, J.: Initial expectations of the doctor-patient interaction as a factor in continuance in psychotherapy, Psychiatry **23**:275, Aug. 1960.

Hollingshead, A.B., and Redlich, F.C.: Social class and mental illness, New York, 1958, John Wiley & Sons, Inc.

Jacobson, G.F.: Crisis theory and treatment strategy: some sociocultural and psychodynamic considerations, J. Nerv. Ment. Dis. **141**:209, Aug. 1965.

Kenniston, K.: All our children, New York, 1977, Harcourt Brace Jovanovich, Inc.

McMahon, J.T.: The working class psychiatric patient: a clinical view. In Riessman, F., and others, editors: Mental health of the poor, New York, 1964, The Free Press.

Myers, J.K., Bean, L.L., and Pepper, M.P.: A decade later: a follow-up of social class and mental illness, New York, 1968, John Wiley & Sons, Inc.

Myers, J.K., and Roberts, B.H.: Family and class dynamics in mental illness, New York, 1959, John Wiley & Sons, Inc.

Opler, M.K.: Culture, psychiatry and human values, Springfield, Ill., 1956, Chalres C Thomas, Publisher.

Redlich, F.C.: The concept of normality, Am. J. Psychother. **6**:551, 1952, Republished in Bergen, B.J., and Thomas, C.S., editors: Issues and problems in social psychiatry, Springfield, Ill., 1966, Charles C Thomas, Publisher.

Riessman, F., and Miller, S.M.: Social change versus the psychiatric world view, Am. J. Orthopsychiatry **34**:29, Jan. 1964.

Riessman, F., and Scribner, S.: The underutilization of mental health services by workers and low income groups: causes and cures, Am. J. Psychiatry **121**:798, Feb. 1965.

Seward, G.: Psychotherapy and culture conflict, New York, 1956, The Ronald Press Co.

Tershakovek, A.: An observation concerning changing attitudes toward mental illness. Am. J. Psychiatry **121**:353, Oct. 1964.

Yamamoto, J., and Goin, M.L.: On the treatment of the poor, Am. J. Psychiatry **122**:267, Sept. 1965.

Additional readings

Adams, P.L., and McDonald, F.: Clinical cooling out of poor people, Am. J. Orthopsychiatry 38:457, April 1968.

Beltrame, T.F.: Meeting the special needs of the Appalachian alcoholics, Hosp. Community Psychiatry 29(6):792, 1978.

Bloch, A.M.: Combat neurosis in inner-city schools, Am. J. Psychiatry 135:1189, Oct. 1978.

Ferguson, M.: The aquarian conspiracy: personal and social transformation in the 1980's, Los Angeles, 1980, Jeremy P. Tarcher, Inc.

Gottlieb, B.H.: The primary group as supportive milieu: applications to community psychology, Am. J. Community Psychol. 7469, May 1979.

Harwood, A.: Ethnicity and medical care, Cambridge, Mass., 1981, Harvard University Press.

Jones, E.: Social class and psychotherapy: a critical review of research. In Banet, A.G., Jr., editor: Creative psychotherapy, La Jolla, Calif., 1976, University Associates, Inc.

Pedersen, P.B., and others, editors: Counseling across cultures, Honolulu, 1981, University of Hawaii Press.

Perlmutter, F.D., and Vayda, A.M.: Barriers to prevention programs in community mental health programs, Adm. Ment. Health 5(2):140, 1978.

Schwartz. L.L.: A note on family rights, cults, and the law, J. Jewish Communal Service 55:194, Feb. 1978.

Segall, M.: Human behavior in cross-cultural psychology: global perspectives, Monterey, Calif., 1979, Brooks/Cole Publishing Co.

Specter, R.E.: Cultural diversity in health and illness, New York, 1979, Appleton-Century-Crofts.

Steele, R.E.: Relationship of race, sex, social class, and social mobility to depression in normal adults, J. Soc. Psychol. 104(1):37, 1978.

Sue, D.: Counseling the culturally different: theory and practice, New York, 1981, John Wiley & Sons, Inc.

Tausignant, M., and Mishara, B.: Suicide and culture: a review of the literature from 1969 to 1980, Transculture Psychiatric Review 18:5, 1981.

Triandis, H., and Draguns, J.: Handbook of cross-cultural psychology, vol. 6, Psychopathology, Boston, 1980, Allyn & Bacon, Inc.

chapter 5

Problem-solving approach to crisis intervention

According to Caplan (1964), a person is constantly faced with a need to solve problems in order to maintain equilibrium. When he is confronted with an imbalance between the difficulty (as he perceives it) of a problem and his available repertoire of coping skills, a crisis may be precipitated. If alternatives cannot be found or if solving the problem requires more time and energy than is usual, disequilibrium occurs. Tension rises and discomfort is felt, with associated feelings of anxiety, fear, guilt, shame, and helplessness.

One purpose of the crisis approach is to provide the consultation services of a therapist skilled in problem-solving techniques. This does not mean that the therapist will have an answer to every problem. However, she will be expected to have a ready and knowledgeable competency in problem solving, guiding and supporting her client toward crisis resolution. The therapeutic goal for the individual seeking help is the establishment of a level of emotional equilibrium equal to or better than the precrisis level.

Problem solving requires that a logical sequence of reasoning be applied to a situation in which an answer is required for a question and in which there is no immediate source of reliable information (Black, 1946). This process may take place either consciously or unconsciously. Usually the need to find an answer or solution is felt more strongly where such a resolution is most difficult.

The problem-solving process follows a structured, logical order of steps, each depending on the one preceding. In the routine decision making required in daily living this process is rarely necessary. Most people are unaware that they may follow a defined, logical sequence of reasoning in making decisions, often only remarking that some solutions seems to have been reached more easily than others. Finding out the time or deciding which shoe to put on first rarely calls for long, involved reasoning, and more often than not the question arises and the answer is found without any conscious effort.

Factors affecting the problem-solving process

Depending on the past experience related to the immediate problem, some people will be more adept at finding solutions than others. Both internal and external factors affect the process at any given time, although initially there may be only a temporary lack of concrete information. For example, when a driver finds himself lost because of a missing road sign, how much finding the right directions means to him in terms of his physical, psychological, and social well-being could affect the ease with which he finds an answer to the problem. Anxiety will increase in proportion to the value he places on finding a solution. If he is only out driving for pleasure, for example, he may feel casually concerned; but if he is under stress to be somewhere on time, his anxiety may increase according to the importance of his arrival at his immediate goals.

When anxiety is kept within tolerable limits, it can be an effective stimulant to action. It is a normal response to an unknown danger, experienced as discomfort, and helps the individual to mobilize his resources in meeting the problem. But as anxiety increases, perceptual awareness narrows and all perceptions are focused on the difficulty. When problem-solving skills are available, the individual is able to use this narrowing of perceptions to concentrate on the problem at hand.

If a solution is not found, anxiety may become more severe. Feelings of discomfort become intensified, and perceptions are narrowed to a crippling degree. The ability to understand what is happening and to make use of past experiences gives way to concentration on the discomfort itself. The individual becomes unable to recognize her own feelings, the problem, the facts, the evidence, and the situation in which she finds herself (Peplau, 1952).

Although problem solving involves a logical sequence of reasoning, it is not *always* a series of well-defined steps. According to Myer and Heidgerken (1962), it usually begins with a feeling that something has to be done. The problem area is generalized rather than made specific and well defined. Next, the memory is searched in an attempt to come up with ideas or solutions from similar problems in the past. March and Simon (1963) refer to this as "reproductive problem solving," and its value greatly depends on past successes in finding solutions.

When no similar past experiences are available, the individual may next turn to "productive problem solving." Here she is faced with the need to construct new ideas from more or less raw data. She will have to go to sources other than herself to get her facts. For example, the driver looking for the road sign may find someone nearby who can give her the needed new data—directions to the right road. If there is no one nearby, she will have to find some other source of information. She may resort to trial and error and with luck and patience find the way herself. Finding a solution in this way may meet a present need, but the information gained may not always be applicable to solving a similar problem in the future.

Problem solving in crisis intervention

John Dewey (1910) proposed the classical steps or stages represented in different episodes of problem solving: (1) a difficulty is felt, (2) the difficulty is located and defined, (3) possible solutions are suggested, (4) consequences are considered, and (5) a solution is accepted. With minor modifications, these steps in problem solving have been persistent over the years. Johnson (1955) simplified problem solving by reducing the number of steps to three: preparation, production, and judgment.

In 1962 Merrifield and associates conducted extensive research on the role of intellectual factors in problem solving. They advocated return to a five-stage model: preparation, analysis, production, verification, and reapplication. The fifth term was included in recognition of the fact that the problem solver often returns to earlier stages in a kind of revolving fashion.

According to Guilford (1967), the general problem-solving model involves the following processes: (1) *input* (from environment and soma), (2) *filtering* (attention aroused and directed), (3) *cognition* (problem sensed and structured), (4) *production* (answers generated), (5) *cognition* (new information obtained), (6) *production* (new answers generated), and (7) *evaluation* (input and cognition tested, answers tested; new tests of problem structure, new answers tested).

Assessment of the individual and the problem

When professional help is sought because a person is in crisis, the therapist must use logic and background knowledge to define the problem and plan intervention. The model for problem solving in the crisis approach will be readily familiar to mental health professionals.

The crisis approach to problem solving involves an assessment of the individual and the problem, planning of therapeutic intervention, intervention, and resolution of the crisis and anticipatory planning (Morley, Messick, and Aguilera, 1967).

The first therapy session is directed toward finding out what the crisis-precipitating event was and what factors are affecting the individual's ability to solve problems.

It is important that both therapist and client be able to define a situation clearly before taking any action to change it. Questions are asked such as "What do I need to know?" and "What must be done?" The more specifically the problem can be defined, the more likely it is that the "correct" answer will be sought.

Clues are investigated to point out and explore the problem or what is happening. The therapist asks questions and uses observational skills to obtain factual knowledge about the problem area. It is important to know what has happened within the immediate situation. How the individual has coped in past situations may affect his present behavior. Observations are made to determine his level of anxiety, expressive movements, emotional tone, verbal responses, and attitudinal changes.

It is important to remember that the therapist's task is to focus on the immediate problem. There is not enough time and *no need* to go into the patient's past history in depth.

One of the therapist's first questions usually is, "Why did you come for help today?" It is important to be emphatic about using the word *today*. Sometimes the individual will try to avoid stating why he came by saying, "I've been planning to come for some time." The usual reply is, "Yes, but what happened that made you come in *today?*" Other questions to ask are, "What happened in your life that is *different? When* did it happen?"

In crisis the precipitating event usually has occurred within 10 to 14 days before the individual seeks help. Frequently it is something that happened the day before or the night before. It could be almost anything: threat of divorce, discovery of extramarital relations, finding out a son or daughter is taking drugs, loss of boyfriend or girlfriend, loss of job or status, an unwanted pregnancy, and so forth.

The next area on which to focus is the individual's perception of the event: What does it mean to her? How does she see its effect on her future? Does she see the event realistically, or does she distort its meaning?

The patient is then questioned about available situational supports: What person in the environment can the therapist find to support the person? With whom does she live? Who is her best friend? Whom does she trust? Is there a member of the family to whom she feels particularly close? Crisis intervention is sharply time limited, and the more people involved in helping the person the better. Also, if others are involved and familiar with the problem, they can continue to give support when therapy is terminated.

The next area of focus is ascertaining what the person usually does when he has a problem he cannot solve: What are his coping skills? Has anything like this ever happened to him before? How does he usually abate tension, anxiety, or depression? Has he tried the same method this time? If not, why not, if it usually works for him? If his usual method was tried and it did not work, why did it not work? What does he feel would reduce his symptoms of stress? Something is usually thought of; coping skills are so very individual. Methods of coping with anxiety that have not been used in years may be remembered. One man recalled that he used to "work off tensions" by playing the piano for a few hours, and it was suggested that he try this method again. Since he did not have a piano, he rented one; by the next session his anxiety had reduced enough to enable him to begin problem solving.

One of the most important parts of the assessment is to find out whether the person is suicidal or homicidal. The questions must be very *direct* and *specific:* Is he planning to kill himself or someone else? How? When? The therapist must find out and assess the seriousness of the threat. Is the person merely thinking about it or does he have a method selected? Is it a lethal method—a loaded gun? Has he picked out a tall building or bridge? Can he tell you when he plans to do it—for example, after the children are asleep?

If the threat does not seem too imminent, the person is accepted for crisis therapy. If the intent is carefully planned and details are specific, hospitalization and psychiatric evaluation are arranged in order to protect the person or others in the community.

Planning of therapeutic intervention

After identifying the precipitating event and the factors that are influencing the individual's state of disequilibrium, the therapist plans the method of intervention. Determination must be made as to how much the crisis has disrupted the individual's life. Is she able to work? Go to school? Keep house? Care for her family? Are these activities being affected? This is the first area to examine for the degree of disruption. How is her state of disequilibrium affecting others in her life? How does her husband (or wife, boyfriend, girlfriend, roommate, or family) feel about this problem? What do they think she should do? Are they upset?

This is basically a search process in which data are collected. It requires the use of cognitive abilities and recollection of past events for information relative to the present situation. The last phase of this step is essentially a thinking process in which alternatives are considered and evaluated against past experience and knowledge as well as in the context of the present situation.

Tentative solutions are advanced about *why* the problem exists. This requires familiarity with theoretical knowledge and the anticipation of more than one answer. In the study of behavior it is important to seek causal relationships. Clues observed in the environmental conditions are examined and related to theories of psychosocial behavior to suggest reasons for the individual's disturbed equilibrium.

Intervention

In the third step intervention is initiated. Action is taken with the expectation that if _____(planned action)_____ is taken, the _____(expected result)_____ will occur.

After the necessary information is collected, the problem-solving process is continued to initiate intervention. The therapist defines the problem from the information that has been given and reflects it back to the individual. This clarifies the problem and encourages focusing on the immediate situation. The therapist then explores possible alternate solutions to the problem to reduce the symptoms produced by the crisis. At this time, specific directions may be given as to what should be tried as tentative solutions. This enables the individual to leave the first session with some positive guidelines for going out and testing alternate solutions. At the next session the individual and therapist evaluate the results, and if none of these solutions has been effective, they work toward finding others.

The therapist may validate observations and tentative conclusions by reviewing the case with another therapist when he thinks that it may be helpful or necessary. Briefly, the therapist identifies the crisis-precipitating event, symptoms that the crisis has produced in the individual, the degree of disruption evident in the individual's life, and the plan for intervention. Planned intervention may include one technique or a combination of several techniques. It may be helping the individual to gain an intellectual understanding of the crisis or helping him to explore and ventilate his feelings. Other techniques may be helping the individual to find new and more effective coping mechanisms or utilizing other people as situational supports. Finally, a plan would be presented for helping the person to establish realistic goals for the future.

Anticipatory planning

Evaluation is made to determine whether or not the planned action has produced the expected results. Appraisal must be objective and impartial in order to be valid. Has the individual returned to his usual or higher level of equilibrium in his functioning? The problem-solving process is continued as the therapist and the individual work toward resolution of the crisis.

Paradigm of intervention

According to Caplan (1964), a crisis has four developmental phases:
1. There is an initial rise in tension as habitual problem-solving techniques are tried.
2. There is a lack of success in coping as the stimulus continues and more discomfort is felt.
3. A further increase in tension acts as a powerful internal stimulus and mobilizes internal and external resources. In this stage emergency problem-solving mechanisms are tried. The problem may be redefined or there may be resignation and the giving up of certain aspects of the goal as unattainable.
4. If the problem continues and can be neither solved nor avoided, tension increases and a major disorganization occurs.

Whenever a stressful event occurs, certain recognized balancing factors can effect a return to equilibrium; these are perception of the event, available situational supports, and coping mechanisms, as shown in Fig. 1. The upper portion of the paradigm illustrates the "normal" initial reaction of an individual to a stressful event.

A stressful event is seldom so clearly defined that its source can be determined

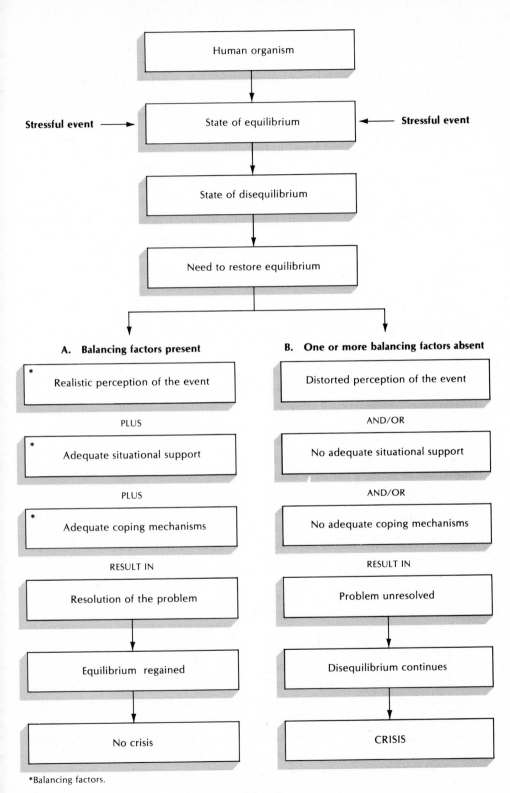

Fig. 1
Paradigm: the effect of balancing factors in a stressful event.

immediately. Internalized changes occur at the same time as the externally provoked stress, and as a result, some events may cause a strong emotional response in one person, yet leave another apparently unaffected. Much is determined by the presence or absence of factors that can effect a return to equilibrium.

In column *A* of Fig. 1 the balancing factors are operating and crisis is avoided. However, in column *B* the absence of one or more of these balancing factors may block resolution of the problem, thus increasing disequilibrium and precipitating crisis.

Fig. 2 demonstrates the use of the paradigm for presentation of subsequent case studies. Its purpose is to serve as a guideline to help the reader focus on the problem areas. An example of its applicability is presented in the cases of two people affected by the same stressful event. One resolved the problem and avoided crisis; the other did not.

Balancing factors affecting equilibrium

Between the perceived effects of a stressful situation and the resolution of the problem are three recognized balancing factors that may determine the state of equilibrium. Strengths or weaknesses in any one of the factors can be directly related to the onset of crisis or to its resolution. These are perception of the event, available situational supports, and coping mechanisms.

Why do some people go into crisis when others do not? In Fig. 2 this is illustrated by the cases of two students, Sue and Mary. Both fail a final examination. Sue is upset but does not go into crisis. Mary *does* go into crisis. Why does Sue react one way and Mary differently to the same stressful event? What "things" in their present lives make the difference?

Perception of the event

Cognition, or subjective meaning, of a stressful event plans a major role in determining both the nature and degree of coping behaviors. Differences in cognition, in terms of the event's threat to an important life goal or value, account for large differences in coping behaviors. The concept of *cognitive style* (Cropley and Field, 1969) suggests a certain uniqueness in the way that people take in, process, and use information from their environment.

Cognitive styles, or the characteristic modes for organizing perceptual and intellectual activities, play an important role in determining an individual's coping responses to daily life stresses. According to Inkeles (1966), cognitive style helps to set limits on information seeking in stress situations. It also strongly influences perceptions of others, interpersonal relationships, and responses to various types of psychiatric treatment.

For example, in stressful situations a person whose cognitive style is identified as

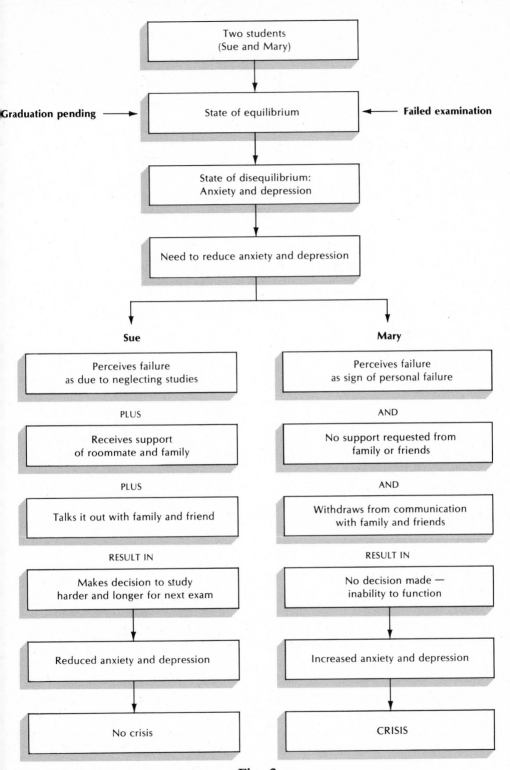

Fig. 2
Paradigm applied to case study.

"field-dependent" is very dependent upon external objects in the environment for orientation to reality. This type of individual tends to use such coping mechanisms as repression and denial. In contrast, the "field-independent" person will tend to prefer intellectualization as a defense mode.

If the event is perceived realistically, the relationship between the event and feelings of stress will be recognized. Problem solving can be appropriately oriented toward reduction of tension, and successful solution of the stressful situation will be more probable.

Lazarus (1966, 1974) focused on the importance of the mediating cognitive process, *appraisal,* to determine the various coping methods used by individuals. This recognizes that coping behaviors always represent an interaction between the individual and the environment, and that environmental demands of each unique situation will initiate, form, and limit coping activities that may be required in the interaction. As a result, people will engage in widely diverse behavioral and intra-psychic activities to meet actual or anticipated threats.

Appraisal, in this context, is an ongoing perceptual process by which a potentially harmful event is distinguished from a potentially beneficial or irrelevant event in one's life.

When a threatening situation exists, first a *primary* appraisal is made to judge the perceived outcome of the event in relation to one's future goals and values. This is followed by a *secondary* appraisal whereby one perceives the range of coping alternatives available either to master the threat or to achieve a beneficial outcome. As coping activities are selected and initiated, feedback cues from changing internal and external environments lead to ongoing *reappraisals* or to changes in the original perception.

As a result of the appraisal process, coping behaviors are never static. They change constantly in both quality and degree as new information and cues are received during reappraisal activities. New coping responses may occur whenever new significance is attached to a situation.

If, in the appraisal process, the outcome is judged to be too overwhelming or too difficult to be dealt with using available coping skills, an individual is more likely to resort to use of intrapsychic defensive mechanisms to repress or distort the reality of the situation. An appraisal of a potentially successful outcome, however, will more likely lead to the use of direct action modes of coping such as attack, flight, or compromise.

If the perception of the event is distorted, a relationship between the event and feelings of stress may not be recognized. Thus attempts to solve the problem will be ineffective, and tension will not be reduced.

In other words, what does the event mean to the individual? How is it going to affect his future? Can he look at it realistically or does he distort its meaning? For ex-ample, Sue sees failing the examination as the result of not studying enough or of concentrating on the wrong material and decides it will not happen again. Mary, on the other hand, thinks that failing the examination makes *her* a failure; she feels threatened and believes she will never graduate from college.

Situational supports

By nature, human beings are social and dependent on others in their environment to supply them with reflected appraisals of their own intrinsic and extrinsic values. In establishing life patterns, certain appraisals are more significant to the individual than others because they tend to reinforce the perception the individual has of himself.

Dependency relationships may be more readily established with those whose appraisals tend to support the individual against feelings of insecurity and with those who reinforce feelings of ego integrity.

These meaningful relationships with others provide a person with nurturance and support, resources vital for coping with a wide variety of stressors. Social isolation, whatever the cause, denies a person availability of social interactions and opportunities to develop meaningful relationships. Sudden or unexpected social isolation results in the loss of usual resource supports. With these lacking, a person is much more vulnerable when confronted with daily living stressors.

Loss, threatened loss, or feelings of inadequacy in a supportive relationship also may leave a person in a vulnerable position. Confrontation with a stressful situation, combined with a lack of situational support, may lead to a state of disequilibrium and possible crisis.

Appraisal of self varies across ages, sexes, and roles. The belief system that forms the basis of the self-concept and self-esteem develops out of experiences with significant others in a person's life. Although self-esteem is fairly static within a certain range, it does fluctuate according to internal and external environmental variables that impinge on it at a specific time and in a specific situation. In order to achieve and maintain a sense of value and self-worth, a person must feel loved by others and capable of achieving an ideal self, one that is strong, capable, good, and loving of others.

When self-esteem is low, or when a situation is perceived as particularly threatening, the person is strongly in need of and seeks out others from whom positive reflective appraisals of self-worth and ability to achieve can be obtained. The lower the self-esteem or the greater the threat, the greater the need to seek situational supports. Conversely, a person will strive to avoid or will withdraw from contacts with those he perceives as threatening to his self-esteem, whether the threat is real or imagined. Any potentially stressful situation can set off questions of self-doubt about how one is perceived by others, the kind of impression being made, and the real or imagined inadequacies that might be disclosed (Mechanic, 1974).

Success or failure of a coping behavior is always strongly influenced by the social context in which it occurs. The environmental variable most centrally identified is the person's significant others. From them a person learns to seek advice, support, and so forth in solving daily problems in living. Confidence in being liked and respected by these peers is based on past testing and reaffirmations of their expected supportive responses.

Any perceived failure to obtain adequate support to meet psychosocial needs may provoke, or compound, a stressful situation. The receipt of negative support could be equally detrimental to a person's self-esteem.

Situational supports are those persons who are available in the environment and who can be depended on to help solve the problem.

Sue talked to her roommate about her feelings over failing the exam; she even cried on her shoulder. She also called home for reassurance from her family. In effect, *someone* had been found for support during this stressful event.

Mary did not feel close enough to her roommate to talk about the problem. She had no close friends whom she trusted. Fearing their reaction, she did not call home to tell her family about failing. Mary did not have *anyone* to turn to for help; she felt overwhelmed and alone.

Coping mechanisms

Through the process of daily living people learn to use many methods to cope with anxiety and reduce tension. Life-styles are developed around patterns of response, which in turn are established to cope with stressful situations. These life-styles are highly individual and quite necessary to protect and maintain equilibrium.

The early work of Cannon (1929, 1939) provided a basis for later systematic research on the effects of stress on the human organism. According to Cannon's "fight or flight" theory, reactions of acute anxiety, similar to those of fear, are vital to readying the individual physiologically to meet any real or imagined threat to self. From his studies of homeostasis Cannon described the mechanisms whereby human and other animal life systems maintain steady life states with the goal always to return to such states whenever conditions force a temporary departure.

Over the years it has not been unusual to find the term *coping* being used interchangeably with such similar concepts as adaptation, defense, mastery, and adjustive reactions. Coping activities take a wide variety of forms including all the diverse behaviors that people engage in to meet actual or anticipated challenges.

In psychological stress theory the term *coping* emphasizes various strategies used, consciously or unconsciously, to deal with stress and tensions arising from perceived threats to psychological integrity. It is not synonymous with mastery over problematical life situations; rather, it is the *process* of attempting to solve them (Lazarus, 1966).

Coleman (1950) defined coping as an adjustive reaction made in response to actual or imagined stress in order to maintain psychological integrity. Within this concept human beings are perceived as responding to stress by either attack, flight, or compromise reactions. These become complicated by various ego-defense mechanisms whenever the stress becomes ego-involved.

Attack reactions usually attempt to remove or overcome the obstacles seen as causing stress in life situations. These may be primarily constructive or destructive in nature. Flight, withdrawal, or fear reactions may be as simple as phsyically removing the threat from the environment (such as putting out a fire) or removing oneself from the threatening situation (running away from the fire area). They might also involve much more complex psychological maneuvering, depending on the perceived extent of the threat and the possibilities for escape.

Compromise or substitution reactions occur when either attack or flight from the threatening situation is thought to be impossible. This method is most commonly used to deal with problem solving and includes the accepting of substitute goals or changing internalized values and standards.

Masserman (1946) demonstrated that, under situations of extended frustration, individuals find it increasingly possible to compromise for substitute goals. This often involves use of *rationalization,* a defense mechanism whereby "half a loaf" does indeed soon appear to be "better than none."

Tension-reducing mechanisms can be overt or covert and can be consciously or unconsciously activated. They have been generally classified into such behavioral responses as aggression, regression, withdrawal, and repression. The selection of a response is based on tension-reducing actions that successfully relieved anxiety and reduced tension in similar situations in the past. Through repetition the response may pass from conscious awareness during its learning phase to a habitual level of reaction as a learned behavior. In many instances the individual may not be aware of *how,* let alone *why,* he reacts to stress in given situations. Except for vague feelings of discomfort, the rise and consequent reduction in tension may pass almost unnoticed. When a novel stress-producing event arises and learned coping mechanisms are ineffectual, discomfort is felt on a conscious level. The need to "do something" becomes the focus of activity, narrowing perception of all other life activities.

Normally, defense mechanisms are used constructively in the process of coping. This is particularly evident whenever there is danger of becoming psychologically overwhelmed. All are seen as important for survival. None is equated with a pathological condition unless it interferes with the process of coping, such as being used to deny, to falsify, or to distort perceptions of reality.

According to Bandura (1977), the strength of the individual's conviction in her own effectiveness in overcoming or mastering a problematical situation determines whether coping behavior will even be attempted in the first place. People fear and avoid stressful, threatening situations that they believe exceed their ability to cope. They behave with assurance in those situations where they judge themselves able to manage and to expect eventual success. It is the perceived ability to master that can influence the choice of coping behaviors as well as the persistence used once one is chosen.

Available coping mechanisms are what people *usually* do when they have a problem. They may sit down and try to think it out or talk it out with a friend. Some cry it out or try to get rid of their feelings of anger and hostility by swearing, kicking a chair, or slamming doors. Others may get into verbal battles with friends. Some may react by temporarily withdrawing from the situation in order to reassess the problem. These are just a few of the many coping methods people use to relieve their tension and anxiety when faced with a problem. Each of these has been used at some time in the developmental past of the individual, has been found effective in maintaining emotional stability, and has become part of his life-style in meeting and dealing with the stresses of daily living.

Sue used her roommate to talk it out; this reduced her tension and anxiety. She was able to solve the problem and decided that for the next exam she would study more, over a longer period of time. Her tension and anxiety were reduced, equilibrium was restored, and she did not have a crisis.

Mary withdrew. She had no coping skills to use, and her tension and anxiety increased. Unable to solve the problem and unable to function, she went into crisis.

References

Bandura, A., and others: Cognitive processes mediating behavioral change, J. Pers. Soc. Psychol. **35**(3):125, 1977.

Black, M.: Critical thinking: an introduction to logic and scientific method, Englewood Cliffs, N.J., 1946, Prentice-Hall, Inc.

Cannon, W.B.: Bodily changes in pain, hunger, fear, and rage, New York, 1929, D. Appleton and Co.

Cannon, W.B.: The wisdom of the body, ed. 2, New York, 1939, W. W. Norton & Co., Inc.

Caplan, G.: Principles of preventive psychiatry, New York, 1964, Basic Books, Inc., Publishers.

Coleman, J.C.: Abnormal psychology and modern life, Chicago, 1950, Scott, Foresman and Co.

Cropley, A., and Field, T.: Achievement in science and intellectual style, J. Appl. Psychol. **53**:132, 1969.

Dewey, J.: How we think, Boston, 1910, Heath Co.

Guilford, J.P.: The nature of human intelligence, New York, 1967, McGraw-Hill Book Co.

Inkeles, A.: Social structure and the socialization of competence, Harv. Ed. Rev. **36**, 1966.

Johnson, D.M.: The psychology of thought and judgment, New York, 1955, Harper & Row, Publishers.

Lazarus, R.S.: Psychological stress and the coping process, New York, 1966, McGraw-Hill Book Co.

Lazarus, R.S., and others: The psychology of coping: issues in research and assessment. In Coehlo, G.V., and others, editors: Coping and adaptation, New York, 1974, Basic Books, Inc., Publishers.

March, J.G., and Simon, H.A.: Organizations, New York, 1963, John Wiley & Sons, Inc.

Masserman, J.H.: Principles of dynamic psychology, Philadelphia, 1946, W.B. Saunders Co.

Mechanic, D.: Social structure and personal adaptation: some neglected dimensions. In Coehlo, G.V., and others, editors: Coping and adaptation, New York, 1974, Basic Books, Inc., Publishers.

Merrifield, P.R., and others: The role of intellectual factors in problem-solving, Psychol. Monogr. **76**(10):1962.

Morley, W.E., Messick, J.M., and Aguilera, D.C.: Crisis: paradigms of intervention, J. Psychiatr. Nurs. **5**:538, Nov.–Dec. 1967.

Myer, B., and Heidgerken, L.E.: Introduction to research in nursing, Philadelphia, 1962, J.B. Lippincott Co.

Peplau, H.E.: Interpersonal relations in nursing, New York, 1952, G.P. Putnam's Sons.

Additional readings

Anderson, M.D.: Care for the worried well, Issues Ment. Health Nurs. **2**(3):15, 1980.

Baldwin, B.A.: A paradigm for the classification of emotional crises: implications for crisis intervention, Am. J. Orthopsychiatry **48**(3):538, 1978.

Brown, G.W.: Meaning, measurement and stress of life events. In Dohrenwend, B.S., and Dohrenwend, B.P., editors: Stressful life events: their nature and effects, New York, 1974, John Wiley & Sons, Inc.

Dohrenwend, B.S., and Dohrenwend, B.P., editors: Stressful life events: their nature and effects, New York, 1974, John Wiley & Sons, Inc.

Dohrenwend, B.S., and Dohrenwend, B.P.: Stressful life events: research issues, New Directions Ment. Health Serv. **6**:57, 1980.

Garber, J., and Seligman, M.E.P., editors: Human helplessness: theory and application, New York, 1980, Academic Press, Inc.

Haley, J.: Problem solving therapy, San Francisco, 1976, Jossey-Bass, Inc., Publishers.

Horowitz, M.J.: Stress response syndromes, New York, 1976, Jason Aronson, Inc.

Kelly, D.: Anxiety and emotions, Springfield, Ill., 1980, Charles C Thomas, Publisher.

Kutash, I.L., and others, editors: Handbook on stress and anxiety, San Francisco, 1980, Jossey-Bass, Inc., Publishers.

Lazarus, R.S.: The self regulation of emotion. In Levi, L., editor: Parameters of emotion, New York, 1975, Raven Press.

May, R.: The meaning of anxiety, rev. ed., New York, 1977, W.W. Norton & Co., Inc.

Mechanic, D.: Some problems in the measurement of stress and social readjustment, J. Human Stress **1**(3):43, 1975.

Pearlin, L.I., and Schooleo, C.: The structure of coping, J. Health Soc. Behav. **19**(3):2, 1978.

Selye, H.: The stress of life, rev. ed., New York, 1976, McGraw-Hill Book Co.

White, R.W.: Strategies in adaptation: an attempt at systematic description. In Coehlo, G.V., and others, editors: Coping and adaptation, New York, 1974, Basic Books, Inc., Publishers.

chapter 6

Situational crises

Whenever stressful events occur in a person's life situation that threaten his sense of biological, psychological, or social integrity, some degree of disequilibrium results, along with the concurrent possibility of a crisis. Several determining factors affect the positive balance of equilibrium, and the absence of one or more could make a state of crisis more imminent.

According to Rapoport (1962), when an instinctual need or a sense of integrity is threatened, the ego usually responds characteristically with anxiety; when loss or deprivation occurs, the response is usually depression. On the other hand, if the threat or loss is viewed as a challenge, there is more likely to be a mobilization of energy toward purposeful problem-solving activities.

Circumstances that may create only a feeling of mild concern in one person may create a high level of anxiety and tension in another. Recognized factors influencing a return to a balance of equilibrium are the perception of the event, available coping mechanisms, and available situational supports. Crises may be avoided if these factors are operating at the time the stressful event(s) is intruding into the individual's life-style.

Studies have been made of behavior patterns that might be anticipated in response to common stressful situations. These have provided valuable clues to anticipatory planning for prevention as well as intervention in crisis situations. Some of these are combat neurosis (Glass, 1957), relocation through urban renewal (Brown and associates, 1965), rehabilitation of families after tornado disasters (Moore, 1958), hospitalization of children and adolescents (Vernick, 1963), crises of unwed mothers (Bernstein, 1960), separation anxiety of hospitalized children (Bowlby, 1960), and death and dying (Kübler-Ross, 1969, 1974). These studies suggest that there are certain patterned phases of reactions to unique stressful situations through which select groups of people can be expected to pass before equilibrium is restored. Preventive techniques of community psychiatry focus on anticipatory intervention; this is to prevent crises that could result from maladaptive responses as individuals attempt to return to equilibrium.

In this chapter stressful events that could precipitate a crisis have been selected on the premise that each could affect some member of a family, regardless of its socioeconomic or sociocultural status. The case studies selected are not to be considered all-inclusive of the many situational crises with which a therapist may come in contact.

It is also important to recognize that the theoretical material preceding each case study is presented as an overview, relevant to the crisis situation. Therapists already trained in crisis intervention will recognize the need for much greater depth of theoretical knowledge than is presented in this chapter. The intent is only to provide guidelines; further study of problem areas is suggested for more comprehensive knowledge.

In order to clarify the steps in crisis intervention, much extraneous case study material has been eliminated. In crisis a person may be confronted with many stressful events occurring simultaneously. He may have no conscious awareness of *what* occurred, let alone which event requires priority in problem solving. The studies may appear oversimplified to anyone who has struggled through the phases of defining the problem and planning appropriate intervention.

The paradigm is a means we devised to keep the reader focused on the problem area and on the balancing factors that influence the presence or absence of crisis. We doubt if it could be successfully used as a form that could be quickly completed after the initial assessment interview; rarely are stressful events so easily defined. It is the very nature of a crisis that interrelated internal and external stresses compound the problem area and distort the causes of objective and subjective symptoms.

One responsibility essential in assuming the role of a therapist in this method of intervention is recognition of the need for knowledge of the generic development of crises.

Prematurity—theoretical concepts

The birth of a premature baby is a stressful situation for any family. Even when anticipated, there is a sense of emergency both at home and in the hospital when labor begins. In the hospital, both staff and parents feel anxiety for the potential welfare of the newborn infant.

Researchers have identified the following four phases or tasks the mother must work through if she is to come out of the experience in a healthy way (Mason, 1963; Kaplan and Mason, 1965).

1. She must realize that she may lose the baby. This anticipatory grief involves a gradual withdrawal from the relationship already established with the child during the pregnancy.
2. She must acknowledge failure in her maternal function to deliver a full-term baby.
3. After separation from the infant as a result of his prolonged hospital stay she must resume her relationship with him in preparation for the infant's homecoming.

4. She must prepare herself for the job of caring for the baby through an understanding of his special needs and growth patterns.

After delivery the infant is hurriedly taken to the premature nursery. The parents have barely had a glimpse of their new son or daughter and certainly have had no opportunity to reassure themselves about his condition. The infant is isolated from all except the medical personnel during his hospital stay, and the parents, with only limited physical contact with the child, cannot allay their anxieties. There is a realistic danger that the baby will not live or that he will not be normal. Often physicians and nurses talk about the baby in guarded terms, not wanting to give false reassurance, so that the feeling of anxiety may last for days or weeks.

The way in which the family members react to this period of stress is crucial in determining whether or not a crisis will develop. These studies of families who have experienced the stress of a premature birth show that some have managed very well; the mother was not apprehensive about caring for the baby, despite the special attention he required. In these families the relationship between husband and wife was found to be good; they seemingly had adjusted to the new member of the family, and their relationship was not threatened by the increased responsibility.

Other families studied appeared to be in a state of crisis, although the premature infant was out of danger. In those cases the relationship between the husband and wife was determined to be unstable. The baby was cared for by an overly apprehensive mother who often seemed unconcerned about important things such as the baby's weight gain, whether or not he was eating adequately, and the immediate prognosis.

It has been hypothesized that women who were most disturbed during the period when there was real danger to the baby dealt with this stress more effectively (Caplan, 1964). Women who showed symptoms of a crisis were those who seemingly denied the existence of any danger. They did not question the information given them or the reassurances of the treating personnel. In fact, they seemed to encourage a conspiracy of silence, avoiding any confrontation with feelings of fear, guilt, and anxiety.

Many emotions develop in parents when a new baby arrives, even when the child is full term. The mother is called upon to meet additional demands on her time and may feel hostility toward the new baby. Usually, however, the strong feeling of a mother's love ensures repression of any resentment she may feel and the guilt it inspires. The usual activities of the father are not as directly interrupted, so that his resentment is usually less than that of the mother and is more often aroused by jealousy of the attention that the mother gives to the baby.

The following case study concerns a young mother of a premature baby. Clues from the initial assessment interview indicated that she was acknowledging herself to be a failure for not delivering a full-term baby. Intervention focused on relieving the immediate causes of her anxiety and depression and assisting her to adapt to subsequent phases in the characteristic responses to a premature birth.

ASSESSMENT OF THE INDIVIDUAL AND THE PROBLEM

Laura and Peter G. were a young couple who had been married for 3 years. Peter, 5 years older than Laura, was the oldest of four children. Laura, a petite young woman, was an only child. They had a 2-year-old daughter and a 2-month-old son, who was born prematurely.

Peter's company had transferred him to another city when Laura was 7½ months pregnant; she went into labor the day after moving into their new home 100 miles from their home town, where both their families lived. She delivered their son in a private hospital with excellent facilities but under the care of an obstetrician previously unknown to her as a result of their recent move. She was upset by the strangeness of the hospital, by the new physicians, and by the precarious physical condition of the son she and Peter had been hoping for. Laura did not want to discuss her fears with her physician because she did not know him, or with the nurses, because they "always seemed so busy." She also thought that since she had had a baby before, she should know the answers to all the questions she had in mind.

After she and Peter brought their son home from the hospital, Laura had episodes of crying and symptoms of anxiety, including insomnia. She felt physically exhausted and increasingly fearful concerning her ability to care for her son. No matter what she did, the baby slept only for short periods and was more fretful when awake than their daughter had been. Because of the baby's small size, Peter was afraid to help with his care, so Laura was responsible for all his physical care.

Peter's mother arrived for a visit "to see how the new baby was doing." She had been critical of Laura's intention to move at the time of Peter's transfer, advising that Laura should wait until after the baby's birth. Laura had now begun to think that she should have followed that advice. Her mother-in-law and she often had talks about the rearing of children. Laura had begun to have confidence in her own mothering abilities as a result of her daughter's good health and average development, but now she was doubtful again because of her apparent inability to care for her new son.

The event that precipitated the crisis was the visit of the mother-in-law, who was critical of Laura's ability to care for her new baby. "I can't understand why the baby cries so much. You must be doing something wrong. My children always slept through the night by 2 months of age and took long naps during the day," were typical of her constant comments. Peter seemed reluctant to take sides against his mother, so Laura received little support from him in dealing with these criticisms. She was finally unable to cope with her feelings of inadequacy, which were intensified by her mother-in-law's visit, and as a result became extremely upset, cried uncontrollably, and was unable to care for the baby at all. Peter's employer commented to him that he seemed upset and asked if there was anything wrong at work. Peter told him that the problem was not his job but Laura's behavior since the birth of the baby. His employer recommended that they seek help at a nearby crisis center.

The goal of intervention determined by the therapist at the crisis center was to assist both Laura and Peter in exploring their feelings about the premature birth of their son, their changed communication pattern, and the lack of support Peter was giving Laura.

INTERVENTION

During the first few weeks, Laura was able to discuss her feelings of inadequacy in the mothering role and to tell Peter of her anxieties about their son, of her fears that he would be abnormal, and of her belief that the premature birth was her fault because she had insisted on moving with Peter at the time of his transfer. Peter, in turn, could tell Laura of his feelings of guilt at not being able to help more during the move and also of the blame he placed on himself because the labor was premature. The therapist assisted them in seeing the reality of the situation. Although the move may have been a factor in the premature onset of labor, there could have been other causes.

Peter discussed his insecurities about the handling of such a small baby; Laura was then able to tell him that she felt the same way, and she feared she might be doing something wrong with this baby. The therapist gave them information about the differences in the behavior of a normal child and the care required for a premature infant. She reassured Laura that she was doing well and that in time the baby would adjust to more regular hours. She encouraged Peter to help his wife so she could get more rest; in turn Laura helped Peter to gain confidence in holding and caring for their new son.

ANTICIPATORY PLANNING

As Peter became comfortable in caring for the baby, he was encouraged to share the responsibility of caring for him in the evenings. This enabled Laura to get more physical rest. Peter's emotional support helped her to relax, and she began to sleep better.

The therapist discussed their need to continue to improve communications between them. It was stressed that they must reestablish a pattern of social activities with each other. They were assured that their new son could survive for a few hours with a competent baby-sitter while they went out to dinner or to play cards with other couples.

Most of the energies and concern during the past 2 months had been concentrated on their son. It was recommended that they also devote some additional time to their 2-year-old daughter. This was a stressful time for her, too! Since her mother and father could not give her their sole attention, she would be competing for time with her new brother, and the feelings of sibling rivalry would emerge. She would need to feel that her position in the family was also unique and important—

CASE STUDY: LAURA

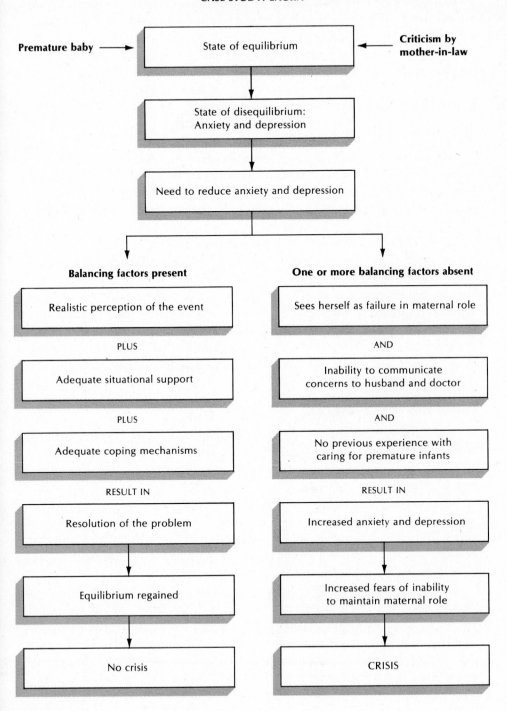

FIGURE 3

that is, a daughter and their firstborn. Time should be planned for her to have some activities with her parents. This would emphasize that she was "old" enough to be included in their activities.

They were warned to expect some acting-out behavior and possibly some regressive behavior in her bids for "equal" attention.

During their last visit Laura and Peter were assured they could return to the center if they felt the need for help with a problem.

SUMMATION OF THE PARADIGM

This case study concerned a young mother unable to cope with problems of an unexpectedly premature baby. Assessment of the stressful events precipitating the crisis indicated that Laura regarded herself as a failure for not delivering a full-term baby. This was reinforced by the criticisms of her mother-in-law and the lack of situational support from her husband.

In the assessment phase the therapist maintained focus on the immediate area of stress that could have precipitated the crisis. After determining a possible cause-effect relationship, a goal for intervention was established. Laura was encouraged to ventilate her feelings of guilt and inadequacy in the present situation. Realistic perception of the event developed as the therapist provided information leading to an intellectual understanding of the relationship between the event and the resulting symptoms of stress. The husband was brought in as a situational support, and new as well as previously successful coping skills were used in resolving the crisis.

Child abuse—theoretical concepts

According to data available from the National Center on Child Abuse and Neglect, an estimated 10.5 children are abused and/or neglected annually for each 1000 U.S. children under the age of 18 years (U.S. Department of Health and Human Services, 1982).

The following major categories of mistreatment of children were represented in these data: (1) physical abuse, (2) sexual abuse, (3) emotional abuse, (4) physical neglect, (5) emotional neglect, and (6) educational neglect. It was also found that 74% of child abuse fatalities occurred in preschool children up to the age of 5 years (U.S. Department of Health and Human Services, 1982).

Child abuse occurs in a wide variety of ways. Recent trends have moved toward greatly expanding its definition from physical abuse alone to include also emotional and sexual abuse, as well as physical and emotional neglect. In general, however, consensus is lacking among professionals for any one single definition of the terms *child abuse* or *child neglect*. Definitions vary greatly because there is much diversity in sociocultural values and practices associated with child rearing, some of which may result in physical and psychological harm to the child.

Child abusers are not limited to any one well-defined group of persons. They can be found among widely differing socioeconomic, racial, cultural, age, and other socially defined groups. Specific differences, however, have been identified among factors related to specific forms of abuse. For example, the physical size, strength, and power of the abuser obviously do not play as great a role in child abuse as in the abuse of adults. Obviously, few are as physically powerless as the infant or small child.

Abuse and neglect of children have been recorded throughout the centuries. It has been suggested that these are by no means new problems, but rather ones that only now are being socially recognized and legally addressed. It was not until 1871 that the first child protective agency, The Society for the Prevention of Cruelty to Children, was established in New York. Nearly a century passed before all 50 states finally enacted legal mandates to report child abuse in 1968.

In 1962 Kempe originated the phrase *battered child syndrome,* which dramatically focused professional and public attention on the abusive actions by parents and/or other adults on select groups of children (Kempe and associates, 1962). This provided a base for the specific labeling and identification of the severest forms of child abuse, for which there is clinically verifiable evidence. Clinical signs include bruises, abrasions, lacerations, broken bones, burns, abdominal and chest injuries, and eye damage. Frequently, examination of new injuries yields clinical evidence of past injuries. Some children experience a single, violent abusive event, others a long series of multiple violent episodes. This label was later superseded by the more comprehensive term *child abuse and neglect* (Helfer and Kempe, 1976).

In 1973 The Child Abuse Prevention and Treatment Act (Public Law 93-247) defined the legal responsibilities of health care providers encountering child abuse or neglect:

> Child abuse and neglect means the physical and mental injury, sexual abuse, negligent treatment or maltreatment of the child under the age of eighteen by a person who is responsible for the child's welfare under circumstances which indicate that the child's health or welfare is harmed or threatened thereby. (U.S. Congress, 1974)

Every state now has written into its statutes a legal definition of child abuse to delineate the range of circumstances to be addressed by the various protective agencies. These definitions vary from state to state, however, which has led to ambiguity and inconsistency in their interpretation and application.

In a comparative analysis of state statutes on child abuse three basic characteristics were found in all legal definitions (Kameron and Kahn, 1976):

1. The behavior violated a norm or standard of parental conduct.
2. The infliction was deliberate and a non-accidental injury.
3. The abuse was severe enough to warrant intervention, whether social, legal, medical, or a combination of any of these.

Although the battered child syndrome may be among the easiest forms of child abuse to prove legally, it has been found to be only a part of the overall problem of abuse of children.

Incidence reports on incest and sexual exploitation of children are admittedly incomplete and, at the most, educated estimates. Case finding is quite difficult, most often coming to the attention of health care agencies when the child is seen for other health care problems such as venereal disease or pregnancy. According to Justice and Justice (1979), sexual abuse, like child abuse, most often involves more than just the victim and the abuser. It also involves another family member or responsible adults who allow the victimization to continue.

In general, incestuous offenders do not exhibit any overtly psychotic or deviant behaviors (Giarretto, 1976). Generally the perpetrator is between 30 and 50 years old, male, and the victim's father more than 75% of the time. Reported female victims outnumber male victims by a wide margin. Investigations of adults who were abused as children reveal that 1 out of every 5 girls and 1 out of every 10 boys had experienced some type of sexual molestation, abuse, or exploitation (Rubinelli, 1980; Salhelz and associates, 1982).

According to Drake (1984), persons who sexually exploit children are usually men who are emotionally dependent with feelings of inferiority and whose lives have been dominated by a significant woman. It has also been found that there is a significantly high correlation between sexual abusers and a history of parental abuse in their childhood. The child frequently knows the abuser and may become involved solely to meet nonsexual needs for attention and affection. Children are particularly vulnerable because of ignorance or fear of losing the caring relationship, or because of ambivalence, shame, guilt, and the fear of not being believed as the "innocent" victim. All of these contribute to an ongoing conspiracy of silence on the part of the child.

Documentation of the psychological and sociological damage resulting from abusive child rearing patterns has been increasing. These, in turn, may lead to intergenerational patterns of abnormal parenting and increased numbers of violent crimes perpetrated by those with histories of child abuse. Violence as the norm is an expectation passed on from victims to the next generation (Silver, 1969; Gelles, 1972).

Other findings suggest that parents most likely to injure a small child are those who themselves were severely punished as children (Kempe and Helfer, 1972).

Three factors intrinsic to child abuse have been identified by the National Center for Child Abuse and Neglect (U.S. Department of Health and Human Services, 1982):

1. A capacity for abuse exists within the parent.
2. One child is perceived as special in some manner by the parents.
3. One or more crisis events occur before the abusive act is committed.

It is of great importance to recognize that what may appear as intentional abuse by an observer may be perceived by the victim merely as a normal way of life. Perhaps the only attention that some children can obtain from a parent or other significant person in their lives is abusive. To a child, love may be inextricably linked with violence. Unfortunately, those with whom they are closest also hold the power to punish, either physically or psychologically (Bandura, 1973).

Several theories have been advanced to help explain why some parents abuse their children. Individually, none provides a comprehensive explanation for child abuse, yet each has contributed significantly to the overall base of information needed to help explain this multidimensional problem. It is becoming increasingly evident that there is a broad scope of causal factors, none of which operates in isolation. Each theoretical model proposes causal relationships to common problem areas. Collectively, this rapidly expanding base of knowledge supports the need for holistic approach to intervention.

Several efforts have been made to categorize the personality traits and characteristics of child abusers in an effort to help explain their behaviors. A major problem has been that, for the most part, data for these studies have been empirical and drawn from clinical practice with identified child abusers. As such, they fail to help explain why other persons with similar personality characteristics and traits and under similar circumstances do not abuse their children.

Personality or character traits that have been suggested as likely to lead to abusive behavior by parents include emotional immaturity, inability to cope with stress, chronic suspicion and hostility, and poor impulse control. Any of these could precipitate rage reactions in the parent when confronted with frustration or undue stress (De Francis, 1963; Pollock and Steele, 1972). When parents with a requisite psychological profile come into confrontation with the demands of a child, an inner-directed rage reaction may be precipitated. As anger and frustration build, such parents will suddenly erupt, striking out physically and/or psychologically at the most vulnerable person within their environment, the child (Halper, 1979; Walker-Hooper, 1981).

It is not uncommon to find the family "scapegoat" as the recipient of such parental acting out behavior. *Scapegoating* is an excellent example of psychological abuse. In order to survive as a unit, some families will allocate the role of "scapegoat" to one member. Most frequently the most vulnerable person is a child because a child is dependent and unable to retaliate against the parent's power (Vogel and Bell, 1960, 1967).

Based on the mechanisms of projection and displacement, scapegoating is often used to divert conflicts between parents. Undesirable traits or feelings are displaced or projected from the parent to the child when tensions become unbearable and parents lack the ability to openly discuss their reactions to stressful situations.

If a child is used to maintain stable relationships between parents, that child becomes the target for blame and is scapegoated for any threats to marital stability. The scapegoat is usually seen as someone who is different or disappointing in some way (Friedrich and Boriskin, 1976).

The abusive-dynamic model constructed by Kempe and others (Kempe and Helfer, 1972; Pollock and Steele, 1972) is based on the presence and interaction of multiple dynamics. Kempe postulates that there are seven dynamics that interact and affect the parent's perception of the child: mothering, imprint, isolation, self-esteem, role reversal, spouse support, perception of the child, and crisis events.

Psychoanalytic theory stresses the vital importance of emotional bonding between the mother figure and the infant during the oral stage of the child's psychosocial development. This provides the child with a healthy base for a future capacity to trust and enter into positive relationships with others.

Mothering imprint is the capacity to nurture and is learned only through one's own childhood experiences. Parents whose needs were not met in a loving, nurturing manner in their infancy tend to lack the capacity for providing nurturance in the care of their children. Overwhelmed by their own unmet dependency needs, they misperceive the dependency needs of their children. Lacking childhood memories of dependency gratification, they are unable to sense their child's needs or to respond empathetically. Rather than feeling sympathy and concern when a helpless infant or child continues to fuss and cry despite their caring efforts, the parents perceive the behavior as criticism. Feelings of failure and powerlessness arise, leading to lowered self-esteem and increased frustration and anger. Unable to redirect these feelings constructively, the parents project blame for the feelings of discomfort toward the cause—the "bad child."

Sometimes an abused child may be seen as special or unique by a parent. This uniqueness may be real, such as a physical or emotional problem. It may also be imagined, or the child is perceived as quite similar to someone disliked or feared in the parent's past memories. In either case, when such a child behaves undesirably or does not live up to the parent's needs and expectations, he creates a negative reflection on parental abilities and cause the threat of loss of self-esteem or self-control to the parent. This child becomes the "bad child," the one who needs to be corrected, to be "straightened out."

Thus disciplinary actions taken by the parents are perceived as positive and corrective rather than abusive behavior. Parents who were raised by similarly abusing parents may see nothing abnormal in their abusive behaviors.

A common victim response to such abuse is to feel at fault and to feel that trying harder to be a "good child" in the future will stop further abusive episodes. This illogical response is supported by the abuser and further blame is projected onto the victim. This vicious cycle continues until broken by circumstances that may be drastic enough to require medical-legal intervention. Examples of such could be the death of a child or injuries requiring professional care, sudden overt socially deviant behavior by the child, or a child runaway.

Role reversal is another dynamic. In this situation the parent attributes adult powers to the child and comes to depend upon the child for emotional sustenance and gratification of the parent's dependency needs. Such persons are seldom able to engage in any meaningful adult relationships or to intuit the needs of others. When this parent is confronted with the need to provide nurturance to another, and is unable to meet his own emotional needs, conflict arises.

Other studies have suggested that abuse may occur when a child is perceived by one parent as winning in a competition for love and caring from the other parent. In this concept the parents are perceived as having developed a strong symbiotic relationship based on caring and love with the advent of a child being a threat to continuation of that relationship. Abuse is for the primary purpose of physically or psychologically eliminating the competition (Justice and Justice, 1976).

Social isolation has been identified as a contributing factor in all theoretical models of child abuse. Persons with low self-esteem and mistrust of others are unable to develop positive interpersonal relationships and to request, accept, or use help from others.

Isolation may also be a learned behavior, one which parents actively teach their children by socializing them to distance themselves from experiences that might promote their learning how to establish positive social relationships.

It may also be due to environmental factors such as socioeconomic deprivation, living in an isolated area, moving into a new neighborhood, or a combination of any such related factors.

Drake (1982) suggests that persons who abuse have a strong tendency to be suspicious of others, most likely because of fear of exposure. Quite frequently such persons will make a great effort to socially isolate their families and to enforce maintenance of a minimum social network. Their goal is to present the appearance of a "normally" functioning family to their community, thereby reducing chances for disclosure and outside intervention.

Whichever the cause, social isolation has been found to reduce a person's access to situational supports and tangible resources. Without these, parents experience increased stress in child rearing and are unable to optimize their coping abilities to deal with resulting feelings of powerlessness, frustration, and anger in their parental roles.

Social explanations of child abuse and neglect stress the negative effects that the environment can have on the family. Exposure to the stresses of prolonged socioeconomic deprivation has been suggested as a major cause. According to Fil (1970, 1975), parents who are under such stress may be unable to maintain the parental mechanism of self-control and express their frustrations with their life-style through abuse of their children.

Others have suggested that a strong relationship may exist between socioeconomic stresses and *neglect,* rather than *abuse.* A major problem in analyzing these types of data is the lack of consensus concerning the definition of abuse versus neglect. Another identified problem is that lower income families are commonly overrepresented in studies of child abuse. This most likely reflects an uncontrolled bias in reporting systems. It is generally the lower income families or those already identified as child abusers, or neglectors, who are most frequently referred to the public services, the major sources for these data.

Case study   *Child abuse*

ASSESSMENT OF THE INDIVIDUAL AND THE PROBLEM

Alice, a 24-year-old divorced mother of 2 small children, was referred to the therapist by the hospital's emergency room physician. Earlier that evening she had brought her 1-year-old daughter Joan to the emergency room. The little girl was bleeding profusely from a deep laceration on her forehead. Alice explained that less than an hour before Joan had climbed over the rails of her crib and fallen, striking her head on the edge of the crib as she fell. Alice said that she hadn't heard Joan fall because she had fallen asleep on the living room couch. They had just moved into the house 2 days ago and she was exhausted from unpacking all day. Her 6-year-old son Mike had awakened her, calling loudly for her to help his sister. She had rushed to the bedroom and found Joan lying on the floor, crying loudly and bleeding heavily from the cut on her head. Mike was vainly trying to pick her up but had only succeeded in dropping her back on the floor. When Alice arrived he too began to cry loudly and cling to her.

Alice said that suddenly all she wanted to do was sit down and cry, too. "I just wanted this all to go away—I wanted all of these problems out of my life. I have never felt so angry and helpless."

She tried to stop the bleeding, but when she couldn't she decided to take Joan to the nearby hospital. She said that she quickly told Mike to put on his bathrobe and get out to the car, but "he began to argue with me—something about getting dressed first—and then started to run out of the room. I suddenly had all I could take! I blew up and slapped him so hard that he flew across the hallway and hit the wall. I was still so angry with him that I just picked up Joan and grabbed him by the arm and dragged him along out to the car. As soon as we all got into the car, though, I began to shake all over. I was horrified at what I'd done to Mike. Sure, I've spanked him before. I was so frightened and felt so alone right then. Right now I'm afraid to be alone with either of them again!"

After the doctor examined Joan and sutured the laceration on her head, he asked to have Mike brought into the room. An examination revealed evidence of new abrasions on the right side of his face and shoulder. Mike responded quietly to his questions about the injuries and said, "Mommy spanked me because I was a bad boy." He was no longer crying and clung tightly to his mother's hand as he spoke. There was no recent evidence of any other injuries.

In view of Alice's obvious emotional state, the doctor decided to admit the children to the hospital for overnight observation and further examination for any signs of past physical injuries indicative of abuse. He strongly advised Alice to meet with a therapist on the hospital's crisis team before going home that night. She agreed and a call was placed for the therapist to meet her at the hospital within an hour.

When he arrived, Alice was waiting, slumped down in a chair in his office. She appeared disheveled, tearful, and physically exhausted. Her tone of voice sounded very depressed, yet defensive, as she began to speak about the incident that evening.

She said that she and the children had just moved to this city a few days ago from a small town in the northern part of the state. She was to start her new job as a receptionist in a large law firm the next week. Divorced for almost a year, she had no family or friends nearby.

When asked about her former marriage she said that she had married when she was an 18-year-old college sophomore and that the marriage had lasted for 5 years. She added that her son Mike had been born only 5 months after the marriage. "That," she said rather cynically, "was definitely a case of 'marry in haste, repent at leisure.' We had 5 long years of trying to make a go of it. Having Joan last year was probably our last big mistake." She said that she became pregnant with Joan soon after Bob, her ex-husband, had finished college and started his law practice. It was a planned pregnancy because they both believed that things in their lives would take a turn for the better as soon as Bob began to build a practice. As it turned out, his practice was slow in building, and it began to seem to her that the need for her additional income would never end. Arguments between them increased until, she said, "One day, heaven help me, I found myself agreeing with Bob when he told me that he wanted a divorce." She added that she had been given full custody of the children.

Bob had remarried less than a year ago, the day after the divorce became final and, just 2 days before moving to this city, Alice learned that a son had been born to his new wife.

When asked about her childhood, she stated that she had been an only child and that her parents had divorced when she was 12 years old. She had remained with her mother, and her father, an attorney, soon moved to a different state and remarried about a year later. She never saw him again, but recalled him as a strict disciplinarian, someone to avoid in stressful situations because "he'd always blow up at me if I were around." He died in an auto accident when she was 15 years old. She recalled that her life with her mother after the divorce had been "rather dull and uneventful." Alice met Bob during her freshman year at college; they soon became engaged and planned to be married after Bob's graduation from law school in about 4 years. She had planned to obtain a law degree, finishing about a year after Bob.

Alice described Bob as being everything then that she thought she would ever want a man to be. She doubted that she could ever love anyone else as much and assumed that he had felt the same way about her.

After she returned to school in the fall of her second year, she discovered she was more than 4 months pregnant, too late for an abortion to be even considered. She recalled that neither she nor Bob was "exactly thrilled by this news" since neither had income to support a child. They were even more concerned about their parents' reaction to the news. At the time, the only solution that seemed feasible to both of them was to get married immediately, and then tell their parents that they had been secretly married the past spring.

As expected, neither of their families was pleased to hear about the "secret marriage" and the impending birth of a grandchild. Their general attitude was that Alice and Bob were still too young and in no financial position to support a family and continue in college. Neither set of parents was financially able to help them any more than they were at present. After much discussion, Bob finally gave in to Alice's decision that she would drop out of school and find a job to help support them both until Bob graduated. Then she would return to school and complete requirements for her degree.

She quickly obtained a part-time job as a receptionist at a law firm and worked for the few months left before Mike was born. After his birth she was asked to return full-time and had remained until just before her recent move to this city. Her new job here was similar and had been obtained through contacts made by her former employers.

As the therapist listened to Alice describe her relationships with her former husband and their children, he noted that a pattern of scapegoating behavior by the parents seemed to evolve whenever she described Mike's role in the family. She frequently described Mike as a child who had "created problems for them from the day he was born."

As she recalled, she and Bob began to have their first "real" arguments about the need to place Mike in a day nursery when she returned to work. Whenever she expressed concern about leaving Mike with "strangers," Bob would get very defensive and angry with her. She remembered him once saying, "It wasn't my idea alone to get married and start raising a family so soon. You're the one who got pregnant! If you'd been careful, you could have been going to school right now, too. That baby's causing problems, too, not just me!"

She said that Mike never was a "cuddly" baby, often bullied the other children at nursery school, and continued to create problems for her and Bob as he grew older.

Their arguments increasingly seemed to center around Mike as he grew older. Bob constantly criticized Alice's decisions about Mike's care, yet never offered any suggestions of his own.

When asked how she and Bob handled this, she responded that Bob always refused to get involved in any disciplinary problems; he always left that to her. She had never seen anything wrong with either spanking Mike or sending him to his room for a while. She added that spankings from her mother and father had never hurt her when she was young so, "whenever Mike deserved one, he got one, too."

She described Joan as being just the opposite of Mike, a child who was warm, loving, and very cooperative. With a sharp laugh she added, "But Mike—heaven help me because he seems to be getting more like his father every day. He's always demanding attention and wanting to have his way about everything."

The therapist then asked her why she had decided to leave her old job and move away from her friends to this city. She responded that since the divorce the town had just seemed too small for her to avoid meetings with Bob and his new family.

After the divorce she had encouraged Bob to keep in close contact with their children and, through them, with her. This continued even after his remarriage. She frequently found herself calling him for advice. In fact, she was surprised to find herself depending on him for advice much more than before their divorce.

Earlier this year she heard that Bob's new wife was pregnant. She said that her immediate reaction was concern for the children, wondering if Bob would continue to visit with them as much after his new child was born, or if he would focus all of his attention on his new family and rarely visit them anymore. The more she thought about this, the more she felt an urgent need to get away from the whole situation before it even happened. As she recalled, "I suddenly felt that I couldn't stand even being in the same town with him when the new baby arrived."

She showed signs of increasing tension and anxiety as she discussed this with the therapist. Suddenly she began to pound her fists on the arms of the chair and sob loudly. "That woman! She'll get to live the sort of life with Bob that I'd always dreamed of. But me, I'm going to have to work the rest of my life and send my children off to strangers because of it. I'll never be able to get back to college and it's just not fair! I have no one anymore to help me. I'm all alone and it's Bob's fault. I hate him! I hate him! Why did he leave me to handle all of these problems alone?"

PLANNING OF THERAPEUTIC INTERVENTION

The therapist felt that Alice had never fully accepted the divorce as final nor dealt with her unrecognized feelings toward Bob. This was evidenced by her continued efforts to draw him back home through repeated requests for his advice in caring for the children and by encouraging his frequent contacts with her, through the children. She was in crisis, precipitated by the news of the early birth of Bob's son and the failure of her usual method of coping with her feelings toward Bob (flight from the situation). This was compounded by the stresses of moving to a new job in a new city far from her usual situational supports. She felt isolated and trapped in a situation not entirely of her own making.

Joan's sudden, unexpected injury was for Alice "the last straw." It served as a catalyst for the eruption of a rage reaction to her overwhelming feelings of frustration and anger about her current life situation. Her comment to the therapist that Mike "was getting more like his father every day" strongly suggested that her assault upon Mike was, in fact, displacement of her feelings of rage toward Bob.

The goals of intervention were to encourage Alice to explore and ventilate her unrecognized feelings about Bob and the divorce, to help her perceive the birth of Bob's new son realistically in relation to her own and her children's future, to provide her with an intellectual understanding of her psychological abuse of Mike caused by her displacement of her anger toward Bob on Mike; and to provide her situational support as she learned new coping skills to deal with her new roles and responsibilities as a single parent.

INTERVENTION

Before the end of the first session the therapist was notified that a more complete examination of Mike revealed two healed fractured ribs and a healed fracture, with no displacement, of his right shoulder. The x-ray technician told the physician that the injuries apparently had occurred at different times within the past 3 years. Alice was informed that the children would have to stay at the hospital for a few days. Alice turned pale and began to cry. She asked the therapist, "Why? They are going to be all right, aren't they?" The therapist informed her of Mike's old injuries and asked if she knew how he had received them. She got up and began to pace the floor saying, "You don't know how difficult it is to control Mike—and Bob was never there!" The therapist asked Alice if she had beaten Mike. She looked at him and replied softly, "Yes. "I didn't mean to—honest—I just got so frustrated with him." It was decided that an immediate priority for her as well as for the children would be to provide her with situational support in her home as soon as possible. The purpose was to ensure protection of the children against any possible further physical abuse and to provide Alice with emotional support until she was better able to cope with the stresses of developing new social networks and adjusting to her new environment. She was given the telephone number and name of a woman who held weekly "self-help" support groups for parents who abuse their children. She was strongly encouraged to call as soon as she returned home, and she stated that she would.

The therapist explored with Alice the possibility of her having a friend or relative visit for a few weeks. Alice strongly agreed with this idea, admitting that she was still fearful of being alone with the children because, "I might blow up again if they made me angry. I'm just not sure how much more I can handle right now."

She decided to telephone her mother, adding in a very depressed tone of voice: "It's for sure there is no point in calling Bob. He'll be much too busy with his new family to help me now." She called her mother from the therapist's office, briefly explained her need for help, and asked her to come for a few weeks. Her mother agreed immediately and promised to be there the next afternoon. Alice's comment before leaving for home was, "You know, suddenly I don't feel quite so alone. Maybe, when I get home, after I call that lady, I can just fall into bed and get some sleep for a change."

When Alice returned for her second session a week later she appeared much more relaxed and less depressed. She said her mother had arrived just as the children came home from the hospital. "Never in my life have I been so glad to see my mother! She has been very helpful, and I never expected her to be so understanding." She had also attended one of the "self-help" groups.

Alice was particularly surprised by her mother's empathy when they discussed Alice's many problems since the divorce. Until then she hadn't realized that her mother, too, had many of the same feelings and problems after she and Alice's father had divorced. She added that the children really enjoyed having their grandmother around and "have been behaving just like angels—I can't believe that Mike has quit bugging me all of the time."

During this session and the next two, through direct questioning and reflection, Alice began to recognize her present crisis as a reflection of her past unrealistic perception of her divorce and Bob's subsequent remarriage.

Throughout her marriage she had always seen herself as being expected to assume the role of a strong, independent decisionmaker so Bob could be free of family problems to devote his full attention to his law studies. She recalled that he had often commented to her and to their friends that his law degree should really have both their names on it, "I couldn't have made it through college if she hadn't taken on most of the family responsibilities and left me free to study."

When asked if she had ever discussed these feelings with Bob, she said that she had tried to at first, but he would get so angry with her and "shout and storm out of the house" that she soon learned that it was easier for her not to argue back. When asked if that made things go any better between them, she said, "probably it didn't, but at least it did help keep the peace. There were times, though, that I wanted to just scream at him and throw things. Instead, I would take it out on Mike. I'd usually get angry with Mike for some dumb thing or other."

With continued direct questioning and reflection Alice gradually began to recognize how, unable to directly confront Bob with her feelings of frustration and anger, she had made Mike a scapegoat for her unhappiness. She had perceived Mike as the cause of arguments with Bob and, therefore, it was Mike who she felt deserved to be punished. She seemed surprised with the realization that his behavior problems with the other children possibly were his reaction to being scapegoated and abused at home. Upon further reflection, she expressed concern for its effect on his future relationships with her as well as with others. At the therapist's suggestion, she agreed to consider seeking a psychological evaluation and, if necessary, counseling for Mike.

She recalled that the year after Bob's graduation had been an unusually happy one for them. They had felt so optimistic about their future that they decided that it would be a good time to have another child.

As things turned out, however, Bob's practice didn't do as well as anticipated and Alice had to continue to work throughout her pregnancy. By the time Joan was born their marriage had greatly deteriorated. They no longer seemed able to communicate anything but their anger and frustration toward each other. Bob began to spend most of his time away from home and, when he finally suggested that they divorce, it seemed the only solution left for their problems.

When questioned directly, Alice admitted to the therapist how much she now regretted the divorce. She added that she always believed that Bob felt the same way, too. It was apparent to the therapist that Alice had still held hopes that Bob would return to her some day, despite his remarriage. His frequent visits with the children, even after his remarriage, had served to reinforce this belief in her mind. It was only when she heard that his new wife was pregnant that she began to experience some doubts and anxiety.

During the third session, through direct confrontation and reflection on her feelings about this news, she suddenly exclaimed, "Betrayed! That's how I felt when I heard the news. I felt like a betrayed wife, angry that he had done such a thing to me and our children—all of a sudden it came to me that, now, he couldn't just pack up and come back to us, even if he wanted to. Someway, I felt, I just had to get away. I just didn't want to be there to see him with a new family. If I stayed, I was sure that my life could never be peaceful again." As soon as she made that last comment, she gave a surprised laugh and said, "Did you hear what I just said? I was acting just like I did during our marriage. I was trying to keep peace by getting out of the situation—by taking a walk, or something like that. Well, I certainly took a walk, didn't I? All the way down to this city!"

She now realized that her choice of flight as a means of coping had indeed proved ineffective since Bob's new son was born two days before she moved. At that time she had regarded her overwhelming feelings of tension and anxiety as normal for anyone moving away from familiar friends and places. She avoided any discussion of her feelings with anyone, afraid that she might have to discuss how she felt about Bob's new baby. She behaved as though she was much too busy with packing and moving arrangements to visit with friends.

After the move she found herself isolated from any situational supports. She avoided telephoning Bob or friends, again using the excuse that she was too busy.

As her tension and anxiety increased, she soon felt too physically and emotionally exhausted to do little more than feed the children their meals and try to keep them from interfering with the unpacking.

After a deep pause, she said, "You know, when I look back, I must have been like a time-bomb waiting for the fuse to be lighted. I realize now that this wasn't the first time I'd ever felt that way. Perhaps it was easier, then, to just take a walk and get away for a while. That way it was easy to avoid dealing with the real cause of my anger—Bob. It was always much easier to talk *at* Bob through Mike's problems than *to* Bob about our problems!''

ANTICIPATORY PLANNING

Providing immediate situational support while encouraging Alice to identify and ventilate her unrecognized feelings about Bob had assisted her in viewing the recent events in her life more realistically.

By the fourth week Alice had made a good adjustment to her new job and was enjoying it very much. She had made several new friends and said that she was really enjoying time spent with her children at home. She said that she had even called Bob and congratulated him on the birth of his new son. An excellent day nursery had been found for Joan, and she had also located an after-school play group for Mike where he could be supervised until she got home from work in the evening.

As suggested by the therapist, she and Mike had visited the guidance counselor at Mike's new school and planned to meet with him regularly until Mike adjusted to the many new changes in his life. Even more important, and on her own, she had decided to attend meetings for divorced single parents, which were held regularly at a nearby YMCA, as well as the "self-help" group.

Reflecting back on her marriage in the final session, Alice summed it up by saying, "Maybe we'd have never married if I hadn't become pregnant. But that was never Mike's fault, and I never should have blamed him when things went wrong. It's Bob and I who are to blame. I'll never know if things might have been different if we had been able to wait longer, but I guess I always will believe that I gave up much more of my life than Bob did to keep it going as well as it did. My anger is with Bob, though. It's not with Mike. I realize now why I felt so angry and frustrated when we divorced. All that I could see was Bob being completely free to start a new life all over again. He never seemed to show any regrets about leaving me and the kids behind. I guess I'd hoped that he would feel guilty, or something, and come back to us.''

After a long pause she added, "Now I know that it wasn't Bob's new baby that upset me so much. It was because, until the very last minute, I'd prayed that Bob would come and beg me not to move away—and he never did—and that hurt the greatest.''

Most importantly, Alice was able to obtain an intellectual understanding of the relationship between her pent-up feelings and her displaced rage reaction toward Mike. She told the therapist that, if nothing else, she would always remember those moments and was quite positive that it would never happen again, "even if I have to stand out in the street and scream until I feel better!''

Before termination Alice and the therapist reviewed and assessed the adjustments that she had made and the insights that she had gained into her behavior.

CASE STUDY: ALICE

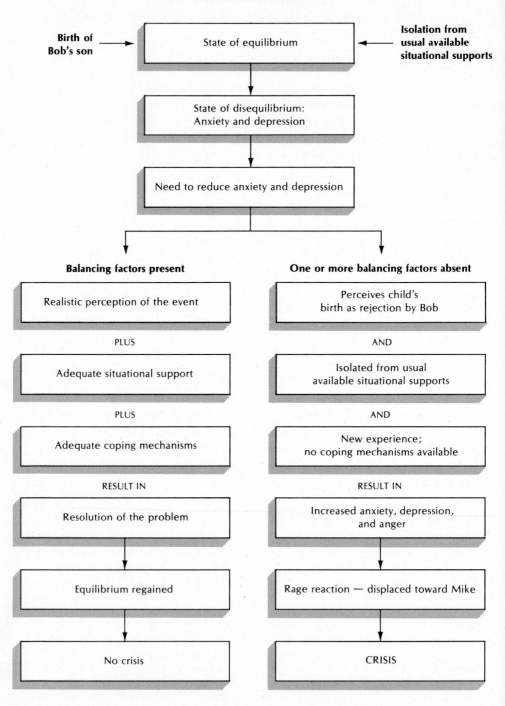

FIGURE 4

Alice was very optimistic about the future, both for herself and for the children. She was assured that she could always contact the therapist if she ever began to feel overwhelmed by problems again.

SUMMATION OF PARADIGM

Alice's crisis was precipitated by the failure of her usual coping method, flight, to deal with her feelings toward Bob over the birth of his new son. This was compounded by the loss of her usual available situational supports because of her move to another city. Overwhelmed by feelings of isolation, frustration, and anger, her perceptions of the event were distorted. As feelings of tension and anxiety increased to intolerable limits, Joan's injury became the "last straw" in a series of stressful events. Alice's feelings erupted into a rage reaction, which was displaced upon Mike. As the family scapegoat in her past relationship with Bob, he was most vulnerable to become the focus of all her negative feelings toward Bob.

A realistic perception of the event developed as Alice was assisted in identifying and ventilating her unrecognized feelings about Bob and her current life situation. She was able to obtain an intellectual understanding of the effects of her past scapegoating of Mike and his vulnerability to becoming the focus of any future rage reactions. The importance of learning alternative, adaptive methods for dealing with stress was emphasized to her.

Status and role change—theoretical concepts

Throughout life a person is constantly in the process of joining and leaving social groups related to family, occupation, recreation, education, church, and so forth. *Status* within each of these groups is determined by the relative rights and duties that society assigns to the position. *Role* is determined by the expectations of society that a person will carry out the duties of his position. If the member's position is changed within the group, his status and role will also change (Linton, 1956).

Allport (1961) cites four interrelated meanings of the term *role*. The first, *role expectation,* is what society expects of the individual. *Role conception* means *how* the individual perceives the effect of the role on his self-concept. He defines the role according to his perception and his needs, which are influenced by life goals, basic values, and congruency with other roles he is expected to perform. *Role acceptance,* like role conception, is a highly subjective matter. Not all roles are willingly accepted, nor are they willingly altered. The political process is one example of the kind of pressure that society can exert to force a role change. Reciprocal role changes will occur for all dependent on the winner's (and loser's) new status.

Role performance depends on role expectation, conception, and acceptance. The performance of the role will meet the expectations of society only to the degree that there has been mutual communication and understanding throughout the process.

The greater the disagreement in any area of understanding, the greater the possibility of failure in the performance.

A person tends to perceive a role from her view of how it relates to her self-concept. The "self" might be defined as the image that a person builds of herself through interpretation of what she thinks others are judging her to be. It is also derived from the reflected values that others place on her and the values that she places on herself in societal roles. As new evaluations are perceived, she is obliged to reconcile these new concepts with preexisting ones. Increasing conflictual appraisals of the self result in increased tension and anxiety, leading to a state of disequilibrium.

A person tries to avoid accepting a role that might threaten the security of the self-concept. Various defensive mechanisms are used to escape conflict and to ensure the integrity of self. Danger occurs when an unacceptable change in role is forced by society and cannot be avoided. For example, in the sudden death of a husband, the existing role of wife ceases to exist; the position is gone and its status with it. Without a husband there is no wife role. Similar loss situations may occur in occupations and other groups; a business closes or a position is abolished, so that the need for certain roles no longer exists.

The individual's feelings of loss are in accordance with the value that she places on the role. Effects of the loss are viewed in relation to the self-image, and this involves consideration of the negative factors that might cause conflicting appraisals from others. The greater the conflict between self-concept and expectations as a result of role change, the more painful is the decision-making experience.

Changes in roles related to loss of status are particularly critical because they represent a direct threat to self-esteem and may encourage the development of a negative self-concept. If defensive coping mechanisms (such as projection or rationalization) prove ineffective in protecting the integrity of the self, anxiety and tension will rise, and the balance of equilibrium will be disturbed.

The following case study illustrates a depressive reaction to a negative change in role status and loss of self-esteem. It was important in the initial interview to determine if Mr. E. was suicidal before intervention was initiated. Intervention focused on clarifying the problem area and assisting him to explore and ventilate unrecognized feelings. The therapist acted as situational support until other supports could be found in his environment.

Case study   *Status and role change*

ASSESSMENT OF THE INDIVIDUAL AND THE PROBLEM

Mr. E. requested help at a crisis center on the advice of his attorney. He was in a state of severe depression and anxiety. He described his symptoms as insomnia, inability to concentrate, and feelings of hopelessness and failure. He was a well-dressed man, 47 years old, who looked older than his stated age because of tense posture, a dull, depressed facial expression, and a rather flat, low tone of voice. Married for 22 years, he had three children, a daughter 13 years old and two sons 8 and 10 years old.

His symptoms had begun about 3 weeks previously when his company closed their West Coast branch and he lost his job. His symptoms had increased in intensity during the past 2 days to the point where he remained in his room, lying in bed, and not eating. He became frightened of his depressed thoughts and feared losing complete control of his actions.

During the initial session he stated to the therapist that he had never been without a job before. Immediately following graduation from college 22 years before, he had started his own advertising agency in New York City. It had expanded over the years, and he had incorporated, retaining controlling interest and the position of company president. On several occasions he had been approached by larger companies with merger proposals. About a year ago one of the "top three" advertising companies offered him the presidency of a new West Coast branch, which he could run with full autonomy, gaining a great increase in prestige and salary. All expenses were to be paid for his family's move to the West Coast.

Mr. E. saw this as a chance to "make it big"—an opportunity that might never come his way again. His wife and children, however, did not share his enthusiasm. Mrs. E. had always lived in New York City and objected to his giving up his business, where he was "really the boss." She liked the structured security of their life and did not want to leave it for one that she thought would be alien to her. The children sided with her, adding personal objections of their own. They had known only city life, had always gone to the same schools, and did not want to move "way out West." Despite resistance from his family, he made the decision to accept the job offer. His business friends admired his decision to take the chance and expressed full confidence in his ability to succeed. Selling out his shares in his own company to his partner, he moved West with his family within a month.

In keeping with his new economic status and the prestige of his job, he leased a large home in an exclusive residential area. He left most of the responsibility for settling his family to his wife and became immediately involved in the organization of his new business. He described her reaction to the change as being "everything negative that she told me it would be." The children disliked their schools, made few friends, and did not seem to adjust to the pace of their peer group activities. His wife could not find housekeeping help to her liking and consequently felt tied down with work in the home. She missed her friends and clubs, was unable to find shops to satisfy her, and was constantly making negative comparisons between their present life-style and their previous one. He felt that there had been a loss of communication between them. His present work was foreign to her, and he could not understand why she was having so many problems just because they had moved to a new location. Her attitude was one of constantly blaming everything that went wrong on his decision to move West and into a new job.

About a month ago the company suddenly lost four big accounts. Although none of these losses had been a result of his management, immediate retrenchment in nationwide operations was necessary to save the company as a whole. The decision was made to close the newest branch office—his branch. There was no similar position available in the remaining offices, and he was offered a lesser position and salary in the Midwest. He was given 2 months in which to close out his office and to make a decision.

Mrs. E.'s attitude toward these sudden events was a quick "I told you so." She blamed him for their being "stranded out here without friends and a job." He said that he was not a bit surprised by her reaction and had expected it. He had been able to "tune out" her constant complaints in the past months because he had been so occupied by his job, but now he was forced to join her in making plans for his family's future and in considering their tenuous economic status. He felt that he had been able to hold up pretty well under the dual pressures of closing out the business and planning for his family's future security. A week ago his wife had found a smaller home that would easily fit into their projected budget during the interim until he decided on a new job. He had felt a sense of relief that she had calmed down and was "working *with* me for a change."

Two days ago, however, their present landlord had sent an attorney, threatening a lawsuit if Mr. E. broke the lease on their present home. His wife became hysterical, blaming him for signing such a lease and calling him a self-centered failure who had ruined his family's lives. "Suddenly I felt as though the bottom had fallen out of my world. I felt frozen and couldn't think what to do next, where to go, and who to ask for help. My family, my employees, everyone was blaming me for this mess! Maybe it *was* all my fault."

Until now, Mr. E. had always experienced a series of successes in his business and home life. Minor setbacks were usually anticipated and overcome with little need for him to seek outside guidance from others. Now, for the first time, he felt helpless to cope with a stressful situation alone. The threat of having to fulfill the lease on a house he could no longer afford not only destroyed his plans for his family, but also broke off what little support he had been receiving from his wife. His feelings of guilt and hopelessness were reinforced by the reality of the threatened lawsuit and the loss of situational support.

PLANNING OF THERAPEUTIC INTERVENTION

Because of his total involvement in his new work, Mr. E. had withdrawn from his previous business and family supports. The sudden loss of his job threatened him with role change and loss of status for which he had no previous coping experiences. Perceiving himself as a self-made success in the past, he now perceived himself as a self-made failure, both in business and in his parent-husband roles.

When asked by the therapist about his successful coping methods in the past, he said that he had always had recourse to discussions with his business friends. He now felt ashamed to contact them, "to let them know I've failed." He had always felt free to discuss home problems with his wife, and they usually had resolved them together. Now he seemed no longer able to communicate at home with his wife. When questioned if he was planning to kill himself he said, "No, I could never take *that* way out. That never entered my mind." After determining that there was no threat of immediate suicide, the therapist initiated intervention.

One goal of intervention was to assist Mr. E. in exploring unrecognized feelings about his change in role and status. His loss of situational supports and lack of available coping mechanisms for dealing with the present stressful situation were recognized as areas in need of attention.

INTERVENTION

In the next 4 weeks, through direct questioning, he began to see the present crisis as a reflection of his past business and family roles. Mr. E. had perceived himself as being a strong, independent, "self-made" man in the past, feeling secure in his roles as "boss," husband, and father. He now felt shame at having to depend on others for help in these roles. Coping experiences and skills learned in the past were proving to be inadequate in dealing with the sudden, unexpected, novel changes in his social orbit. The loss of situational support from his wife had added to his already high level of tension and anxiety. This resulted in the failure of what coping skills he had been using with marginal success and in precipitation of the crisis.

After the fourth session Mr. E.'s depression and feelings of hopelessness had diminished. His perception of the total situation had become more realistic, and he realized that the closing of the branch office was not the result of any failure on his part. It was, in fact, the same decision that he thought he would have made had he been in charge of the overall operation. He further recognized what great importance he had placed on the possibility that this job would have been his "last chance to make it big." His available coping skills had not lessened in value but had, in fact, been increased by the experience of the situation.

By the fifth week Mr. E. had made significant changes in his situation, both in business and in his family life. He had been able to explore his attitudes about always feeling the need to be "the boss" and a sense of shame in being dependent on others for support in decision making. He was now able to perceive the stressful events realistically and to cope with his anxieties.

He met with his former landlord and resolved the impending lawsuit, breaking the lease with amicable agreement on both sides. His family had already decided to

CASE STUDY: MR. E

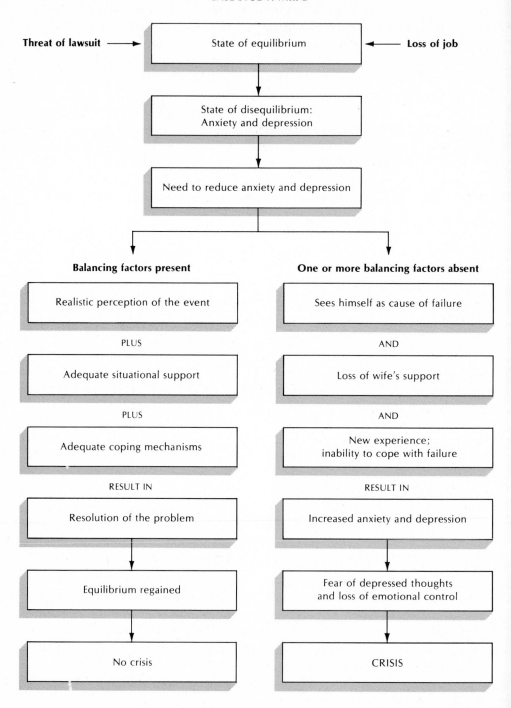

FIGURE 5

move into a smaller home, and his wife and children were actively involved with the planning. He had contacted business friends in the East and accepted one of several offers for a lesser position. He would return East alone, his family choosing to follow later when he had reestablished himself. His wife and children made this choice rather than repeat the sudden move into an unsettled situation as they had a year ago.

He felt pride that his friends had competed for his services rather than giving him the "I told you so" that he had been dreading.

ANTICIPATORY PLANNING

Before termination Mr. E. and the therapist reviewed the adjustments and the tremendous progress Mr. E. had made in such a short period of time. It was emphasized that it had taken a great deal of strength for him to resolve such an extremely ego-shattering experience. He was also complimented on his ability to recognize the factors he could change, those he would be unable to change, and his new status in life.

He viewed the experience as having been very disturbing at the time, but felt he had gained a great deal of insight from it. He believed that he would be able to cope more realistically if a similar situation occurred in the future. He was quite pleased with his ability to extricate himself from a seemingly impossible situation.

In discussing his plans for the future, he stated that he no longer believed he had lost his chance for future advancement. He was realistic about past happenings and the possibility that such a crisis could occur again. He was relieved about his family's rapid adjustment to the lesser status of his new position. They were happy to be returning to family and friends on the East Coast.

He expressed optimism about again rising to a high position in business, concluding with, "I wonder if I could ever really settle for less."

SUMMATION OF THE PARADIGM

Mr. E.'s crisis was precipitated by a sudden change in role status (loss of his job) and threatened economic, social, and personal losses. Assessment of the crisis situation determined that he was depressed but not suicidal. Because he was overwhelmed by a sense of failure in both business and family roles, his perceptions of the events were distorted. Having no previous experience with personal failure of this scope, he was unable to cope with his feelings of guilt and depression. His wife's actions reinforced his low self-esteem, and she withdrew as situational support.

Realistic perception of the event developed as the therapist assisted him in exploring and ventilating unrecognized feelings; he was able to gain insight into relationships between his symptoms of depression and the stressful events. Mrs. E. resumed her role of situational support as his new coping skills were successfully implemented in resolving the crisis.

Rape—theoretical concepts

The word *rape* arouses almost as much fear as the word *murder*. In a sense it kills both the rapist and his victim. The rapist dies emotionally because he can no longer express or feel tenderness or love, and his victim suffers severe emotional trauma.

Women have nightmares about being sexually assaulted; they anguish over what to do. They can either resist, hoping to fend off the rapist, or they can obey his commands, hoping he will leave without seriously injuring or killing them.

Rape is defined in numerous ways, usually including terms such as *forcible carnal knowledge* (McDonald, 1971:24), *unlawful carnal knowledge* (Amir, 1971:48), and *against the will* or *without the consent* (McDonald, 1971:75) of the victim. For our purposes rape is defined as forcible carnal knowledge of a woman without consent and against her will.

Rape, although an overtly sexual act, is properly considered an act of violence with sex utilized as the weapon (Burgess and Holmstrom, 1974). Viewing the victim of rape as a victim of violence might assist in a more objective and nonjudgmental approach to the victim. The victim of any other type of physical violence is never treated with the same type of emotional, superstitious approach that the victim of rape must endure.

The victim of rape is the victim of medical and cultural myths. The medical myth insists that a healthy adult woman cannot be forcibly raped with full penetration of the vagina unless she actively cooperates (Amir, 1971).

The medical myth does not seem to consider emotional reactions, such as fear and panic, or logic reactions, such as submissiveness, to ensure life. Neither does the use of weapons, fists, or threats by the offender seem to have a role in the medical myth. The medical myth must spring from the cultural myth that "whatever a man does to a woman she provokes" (McDonald, 1971:74). The low esteem that society in general holds for women is reflected in both the medical and the cultural myths.

Sociological studies reflect that the most typical female victim is between 15 and 24 years of age, of the same race as the offender, and of the lower socioeconomic group of the society. The initial contact for the rape or the rape itself occurs in the approximate neighborhood of the offender and the victim (Amir, 1971).

The victim's emotional reactions to rape have been classified into phases by McDonald and by Burgess and Holmstrom. McDonald (1971) classifies the emotional reactions of victims into phase I, acute reaction; phase II, outward adjustment; and phase III, integration and resolution. Burgess and Holmstrom (1974) classify the rape trauma syndrome into the acute phase: disorganization, and the long-term process: reorganization.

McDonald's "acute reaction" and Burgess and Holmstrom's "acute phase" are very similar. The victim is seen in a disorganized, emotionally active state, weeping, distraught, and unable to think clearly, or, conversely, as emotionally contained with only occasional signs of emotional pressure, such as inappropriate smiling and increased motor activity.

McDonald's "outward adjustment phase" is described as a period where the victim goes through a denial of the emotional impact of the rape. She goes back to work, restores her social life, rejects any attempts at assisting her, and in general attempts to carry on as if nothing had happened.

Burgess and Holmstrom's "long-term process: reorganization" seems to contain elements of McDonald's "phase II" and "phase III." The emphasis in both studies is on the necessity of emotional confrontation with the experience, changes in life space because of the trauma, the resultant dreams, and deterioration of sexual relationships.

The treatment of the rape victim is not well studied or documented. McDonald emphasizes traditional short-term psychotherapy, whereas Holmstrom and Burgess (1975) emphasize the crisis intervention model. Perhaps McDonald's finding of depression in the third phase and Burgess and Holmstrom's lack of emphasis on depression are the result of the different modes of treatment utilized. Crisis intervention seems to be an ideal model for use with rape victims. Rape is a sudden, overwhelming experience for which the usual coping mechanisms probably are inadequate. The victim needs an opportunity for emotional catharsis, reality testing for self-blame, active support on a short-term basis, and someone who will assist in identifying the situational supports available. Crisis intervention seems to be well defined to reach this group of people.

Crisis intervention is also increasingly available in the area where rape victims are initially brought to the attention of the health care system—the emergency room. Prompt referral and active intervention in the emergency room may well prevent deterioration of the victim's emotional status (Burgess, 1973).

The crisis precipitated by rape seems to be approachable by the generic type of crisis intervention. There are recognized patterns of behavior; a characteristic course of behavior results, and specific interventions seem to be effective with the majority of the victims. The exceptions to the generic approach are those victims with compounded reactions because of a history of physical, psychological, or social problems. In those instances the usual physician, therapist, or agency probably should handle the case.

To be a genuine victim in our society means that one must have people available who can accept and acknowledge that something extremely disruptive has occurred in one's life. In other words, the victim's claim to having been victimized needs to receive confirmation from others.

There are three basic types of rape. The first type is rape involving persons who know one another, for example, neighbors, separated husbands and wives, fathers and daughters, and prostitutes and dissatisfied clients. The second type of rape is gang rape, in which two or more men, usually young men, rape one woman. These encounters follow different patterns. It is the third type, the stranger-to-stranger rape, that women fear most, and it is this type of rape that follows an identifiable pattern.

First, a potential rapist looks for a woman who is vulnerable to attack. Rapists differ in defining who is vulnerable. Some look for victims who are handicapped or who cannot react appropriately or swiftly to the threat of rape. Such a man might prey on retarded girls, old women, sleeping women, or women who are intoxicated.

Other rapists look for environments that are easily entered and relatively safe. They make certain that the victim is alone and that they will not be interrupted. This type often commits his crime in the run-down sections of town, where many women live alone.

Rapists often select their victims long before they approach them, and they usually are very consistent in how they do it; they repeat the same pattern over and over again. Rapists seem to have a sixth sense for identifying women who live alone, and they are especially good at finding streets, laundromats, or theater rest rooms that are isolated but that draw unsuspecting victims.

Housing that is easy to enter and the isolation of the victim are two obvious factors that make women particularly vulnerable to rape, but women who are usually friendly and who like to help others are also courting danger. Teachers, nurses, volunteers, and other women who have learned to serve others, to be charitable, and to give of themselves are especially vulnerable to sexual exploitation.

A woman's first act of resistance should be to refuse to help—or be helped by—strange men. It is not wise to stop on a street to give a man a light or to explain street directions. It may be rude but much safer to state firmly while continuing to walk, "I don't have a match," or "I don't know." Do not smile and say, "I'm sorry but . . .," and so forth.

Women should refuse to let a stranger in their apartments or homes to make an emergency phone call or for any other reason. These may be ploys, and there are hundreds of clinical case histories and police reports to validate this method of entry for the purpose of rape.

After finding a vulnerable target, the rapist proceeds, in essence, to ask his victim, "Can you be intimidated?" If she can, he then threatens her life. For example, a rapist may approach a victim on the street and ask her for a light. If she provides it, he may ask her an intimate question. If she reacts submissively or fearfully, he knows he has intimidated her and that she likely will submit to his demands.

This testing phase is crucial for the rapist. If he guesses incorrectly about whether a woman can be intimidated, he will lose the opportunity to rape her, and if he is incorrect about the victim's situation, he may be caught, convicted, and sentenced to a penitentiary. The rapist tests his victim's responses to threats for intimidations such as: "Don't scream!" "Don't shout!" or "Take your clothes off!"

The safest stance for a woman alone either on the street or in her home is to be aloof and unfriendly. This is her first line of resistance to rape.

When a rapist attacks a woman without warning, that is, climbs into her bedroom while she is asleep, or pulls her into a dark alley, she must decide whether to use direct methods of resistance or to submit.

In the third, or "threat," stage of rape we find the rapist telling his victim what he wants from her and what he will do to her if she refuses to cooperate. Most important, he tells her what reward she will receive if she submits. Typically he says he will kill her if she does not cooperate and that he will not hurt her if she does. If the victim is terrified, immobilized, or hysterical, the rapist may reassure her. He will repeatedly promise her that nothing will happen to her if she does as he tells her. He may express concern for her health or future relationships with her husband or boyfriend.

The final stage of rape is the sexual transaction itself. Vaginal intercourse occurs in less than half of rape victims—anal or oral intercourse is common. In this stage we see the rapist's fantasy life in full blossom. Here he imprints his unique personality on the crime. Some rapists will create a false identity and describe a nonexistent person to the victim; others will reveal their split personalities by telling the victim, "It isn't really me doing this," or "I can't help it."

Most rapists fall into two categories. One type includes those who are usually victims of what analysts call ego splits. They are married, young, employed, and living a life that you could not describe as typical of a person who is mentally ill. However, their family life is disturbed; they cannot relate successfully to their wives or parents, and as youngsters they had problems with an older sister, cousin, or aunt.

After the crime these men will deny their behavior. Typically they will say, "I don't remember," "It wasn't me," or "I felt like I was watching a movie." If they do not harm their victims, these rapists often get a suspended sentence or are sent to reformatories where they can get work releases and return to the communities in a matter of months. The courts generally give them a second chance on the condition that they receive psychotherapy. Most rapists fall into the first category.

The other type of rapist is a predator. Often he is a man who goes into a place to rob it. In the course of the crime he enters a bedroom where he finds a lone woman sleeping. On the spur of the moment he decides to rape her. These men are out to exploit or manipulate others, and sometimes they do it through rape.

The rapist who requires his victim to pretend to respond sexually has often failed to please his wife or lover. On a deeper level he may be trying to maintain his shaky defenses about his own sexual inadequacy.

Most rapists have narcissistic and self-centered relationships with women. They have only a minute awareness of their partner's social needs or of the social situation itself.

A rapist also writes his diagnostic signature in the sign-off, or termination, stage of rape. A rapist who assumes the victim will report the crime terminates the rape by trying to confuse the woman. He will say, "Don't move until you count to 100." Then he will go into another room and wait to see if she moves. A minute later he will reenter the room, and if the victim has moved, he will berate her for failing to follow his directions. He may do this several times. Other offenders act guilty or apologetic when they leave. They plead for the victim not to call the police. Still others threaten future harm if she calls for help.

Unfortunately most rapists can neither admit nor express the fact that they are a menace to society. Even convicted rapists who are serving long prison terms deny their culpability; they tenaciously insist that women encourage and enjoy sexual assault. These men will tell you they are the greatest lovers in the world.

Case study   *Rape*

ASSESSMENT OF THE INDIVIDUAL AND THE PROBLEM

Ann, an attractive 26-year-old legal secretary, was brought to the crisis center by her employer. That morning on her way to work, she had been raped by a man. She returned to her apartment after being raped, showered, changed her clothes, and calmly went to work.

At approximately 11:30 AM she matter-of-factly announced to her employer that she had been raped and told him the details. He was shocked and horrified. He asked her to go to the hospital for treatment and to notify the police. She stated very unemotionally that she was "fine" and had only numerous superficial cuts on her breasts and abdomen and would continue working. By midafternoon she appeared to her employer to be in a state of shock and was acting disoriented and confused. He drove her to the crisis center where she was seen immediately as an emergency by a female therapist who had expertise in working with rape victims.

The therapist offered Ann a cup of coffee, and she accepted. While they were drinking their coffee, the therapist quietly asked Ann to tell her what had happened. Ann began to sob. The therapist handed her some tissues, put her arms around her shoulders, held her close, and told her that she understood how she was feeling. Gradually Ann calmed down and stopped crying. She then said, "I feel so filthy—I feel I should have resisted more—I am so confused." She was reassured that these feelings were normal and was asked to tell what happened.

Ann stated that she always got up early and took the bus to work since it was very convenient, and she arrived before anyone else was in the office. She liked to get her desk "in order" for the day and make the coffee so that she could serve coffee to the attorney she worked for when he arrived. She smiled slightly and said, "He isn't fit to talk to until he has finished his second cup of coffee in the morning . . . he commutes in from a suburb, and he has to battle the traffic for at least an hour or an hour and a half." The therapist smiled and asked her to continue. She took a deep breath and stated that this morning she had gotten up as usual and rode the bus to work. As she was walking from the bus stop to her office building, approximately three blocks, a man walked toward her. He was tall, attractive, and well dressed. When he approached her, he smiled and said, "Can you tell me where Fifth Street is?" She returned his smile and said, "You are going the wrong way. It's the next street up" (pointing in the direction she was walking). He said, "thank you" and, turning around, fell into step with her and started talking about the weather—"what a beautiful morning"—and other "small talk." They had walked approximately 100 yards when he suddenly pulled out a knife, shoved her against a car, put the knife to her throat, and said, "Don't scream or I'll kill you. Get in the car." Ann began to tremble and tears rolled down her cheeks. The therapist said, "How frightening! What did you do?" Ann said, "I was so shocked and terrified, I thought he *would* kill me. So when he opened the car door, I got in."

Ann continued to tell what had happened. He made her slide over to the driver's seat, keeping the knife firmly at her waist, ordered her to start the car, and told her where to drive (an isolated area near the river). He then made her get in the back seat and undress. He started caressing her and talking obscenities to her, telling her how he was going to make love to her "like no other man could." Ann said that she began to cry and plead with him, but it only seemed to make him angry. He began making small cuts on her breasts and abdomen and kept saying he would kill her if she did not "cooperate." Ann said that he acted "spaced out" and had a glazed look in his eyes, as if he was not really raping her *personally*—just somebody.

Ann stated that after he raped her, he seemed to "come to" and started to cry, saying, "I'm so sorry—I didn't mean to hurt you—please forgive me—I just can't help it—please don't tell anyone." Ann got dressed, and he helped her into the front seat and kept asking her if she was all right and generally expressed concern for her well-being. He asked if he could drive her someplace, and Ann asked him to drop her off approximately four blocks from her apartment, telling him she was going to a girl friend's to "clean up." He dropped her off and again begged her not to tell anyone and to please forgive him. Ann said that when she was certain he had driven away, she walked to her apartment in a daze. All she could think about was taking a shower to "get clean again" and to change her clothes completely to try to erase her feelings of degradation. She stated that she thought she should go to work "to keep her mind off it." It was only later in the afternoon as she "relived" the events in her mind that she began to feel terribly guilty over not "resisting" or "fighting back" when he first pulled the knife. She said (with a tone of great remorse), "I didn't even scream!"

PLANNING OF THERAPEUTIC INTERVENTION

The therapist felt that Ann should go to the hospital immediately for treatment of her numerous cuts and to determine the presence of spermatozoa in the vagina and then report the incident to the police. After this was done, she should return to the center to meet with the therapist and continue her mental catharsis. The therapist explained to Ann that someone from the rape hot line would go with her to the hospital and remain with her constantly at the hospital and while she gave her report to the police. She was assured that the therapist would contact the hospital to arrange that Ann be examined by a female physician and that she would be interrogated by a female police officer. Ann agreed to go, and a member of the rape team was called to be with her and then to return her to the center.

INTERVENTION

When Ann returned, she was pale and trembling but apparently in control of her emotions. Again she was offered coffee, which she accepted, and she and the therapist discussed how things "had gone" at the hospital and with the police interrogation. Ann stated it was definitely *not* pleasant but that it was not as bad as she had thought it would be and added, "Thank God I didn't take a douche!"

The therapist asked Ann if there was a friend or family member that she would like to contact and possibly have spend the night with her since she was still very frightened by her experience. Ann turned even paler and exclaimed, "Oh my God—Charles!" She was asked, "Who is Charles?" She replied, hesitantly, "My fiance." The therapist asked Ann if she could call Charles and tell him what happened. Ann began to cry and said, "I am so ashamed—he will probably hate me— he probably will never want to touch me again—what have I done!" She was comforted by the therapist and told that *she* had done nothing wrong. She continued to cry and berate herself. The therapist gave her a mild sedative and asked her to lie down and rest. Twenty minutes later Ann asked the therapist if she would call Charles and tell him what had happened, but she said that she did not want to see him until she knew how he felt about her being raped. The therapist agreed and asked for Charles's telephone number.

The call was placed to Charles, and a brief explanation was given by the therapist about Ann being raped and that she was physically unharmed but psychologically very traumatized. Charles responded with concern and anger and asked if he could see Ann. He was told to come to the center and to ask for the therapist.

Charles arrived and was extremely upset and angry. The therapist took him to her office and explained fully what had happened to Ann and what had been done for her. He started to cry and to curse, stating, "My God—poor Ann" and "I'll find that dirty bastard and kill him!" The therapist allowed him to ventilate his feelings of pity and anger, and he began to calm down. When he seemed calmer, he was asked, "Does this change your feelings for Ann?" He appeared startled and said, "No, I love her. We are getting married!" He was told that Ann was afraid he would not love her anymore, and so forth. He replied, "It wasn't her fault. Of course I still love her!"

It was explained that after being raped women usually felt "guilty," "unclean," and very fearful of intimacy with another man, even though they loved them very much. The therapist added that Ann needed his strength, love, and constant reassurance that nothing had changed between them. He listened and said, "I'll do anything I can to help her forget this."

The therapist asked if he sometimes stayed overnight at Ann's apartment, and he answered, "Yes, often." He was asked if he would spend the night with her (if she agreed) and hold her (if she would let him), touch her, reaffirm his love for her, and speak about their coming marriage but not attempt sexual intercourse unless she asked him; he agreed and asked to see Ann. The therapist asked for a few minutes alone with Ann first.

Ann was lying on the couch staring at the ceiling when the therapist entered. She turned her head and looked fearfully at the door. The therapist smiled, sat down by Ann, held her hand, and said, "I like your Charles. He is a fine young man—he will probably break down that door if I don't let him in to see you!" Ann said, "What did he say?" The therapist told her that he had stated he loved her very much and that he would do anything to help her forget, that it was not her fault, and that he would like to "kill the bastard who hurt you." Ann said, hesitantly, "Are you sure?" The therapist replied firmly, "Positive! Now comb your hair and put some makeup on, so I can let him in!" Ann smiled weakly and complied.

Charles entered the office, took Ann in his arms, and held her gently, stroking her hair and face, saying, "I'm so sorry, my love—let me take care of you—everything is going to be all right—I love you—you are the most precious thing in my life." Ann cried softly on his shoulder. The therapist said, "Why don't you two go home and get some rest, and I'll see you both next week." Ann and Charles agreed and left with their arms around each other and Ann's head on his shoulder.

(*Note:* The therapist had listened to Ann's account of the rape and modus operandi with increasing feelings of helplessness and anger because in the past 3 months she had worked with two other rape victims who had described the exact same details but with one major difference, the first victim had only one minute cut on her throat, which she received when he pushed her against the car; the second had several small superficial cuts on her breast; and now the third victim [Ann] had numerous cuts on her breast and abdomen. The rapist was obviously becoming increasingly more violent with each rape.)

ANTICIPATORY PLANNING

The next sessions were spent in collateral therapy with Ann and Charles. The focus was on ventilation of their feelings and helping Ann begin to express anger toward her rapist. By the end of six sessions they had resumed their normal sexual activities and had advanced their wedding date 3 months. Charles felt he was really living at Ann's apartment because he wanted to be with her as much as possible; therefore they agreed to get married sooner than they had planned.

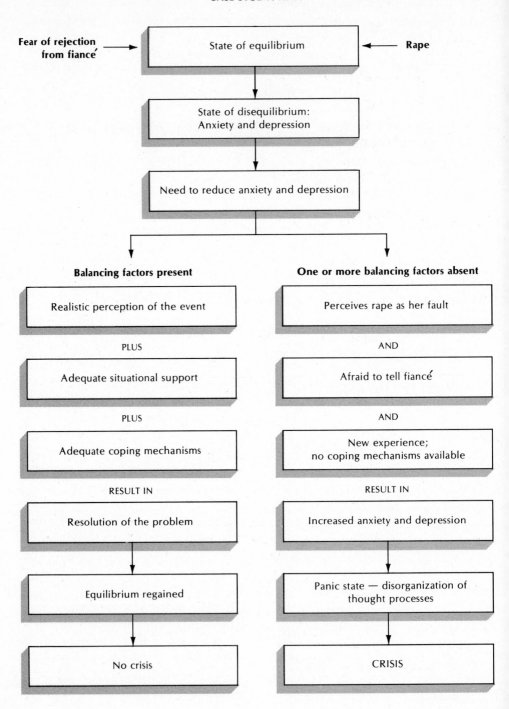

CASE STUDY: ANN

Fear of rejection from fiancé → State of equilibrium ← **Rape**

State of disequilibrium: Anxiety and depression

Need to reduce anxiety and depression

Balancing factors present | **One or more balancing factors absent**

Realistic perception of the event | Perceives rape as her fault

PLUS | AND

Adequate situational support | Afraid to tell fiancé

PLUS | AND

Adequate coping mechanisms | New experience; no coping mechanisms available

RESULT IN | RESULT IN

Resolution of the problem | Increased anxiety and depression

Equilibrium regained | Panic state — disorganization of thought processes

No crisis | CRISIS

FIGURE 6

SUMMATION OF THE PARADIGM

Since rape is so emotionally traumatic, Ann was treated as an emergency situation by the therapist. The sooner intervention begins with a rape victim, the less psychological damage will occur.

Most women are totally unprepared for rape; therefore, it is a new traumatic experience to cope with, and previous defense mechanisms are usually ineffective to resolve the crisis.

Ann greatly feared total rejection by her fiance (a very real and common occurrence). This is why the therapist saw both Ann and Charles in collateral sessions; thus both would have a chance to explore and ventilate their feelings together.

The event, rape, was perceived by Ann as being her fault because she did not resist immediately and did not scream. Again these feelings are common in women who have been raped. Usually everything occurs so rapidly, and the ever-present fear of being killed or seriously injured tends to immobilize the victim.

ADDENDUM

Four months later a patient was referred to the center because he was on probation for rape, and he became the same therapist's patient. When questioned about how and why, as he described his modus operandi, the therapist *knew* he was the one who had raped Ann and the two other victims. After the rapist discussed his feelings—guilt, shame, and helplessness in controlling his actions—the therapist asked about his background and family. This new patient, Phillip, described his childhood as one deprived of affection. His mother had left his father, and he was reared by an "old-maid aunt" who was very cold, undemonstrative, and—to him—uncaring and rigid.

When questioned about his present living circumstances, he stated that he was married (happily) and had three small children. When asked why he felt the need to rape, he stated, "I don't know." He began to cry and said, "Please help me—I can't help myself."

When the therapist asked if his wife knew that he was on probation for rape, he said, very hesitantly; "No, but I *know* she thinks something is wrong with me." The therapist told Phillip that she had worked with three of his victims, and she felt that he was becoming increasingly more violent, as evidenced by the increasing use of the knife and the sight of blood to stimulate him.

Phillip stared intently at the therapist and said with amazement in his voice, "My God, don't you hate me? I hate myself." The therapist was able to admit that her bias was toward his victims but that she felt he needed help because she was afraid he might kill his next victim. He admitted that he did not know whether he *would* or *would not* kill someone.

The therapist then asked him what his wife and children would feel if they found out he was a potential murderer. He shuddered and said, "Help me! I don't know what to do!" The therapist stated that he should tell his wife about being on probation and about the rapes, and then the therapist would do all she could to get him help. He agreed and called his wife and asked her to come to the center.

His wife arrived, and Phillip, with the therapist present, told her what he had done and the possibility of what he could do in the future. She began to cry and said, "I've *known* something was wrong, but I didn't know what." She turned to the therapist and asked, "What can we do?" The therapist was very candid and stated that Phillip should be at a well-known maximum security prison where he could receive consistent, intensive psychiatric therapy in order to protect the reputation of their family and to protect the community.

They agreed with this decision. The therapist then called the judge and told him the facts. He agreed that maximum security was needed and said he would send a car to transport Phillip to the facility.

It must be noted that *rarely* does a therapist work with rape victims and then with their offender. It was extremely difficult to remain "cool, calm, and collected" while Phillip related his modus operandi; however, he too was a "victim" and needed help, and help he did receive.

Physical illness—theoretical concepts

Diseases are known to have their places as well as their times. Primitive societies have been characterized by health problems related to recurrent famines, and urban societies, until recently, by epidemics of infectious disease. Modern industrial societies are characterized by a new set of diseases: obesity, arteriosclerosis, hypertension, diabetes, and widespread symptoms of anxiety. Arising from these are two of the three greatest disablers of our own place and time: coronary heart disease and stroke. In recent years increasing concern has focused investigation not only on the etiology and epidemiology of cardiac disease but on factors affecting the process of recovery.

The unexpected recognition that one has heart disease is usually a crisis event for an individual. The disease could also be a chronic condition, persisting throughout life and precipitating a series of crisis both for the patient and for his family.

The conceptualization of the recovery process in heart disease as a response to crisis provides strategic advantages in approaching the problem. It leads to focusing on the kinds of adaptive and maladaptive mechanisms that patients employ in coping with this illness, on the stages of recovery, and on the resources that patients use and require at each stage. Viewing response to coronary heart disease as a problem that can be approached through crisis intervention permits the utilization of concepts and formulations inherent in crisis theory.

In a discussion of the rehabilitation of patients with cardiac disease, a report by the World Health Organization in 1966 distinguished between phases of the recovery process in terms of time and coping tasks. The first phase is categorized as one in which the patient spends approximately 3 weeks in bed, with minimal physical activity. In the next phase the patient spends approximately 6 weeks at home with a variety of sedentary activities. In the third phase, which lasts from 3 to 6 months, the patient makes a gradual reentry into the occupational world.

Lee and Bryner (1961) conceptualize phases according to the kinds of care the physician must provide for the patient at each point of the process. They specify (1) evaluation of the patient and his environment, (2) management of the patient, and (3) reestablishment of the patient in his community.

In other formulations of recovery phases, emphasis is on the kinds of therapeutic or rehabilitative relationships that predominate at each point. Hellerstein and Goldstone (1954) describe the first, or acute, phase as one in which the relationship between the physician and patient is of the utmost importance. The convalescent phase then follows, with the relationship between the patient and family and friends becoming primary. During the recovery, or third, phase the employer or vocational counselor becomes the vital participant in the rehabilitation of the patient with cardiac disease.

Phases have also been viewed in terms of the emotional adaptation of the patient. Kubie (1955) suggests that the first phase is marked by initial shock and the second by appreciation of the full extent of the disability. In the third there is "recovery from the lure of hospital care," and in the fourth and final phase there is "a facing of independent, unsupported, competitive life."

Among the most obvious and critical determinants of the outcome of the recovery process are the severity of heart damage, the degree of impairment, and the physiological resources of the patient. While cardiac damage has much to do with setting limits on performance and affecting levels of adjustment, studies of physiological factors alone contribute only partially to understanding the recovery process. Research on the importance of the premorbid personality of the patient as a determinant of adjustment to illness suggests that this is a second important factor in the recovery process.

Other important factors bearing on the recovery process include the various psychological mechanisms that the patient uses in handling illness. If the recovery process is viewed as a response to a crisis situation, then the individual mechanisms used by patients appear particularly important in the resolution of the crisis. The significance of emotional response to disease has often been underlined in discussing the elements that determine recovery. McIver (1960) states, "The way in which a crisis is handled emotionally may significantly influence the eventual outcome of a case in terms of the extent of recovery and the degree of rehabilitation achieved." Reiser (1951) emphasizes that it is essential to deal with the anxieties associated with the diagnosis and symptoms of heart disease if the therapy of cardiac disease is to attain its optimal effect.

A common view held is that during the acute phase of any serious illness the patient's emotional state is characterized by fear, since the illness threatens his total integrity as well as his sense of personal adequacy and worth to others.

Compared with other serious illnesses, heart disease has several unique features. Associated as it is with sudden death, it is viewed by the patient and family as an immediate and severe threat to life. Hollender (1958) has written that even in the most stable patients the onset of heart disease is associated with an onslaught of anxiety. During the first days of illness the patient with heart disease must assume a passive role, and some believe that this tends to compound anxiety. Physical restriction usually increases feelings of helplessness, vulnerability, and depression. The patient is then handicapped in utilizing defense mechanisms that should ultimately help him to adjust to an altered status.

Although coping responses vary widely, there appears to be a core of relatively uniform responses of adjustment. For example, depression and regression have often been reported as the initial reaction to the illness. Some patients display aggression and hostility, placing the blame for the illness on external factors. Some deal with the threat to life by denial of the illness.

It has been suggested that certain coping responses are appropriate at one stage of recovery but are inappropriate at another. When patients at the same stage of recovery are compared, similar responses may function in different ways: constructively for some patients but hindering recovery for others. There is disagreement at present about the role denial plays in recovery. Some regard denial, which may lead to noncooperation with the physician, as a response of self-destruction. Others consider that denial arises from a belief in the integrity of the self and the invulnerability of the body. It is regarded as constructive and associated with the maintenance of health.

Since each patient will react as an individual in this life-threatening situation, it would be well to remember that the therapist will, in all probability, see a variety of coping responses being utilized. It is not the therapist's role to change the patient's pattern of coping but to understand that this reaction to illness is part of the patient's defense.

King (1962) has stated that ''Man's basis for action in health and disease is a composite of many things. One crucial variable is the way that he sees or perceives the situation . . . and all of the social ramifications that accompany it.'' These perceptions are conditioned by socialization in a sociocultural context. How the patient responds to the disease is influenced by what she has learned. The content of the learning is in turn determined by the norms and values of the society in which she lives. The meaning of the disease, attitude toward medical practitioners, willingness to comply with medical advice, and the patient's management of her life after a heart attack are all influenced by the attitudes and beliefs that she has learned.

Pertinent to the recovery process is the conceptualization of the "sick role," which Parsons (1951) describes as a social role, with its own culturally defined rights and obligations. While a person may be physiologically ill, she is not recognized as legitimately ill unless her illness fulfills the criteria or standards set by the society. Once defined as legitimately able to be in the "sick role," she is expected to meet certain expectations of others. The person is expected, for example, to make an effort toward becoming well and to seek help. In turn she has the right to expect certain kinds of behavior in others toward her, including a willingness to permit her to relinquish her normal social role responsibilities.

Willingness to accept the sick role may mean that a patient with heart disease is likely to follow the regimen of her physician and to care for herself in ways that will maximize her recovery. At the same time, reluctance to accept the sick role may also influence the recovery process favorably. Such a patient may be anxious to avoid being defined as sick. Like the willing patient, she too may follow the therapeutic regimen in order to shorten the period of incapacity. On the other hand, reluctance to view herself as sick may lead a patient to comply minimally with medical advice and to attempt full activity before she is physically able to do so.

In essence, social and cultural standards and expectations may have a strong influence on the kinds of action a patient with cardiac disease may take concerning her own health status.

Case study   *Physical illness*

Mr. Z., aged 43, was chairing a board meeting of his large, successful manufacturing corporation when he developed shortness of breath, dizziness, and a crushing, vice-like pain in his chest. An ambulance was called, and he was taken to the medical center. Subsequently he was admitted to the coronary care unit with a diagnosis of impending myocardial infarction.

Mr. Z. was married, with three children: Steve, aged 14; Sean, aged 12; and Liza, aged 8. He was president and the majority stockholder of a large manufacturing corporation. He had no previous history of cardiovascular problems, although his father had died at the age of 38 of a massive coronary occlusion. His oldest brother had died at the age of 42 from the same condition, and his other brother, still living, was a semiinvalid after suffering two heart attacks—one at the age of 44 and the other at the age of 47.

Mr. Z. was tall, slim, suntanned, and very athletic. He swam daily, jogged every morning for 30 minutes, played golf regularly, and was an avid sailor who participated in every yacht regatta, usually winning. He was very health conscious and had annual physical checkups, watched his diet, and quit smoking to avoid possible damage to his heart, determined to avoid dying young or becoming an invalid like his brother.

When he was admitted to the coronary care unit, he was conscious. Though in a great deal of pain, he seemed determined to control his own fate. While in the coronary care unit he was an exceedingly difficult patient, a trial to the nursing staff and his physician. He constantly watched and listened to everything going on around him and demanded complete explanations about any procedure, equipment, or medication he received. He would sleep in brief naps, and only when he was totally exhausted. Despite his obvious tension and anxiety, his condition stabilized. The damage to his heart was considered minimal, and his prognosis was good. As the pain diminished, he began asking when he could go home and when he could go back to work. He was impatient to be moved to a private room so that he could conduct some of his business by telephone.

Mr. Z. denied having any anxiety or concerns about his condition, although his behavior in the unit contradicted his denial. Recognizing that Mr. Z. was coping inappropriately with the stress of illness, his physician requested as consultant a therapist whose expertise was crisis intervention to work with Mr. Z. to help him through the crisis period.

The therapist agreed to work with Mr. Z. for 1 hour a week for 6 weeks. Their first session was scheduled the second day of his stay in the coronary care unit.

ASSESSMENT OF THE INDIVIDUAL AND THE PROBLEM

The therapist reviewed Mr. Z.'s chart and talked with his physician before the first session in order to gain an accurate assessment of Mr. Z.'s physical condition and to gain some knowledge of factors (socioeconomic status, marital status, family history, and so on) to assist in assessing his biopsychosocial needs.

In the first session the therapist observed Mr. Z.'s overt and covert signs of anxiety and depression and determined, through discussion with him, his perception of what hospitalization meant to him, his usual patterns of coping with stress, and available situational supports. Through direct questions and reflective verbal feedback she was able to elicit the reasons for his behavior and reactions to his illness and to his confinement in the coronary care unit.

Observing his suntanned, youthful appearance and the general physical condition of a very active and persistent athlete, the therapist questioned him about his life-style and patterns before his hospitalization. Mr. Z. was quite adamant about his "minor" condition and the possibility of curtailed activity. He stated that he was very aware of his family's tendency toward cardiac conditions, but added, "I have always taken excellent care of myself to avoid the possibility of becoming a cardiac cripple like my brother." Apparently he was not too concerned about the prospect of dying; in fact, he might prefer it to the overwhelming prospect of being a useless, dependent invalid.

He expressed concern about the length of time he might have to spend in the hospital. When questioned about his concern he stated: "I *have* to be in good shape by the second of December [approximately 3½ months]: I've entered the big yacht race, and I plan to win again!"

When he was asked how his wife and children were reacting to his illness and hospitalization, Mr. Z.'s facial expression and general body tension relaxed noticeably. He smiled and said, "My wife, Ann, is simply unbelievable; she takes everything in stride. She is always cool, calm, and collected. She even met with the board of directors and told them to delay any major decisions until I return—but that any minor decisions she could handle!

The therapist asked if she could meet his wife. Mr. Z. replied that his wife would be in to see him soon and suggested she stay and meet her.

After meeting with them briefly, the therapist asked Mrs. Z. to stop by her office before leaving.

Session with Mrs. Z. Mrs. Z. arrived at the office and sank gratefully into a chair, losing the bright, cheerful, and optimistic manner she had maintained while with her husband. Observing her concerned expression and slumped posture, the therapist inquired, "You are very concerned about your husband, aren't you?" Mrs. Z. readily admitted that she was concerned but did not want her husband to know. When asked what specifically concerned her, she replied: "Jim's inability to accept any type of forced inactivity and his refusal to accept the possibility that he might have to change his hectic life-style. He can't *bear* the thought of being ill or being dependent upon anyone or anything!"

The therapist explained that it is difficult for many patients to accept a passive, dependent role while ill and that it takes time for them to adjust to a changed life-style. She then explained to Mrs. Z. that the physician had arranged for Mr. Z. to have therapy sessions for the next 6 weeks to help him through his crisis. Mrs. Z. seemed relieved that someone else recognized the problems confronting her husband and would help him as he worked through his feelings about his illness and unwanted, though inevitable, change in life-style.

The therapist suggested that Mrs. Z. might also need some support, as she too had to adjust to Mr. Z.'s illness. They agreed to meet for an hour each week so they could work together toward a resolution of the crisis. A convenient time was arranged each week when Mrs. Z. came to visit her husband.

PLANNING OF THERAPEUTIC INTERVENTION

Mr. Z.'s denial of the possibility that he might die like his father and oldest brother or that he might become an invalid, "useless and dependent," like his other brother was considered of prime importance. It was felt that the first goal of intervention was to assist Mr. Z. to ventilate his feelings about his illness and hospitalization. A second goal was to assist him to perceive the event realistically. A third goal established was that of giving support to Mrs. Z. and assisting her in coping with the stress induced by her husband's hospitalization.

INTERVENTION

It was felt that Mr. Z.'s high anxiety level would interfere with his ability to express his feelings about his illness and his hospitalization. In an attempt to reduce his anxiety, the therapist made two recommendations to his physician, which were accepted. The first recommendation was that Mr. Z. be moved out of the coronary care unit to a private room as soon as possible. The environmental surroundings in the coronary care unit, with its overwhelming and complex equipment, strange sounds, and constant activities of the staff, apparently increased Mr. Z.'s anxiety. Because of the stressful situation, he was not getting sufficient rest. After his move to a private room later that afternoon, he began to relax noticeably, became much less demanding of the staff, and began sleeping and eating better.

The second recommendation was that he be permitted to use the telephone for 30 minutes three times a day. Thus he was able to conduct some of his business from his bed. This apparently made him feel less dependent, and the increased mental activity relieved some of his anxiety about becoming a "helpless" invalid.

In the next sessions Mr. Z. began to discuss—hesitantly at first, and then more freely—his feelings about his illness and his reaction to hospitalization. He discussed his father's sudden death when he was in his teens and how lost he would have felt if his older brother had not stepped in and taken over. All three brothers were very close, and the death of the oldest one, while Mr. Z. was in college, reactivated the grievous loss he had felt for his father. He was just beginning to accept his oldest brother's death when, a year later, his other brother had a severe heart attack and was unable to continue in the family business. As Mr. Z. saw it, his brother was a "helpless" invalid. Mr. Z., the youngest son, then became the major stockholder and president of the corporation.

He stated that while he certainly didn't *want* to die, he was less afraid of dying than he was of becoming useless, helpless, and a burden to his family.

Through discussion and verbal feedback, it was possible to get Mr. Z. to view his illness and the changes it would make in his life in a realistic perspective. No, he was *not* an invalid. Yes, he *would* be able to work and live a normal life. No, he would not have to give up sailing, just have someone else do most of the crewing. Yes, he would be able to resume his activities but would continue them at a more leisurely pace: instead of scheduling 15 things to do in a day, schedule 7, and so forth. Gradually he became more accepting as he began to realize that the impending myocardial infarction was a warning he should heed and that with proper care and some diminishing of his usual hectic pace he could continue to live a productive and useful life.

The therapist continued to meet with Mrs. Z. to give her support and began anticipatory planning for her husband's convalescence at home. She discussed with her Mr. Z.'s strong need to feel independent and in control of all situations and encouraged her to continue to let her husband make decisions for the family. She assured Mrs. Z. that he would be able to continue a relatively normal life and that she did not need to protect and "coddle" him, something he would greatly resent! When asked how their children were reacting to their father's hospitalization, Mrs. Z. replied: "At first they were terribly concerned and silent; now they are beginning to ask, 'When is he coming home, and what can we do?' " It was obvious that Mr. Z. had strong situational support in his family!

Mr. Z.'s recovery progressed fairly smoothly, and he began to ambulate and take care of his basic needs. While more accepting of his need for some assistance, he still became upset and impatient if the staff intervened to assist him in routine care.

Mr. Z. was discharged after the fourth week, with instructions for his convalescence at home. The therapist continued to meet with Mr. and Mrs. Z. at their home during the fifth and sixth weeks to assist the family toward stabilization as Mr. Z. adjusted to his new regimen of reduced activity and to provide anticipatory planning for their future.

ANTICIPATORY PLANNING

By the end of the fifth week, with the strong support of his family and the therapist, Mr. Z. was able to view his illness and his feelings about curtailing some of his hectic activities in a more accepting and realistic manner. His family still consulted him for advice and opinions about family decisions. This made him feel he was still an active, participating member of the family.

He was able to conduct a large part of his business from his home by having board meetings there and by holding periodic telephone conversations to his office. His secretary came to his home 3 days a week to take dictation and to secure his signature when needed on documents. Thus he still remained in control of his business life, which contributed greatly to his self-esteem.

The children and Mrs. Z. were encouraged to continue in their usual daily activities so that Mr. Z. would not feel that his being at home was disrupting to their lives. It also helped Mrs. Z. to cope with her feelings and her desire to protect her husband from stress. Gradually she was able to realize that he was capable of coping with some stress and that he was not as fragile as she had believed him to be.

Before termination the therapist and Mr. Z. reviewed the adjustments he had made and the insights he had gained into his own behavior. He was able to intellectually understand his reasons for his denial and dependence/independence conflicts.

He was very optimistic about his future and felt that he could adjust to a re-

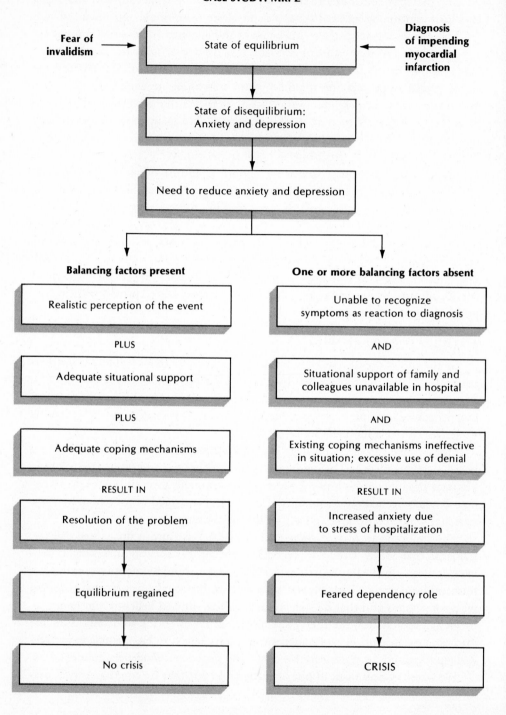

duced-activity schedule. He still, rather wistfully, was hoping his physician would approve his entering the yacht race.

He was realistic about his physical condition and the possibility that a coronary attack could occur again, stating, "At least now I've learned to relax and roll with the punches."

Mrs. Z. and the children felt they would be able to cope with the occasional bouts of frustration and temper flare-ups of Mr. Z. They were now aware of how difficult it was for him to make the many adjustments necessary to his new way of life.

SUMMATION OF THE PARADIGM

Mr. Z.'s fear of becoming a "cardiac cripple" like his brother distorted his perception of the event. He was unable to relax and be dependent in the coronary care unit. His anxiety and tension made him unable to accept the fact that he had had a myocardial infarction. His family and his colleagues—his usual situational supports —were unable to be with him because of rules of the hospital and his restricted activity. He used denial excessively because he was unable to accept the fact that he might have to change his life-style. Since this was his first hospitalization and the first time he had to be in a dependent role, his anxiety increased considerably.

ADDENDUM

Several months later the physician informed the therapist that he had permitted Mr. Z. to enter the yacht race as a passenger, not as crew, and that his yacht had finished third.

Alzheimer's disease—theoretical concepts

The term Organic Brain Syndrome (OBS) is used to describe symptoms of emotional, perceptual, and cognitive dysfunction arising from disturbances in previously unimpaired brain structure and mental functioning. These symptoms may be caused by physical or chemical insult to the brain, overload or deprivation of sensory input, overwhelming stress and anxiety, or by degenerative disease of the brain by causes as yet generally unknown (Mace and Rabins, 1981; Seltzer and Frazier, 1978; Heller and Kornfeld, 1975).

OBS is one of the most prevalent causes for abnormalities in judgment, intellectual functioning, and behavior. It is usually classified into two major categories, acute and chronic. The generally accepted distinguishing factor between them is reversibility of symptoms as a result of appropriate medical intervention (Lipowski, 1980). When symptoms are reversible, the diagnosis is "acute organic brain syndrome"; when irreversible, it is termed "chronic organic brain syndrome."

When no particular pathological process can be identified directly as the cause of chronic, or irreversible, brain syndrome, the condition is considered to be primary and classified according to age of onset. A diagnosis of "primary degenerative dementia, presenile" indicates that the condition occurred before the sixth decade in life, and one of "primary degenerative dementia, senile" indicates that it occurred after that age. However, according to Seltzer and Frazier, this has always been somewhat of an arbitrary designation.

Of those conditions for which no primary, underlying cause can be identified, Alzheimer's disease appears to be the most frequent. Definitive diagnosis still depends on the presence or absence of specific abnormalities within the structure of the brain tissue, which can be obtained only by brain biopsy. This is not a routine procedure since, at present, no specific treatment is available even if a diagnosis is confirmed (Mace and Rabins, 1981; Reisberg, 1981).

Alzheimer's is a slow, progressive condition, characterized by a steady, irreversible decline in intellectual functioning. Its incidence is equally distributed along sexual, socioeconomic, racial, and ethnic lines (Reisberg, 1981).

There are approximately 1.5 million victims of Alzheimer's disease in the United States; it occurs in about 5% of the population over 65 years of age and 20% of those over 85. The economic consequences of this disease have been estimated to be about 25 billion dollars a year in this country alone (Hubbard, 1984). According to Mace and Rabins, approximately 50% of all dementias are caused by Alzheimer's disease.

The initial symptoms of Alzheimer's disease are very insidious and often imperceptible as organic changes start to occur in the brain and a decline in many areas of intellectual and physical abilities begins. Initially no objective or subjective symptoms are reported. As the disease progresses, the earliest noticeable symptoms are generally related to memory impairment. While motor activities are not affected at this time, subjective awareness of memory loss begins to interfere more and more with the person's daily living activities.

It is a rare person among us who has not occasionally misplaced needed items, forgotten familiar addresses and telephone numbers, and even forgotten the name of closest friends. If this does not happen too often, the usual response can be momentary embarrassment or irritation. We blame it on being tired, or under stress, or just having "too much on our minds to remember"; but there is always a sense of self-confidence that the memory will be recalled.

For the Alzheimer's patient, however, such forgetfulness begins to become chronic, something that cannot be shrugged off so easily as only temporary. As subjective awareness and concerns over memory loss increase, self-confidence in an ability to recall lost memories diminishes. For many, the development of written check lists and notes of "things to do" become a way of life. Eventually, however, these no longer suffice as memory supports as they, too, become lost and forgotten.

As memory loss increases, signs of early confusional behavior begin to be exhibited. A person easily becomes lost in unfamiliar places and needs to depend increasingly on others for help in "finding his way" when away from home or other familiar locations. Changes to new environments create much anxiety, particularly when combined with stressful events such as an illness requiring hospitalization. The person's forgetfulness begins to be noticed by others and can no longer be seen simply as temporary or "normal" behavior. At the same time, recent memory loss becomes much more subjectively noted. Ability to concentrate decreases, and the use of denial as a defense mechanism increases.

From this stage in intellectual decline identifiable overt symptoms of Alzheimer's disease begin and regression continues into a late confusional stage. The person is still able to handle his own immediate physical needs, yet motor skills gradually decrease. Language becomes affected, and it becomes increasingly difficult for the person to find "the right words." The ability to concentrate diminishes greatly and the ability to handle finances, cooking, and other daily decision-making activities suffers accordingly. The individual becomes more withdrawn and anxious. Frustration and anger increase as the use of denial becomes less effective. No longer can he deny to himself or to others that something is wrong with him.

Inevitably, whether slowly or rapidly, regression continues into a period of early dementia. At this stage such persons can survive no longer without assistance from others. Now there is time disorientation and, frequently, forgetfulness of familiar family names. While the person is still capable of handling the basic functions of daily living (such as feeding himself, bowel and bladder control, and bathing), caretaking needs increase greatly as intellectual and motor skills continue to decline. For many, this is a period of rapid decline as the disease progresses toward the stage of middle dementia.

By now there is evidence of symptoms of hallucinatory types of perceptions, which are responded to with fear, agitation, and even violence. Familiar faces may be recognized, but name recall is nearly nil. Variable awareness of recent events and past memories may be sketchy and incomplete.

As motor skills decrease, bowel and bladder incontinence begins. Constant attendance becomes necessary for all activities of daily living. Caretaking activities may exceed the abilities of family and friends; institutionalization may be the only family recourse.

In the final, late dementia stage of Alzheimer's disease the person becomes increasingly "vegetative" and requires total care. Speech decreases to one or two words, all intellectual skills disappear, and motor skills decline until full assistance is needed to eat, drink and even to turn in bed. Eventually there is coma and, finally, death.

Alzheimer's disease usually leads to death within 7 to 10 years. However, some deaths may occur within as little as 3 to 4 years while others may not occur for 15 years (Mace and Rabins, 1981).

A diagnosis of Alzheimer's disease for a family member means that the whole family, as well as the patient, must learn to live with the condition. Insidious in its onset, a misdiagnosis of early symptoms can create added stress for everyone concerned. Too often the early symptoms of memory loss, depression, passive dependency, and emotional lability are misunderstood or passed off as transient reactions to situational stress.

As the disease progresses, a person with Alzheimer's disease becomes impaired in his abilities to control the appropriate expression of his own emotions and comprehend the effect of his behavior on others. He is emotionally labile, overreacts, and often appears insensitive to other's feelings. Emotional changes often appear as exaggerations of previously established behavioral characteristics. For example, the passive and withdrawn person may become even more dependent, suspicious, and depressed; the characteristically independent-aggressive person may appear demanding, hysterical, and even manic in behavior.

As organic changes in the brain occur, dependency on others will increase. This may not be too disturbing for one whose past personality characteristics were those of passive dependency. However, for one whose personality characteristics emphasized independent-aggressive behaviors, feelings of frustration and anger will increase as dependency needs increase. This can lead to what has been termed a *catastrophic reaction,* which is best described as an emotional overreaction, one that is obviously out of proportion to an anxiety provoking situation. It occurs as intellectual impairment increases and emotional control decreases. This is a fairly common response as the affected individual is increasingly confronted with failure in achieving what formerly were, to that person, "simple tasks." Often believing that the individuals concerned have full control over their behavioral changes, family and friends may respond inappropriately in turn. Such a reaction may only serve to increase stress and, consequently, the severity of the symptoms exhibited.

Family members will almost invariably need to cope at some time with feelings of fear, anger, guilt, shame, isolation, and persistent feelings of grief and mourning. These feelings may arise intermittently and in varying degrees, dependent on each member's past experiences, values, personal resources, and current life situation.

Any unusual problems arising with the patient may, in fact, be a symptom of family dysfunction. It would not be unusual for family members, no longer able to relate to each other openly and directly, to relate through problems as they arise in the patient. It is as though there is a need for the patient to have problems in order for family members to continue to relate. This, of course, only serves to reinforce problematic behaviors by the patient.

Once the diagnosis of Alzheimer's disease has been confirmed and denial of the illness diminishes, each family member begins to face the reality of its consequences for herself as well as for the patient. Each member strongly feels a need to find a satisfactory reason or meaning for the occurrence of the illness. Until one is found, real or imagined, feelings of helplessness, powerlessness, and insecurity exist. It is realistic for family members to be anxious, confused, and fearful and to feel "alone" with the situation. It is not at all unusual for them to be completely uninformed when a diagnostic label like this is attached to one of their members. Their only source of knowledge could be one of hearsay misinformation. It may also be that there has been misperception of correct information provided them at the time of the diagnosis.

One natural outcome is feelings of anger and aggression, which can mobilize members toward constructive actions, thereby reducing feelings of helplessness and powerlessness. Another outcome may be that of outwardly destructive behavior, which leads to increased feelings of helplessness and anger, compounded by feelings of guilt. Depression and discouragement are the most common feelings for close relatives or friends of those with chronic, irreversible diseases. Anger and frustration leading to rage reactions or internalized toward feelings of suicide are not uncommon during the progressive course of the illness.

As a family develops, highly structured roles, functions, and expectations are established for each member. None is created in isolation, and all are reciprocal. A change in any one member will almost inevitably result in changes throughout the structure of family roles. Equilibrium within the family system depends largely on all members' continuing acceptance and performance of their unique roles, responsibilities, and expectations.

Family members are faced with the need to identify the meaning of the functional loss of one of their members and what it will mean to each member as family roles are redefined and functions redistributed. Until these are dealt with, conflict and chaos are inevitable outcomes. The family system will become less cohesive and could eventually break up or disintegrate altogether. Any one role change, subtle or otherwise, will almost invariably lead to change in those of other members. Welcome or unwelcome, planned or unplanned, a role change can affect each member's usual ways of thinking, feeling, and behaving. Feelings in particular strongly affect perceptions and the thinking processes.

Not everyone involved in learning that a family member has an irreversible illness will respond in the same way. The degree to which an individual reacts is, in great part, determined by how much she perceives the illness interfering in her daily life.

If a parent is affected and children are involved in the care-taking process, role reversal becomes an inevitable problem with which they must deal. This will occur as responsibilities and control—from the more abstract, intellectual decision-making responsibilities to, eventually, basic physical functions—gradually must be taken from the affected person. This is particularly difficult for many to accept because of the relatively early age at which Alzheimer's disease occurs and the insidious nature of its onset and progress. It would not be unusual to find strong feelings of ambivalence, anger, and reluctance to accept the loss of the child role and the reversal of dependency roles with the parent. These feelings are compounded by the fact that the parent may appear, physically, quite well and capable of self-care until the later stages of the illness. To accept the reversal in roles is also to acknowledge anticipation of an ultimate desertion by death.

Family members experience many conflicting and unique feelings as the disease progresses. Emotions may run the gamut from hopeful optimism to hopeless despair. All these emotions are as highly complex and variable as is each member's perception of the situation and its effect on her own life.

There may be feelings of frustration and anger as caregivers' patience wears thin and the caregiving chores continue to increase. It is not uncommon at all to observe the attitude switch from "What did *she* ever do to deserve this?" to "What did *I* ever do to deserve this?"

Denial is not an uncommon initial response when a person is overwhelmed with a stressful situation. However, for those who do not cope through use of denial, it would not be unusual to find the grief process beginning in anticipation of the loss. The more a person is emotionally invested in the "loved one," the more threatened that person may feel in anticipation of the loss.

The four phases of grief and mourning are a response to any situation involving loss, not just the death of a loved one. Families of patients with Alzheimer's disease are faced with prolonged periods of grief and mourning. This greatly differs from an overwhelming feeling of grief that gradually lessens as time passes after a loved one's death. Grief and mourning for death is sanctioned by our society, but overt, prolonged grief and mourning for a chronically ill person, particularly one who looks physically well, is rarely accepted as "death" connected. More often such mourning may be perceived as self-pity or weakness.

When the stresses of caring for the affected person become so great that a family or a personal crisis is precipitated, professional counseling may be required to avert maladaptive problem-solving behavior.

Case study   *Alzheimer's disease*

ASSESSMENT OF THE INDIVIDUAL AND THE PROBLEM

Frank was referred to a community crisis clinic by his family physician because of his increasing symptoms of tension, anxiety, and depression. When he arrived, he appeared quite tense with visible hand tremors. The receptionist contacted a therapist, and Frank was directed to his office.

When asked by the therapist why he had come to the clinic that day, he replied in a very depressed tone of voice, "My whole world is collapsing around me. My wife, Molly, is sick, but I've been able to handle it—until now. My daughter has always been such a help, but now she is walking out on us. I just can't handle much more; I can't do it alone."

He became increasingly agitated as he spoke, his voice rising in anger. After a long pause, he seemed to regain his composure. In response to direct questioning by the therapist, he slowly described the problems that had led up to this visit to the clinic for help.

Frank said that he and his wife, Molly, who were both 50 years old, had been married for 20 years. They had one daughter, Ann, who was 17 years old and had just graduated from high school. He described his family life as "good—no more problems than most people," until about a year ago when Molly had to quit her job. She had worked for the same person all of their married life. When that person had retired a year ago, Molly was reassigned to a new office in the same company. Within a few days she had begun to complain that her new boss was very disorganized and seemed to go out of his way to find fault with her work. She said that she had even been accused of such ridiculous things as misplacing records and forgetting to tell him of his appointments. She had started going to work earlier and staying later in an effort to "get the boss organized," but he continued to criticize and complain about her work.

Frank said that Molly became increasingly irritable, preoccupied, and forgetful at home during that time. It seemed as though she were scapegoating him and Ann for all of her problems at work.

Finally, she came home one day and told him that she had been given the option of either resigning or of being demoted to a lesser position. With Frank's encouragement, she decided to resign and take a few week's vacation before looking for another job.

Frank had hoped that, with time and some rest, she would "pull herself together, and eventually become her cheerful, organized self again." This, however, was not to be the case.

As the weeks passed, Molly seemed to become even more disorganized and forgetful. She never again spoke of looking for a new job. She argued increasingly, accusing him and Ann of misplacing her personal items, losing telephone messages, and so on. Bills were left forgotten and unpaid in her desk until Frank learned to watch for them in the mail.

Neither he nor Ann seemed able to reason with her any longer about these incidents. Any references to her forgetfulness were met with denial and angry responses. Finally, they learned to cope as best they could with her erratic, irresponsible behaviors. Over time, they gradually took over many of her household responsibilities.

Molly first displayed overt signs of confusion, disorientation, and memory loss about 6 months before Frank came to the clinic, when she was hospitalized for elective surgery. Nurses had found her late at night wandering down the halls in her barefeet, "looking for my bedroom." When the nurses suggested that she had lost her way, she became verbally abusive to them for saying that to her. Before dawn she was found fully dressed and sitting on a chair in the hallway. When questioned, she replied that she was "waiting for Frank to drive me to work." Further questioning revealed that she was disoriented as to place, could not recall the day of the week or her physician's name, and had forgotten why she had come to the hospital.

Following this episode further tests and examinations were completed and a diagnosis of Alzheimer's disease made. Findings suggested that Molly had progressed into the early confusional stage.

When asked how he and Molly responded to this news, Frank said that their initial feelings were quite mixed. "We were glad to finally find a physical reason for her behavior changes but were shocked and really couldn't believe that there was no known cure for it. It made me really angry that this could happen to any of us."

When it was strongly suggested that Frank contact a local Alzheimer's disease group for ongoing support and information about Molly's care at home, Frank saw no immediate need to do so. To him, Molly appeared quite healthy. As he perceived it, all that he and Ann would need was "a little more patience with Molly when she forgot things or lost her temper." Over time they had learned to help her avoid stressful situations, even though it sometimes made life more stressful for them. Gradually, however, relationships between him and Ann distanced as he spent increasing amounts of time away from home at his job.

At first Ann never complained of having to spend increasing amounts of time at home with her mother. Neighbors and friends visited often and she could still leave Molly alone for brief periods of time. But, as Molly's memory loss increased, Molly's frustration tolerance decreased. Her unprovoked irritability became much more frequent and, soon, visitors rarely came to see them.

At the same time, Ann found herself having to assume an increasing number of the household roles and responsibilities formerly held by her mother. Any attempts to bring in a housekeeper or a companion for her mother were met with overt antagonism from Molly.

Two evenings ago Frank had come home late and was confronted by a tearful, angry Ann. She told him that she "couldn't take it anymore" and was going to move out if he didn't find someone else to take care of her mother. He said that her outburst really took him by surprise. When he asked her the cause of this sudden change in attitude, she angrily responded, "Sudden? There is nothing sudden about this! For weeks I've been telling you how I feel, but you never listen to me anymore. You're always too busy at work, and when you come home you seem to ignore just how much mother has changed. She's become like a spoiled, demanding little child. I feel more like a live-in babysitter than like her daughter. I have no life of my own anymore—and you don't seem to care what happens to me!" The conversation was abruptly ended by Ann leaving the house and slamming the door behind her. She called Frank about an hour later to say that she was going to spend the night at a friend's house. She added that she still had a lot to think over but would be home the next morning.

Frank said that he never slept that night, his mind in a turmoil of thinking about what Ann had said. He felt shocked and overwhelmed with strongly ambivalent feelings toward Molly who slept quietly upstairs in their bedroom. He said that he "suddenly faced reality—and hated it." He felt completely alone and trapped with no way out of the whole situation. As he described it, "By morning I had the shakes, couldn't concentrate on anything, and felt like hell."

When Ann came back the next morning, neither mentioned what had been said the night before. He left for his office as quickly as he could.

For the next several hours he drove his car randomly about the city, thinking about what had been happening to his life for the past year. It was only then, he said, that he finally faced the reality that he had lost forever the Molly that he had loved and married. And now he was in danger of losing Ann, too. He suddenly felt so overwhelmed with grief that he pulled the car to the side of the street and parked. He felt so sick and trembled so severely that he was afraid to drive. As soon as he felt able, he drove directly to his physician's office, where he was seen immediately. It was from there that he had been referred to the clinic.

PLANNING OF THERAPEUTIC INTERVENTION

It was the therapist's assessment that, until his confrontation with Ann, Frank had successfully used denial to cope with Molly's illness. This was supported by his avoidance of opportunities to obtain more information about Alzheimer's disease from one of the local support groups.

As Molly's symptoms became more overt, he avoided having to "do something about it" by extending his time at work and away from home. When Ann had tried to communicate to him her need for help and understanding, he effectively managed to "tune her out." As a result, he was not consciously lying when he said that he was shocked at the "sudden change in Ann's attitude."

Frank's crisis was precipitated by the threatened loss of his daughter, compounded by unresolved feelings of grief and mourning for the anticipated loss of his wife.

The goals of intervention were to assist Frank to identify and ventilate his unrecognized feelings about his wife, to help him obtain appropriate situational support for himself and Ann as he dealt with plans for Molly's future care, and to help him obtain an intellectual understanding of role reversal as it was affecting Ann's relationship with her mother.

INTERVENTION

During the first session it was determined that Frank was not suicidal. When asked to describe himself as he "usually was," he said that he was a person who prided himself on being able to maintain control over his life. He believed that, to be successful, a person should be able to set goals and, with good planning, achieve them. Reflecting further on his feelings about Molly, he admitted to the therapist that, deep down, he'd always believed that Molly could have controlled her behavior if she really wanted to do so. He had felt that her failure to do so was, in some way, a personal rejection of him. No longer able to communicate with her about his feelings, he'd used denial and avoidance to cope.

As Molly's condition deteriorated, he'd felt more angry and frustrated with her and used his work to justify the increasing amount of time spent away from home.

With further discussion and reflection about Molly's behavioral changes, it became very apparent that Frank had little factual information about Alzheimer's disease. His anxiety had been so high when first informed by the doctors that he remembered hearing little other than that her memory loss would continue to get worse and that there was no cure.

As Molly's increasing episodes of unprovoked anger increased, their few remaining friends had gradually begun to avoid contact with her. Recalling this now with the therapist, he acknowledged that, in fact, this had been a relief for him. He no longer had to worry about what she might do or say to their friends if she became upset.

What he had failed to realize, though, was the added stress that this had placed on Ann. Upon further questioning and reflection he said, "Could it be that I didn't listen to Ann because I didn't want to know? I didn't want to hear how bad things had really become?" He paused, and then said softly, "The Molly that I loved so much left me long ago. I miss her so much and wish that she could come back, even for a little while. There's so much I want to say to her. While I stay away from home, I can make believe that she's still there, waiting for me—going home hurts so very much."

It was suggested that he now contact the local Alzheimer's disease group to learn about alternative ways available to him for Molly's care at home. He was made to realize that, unless he began to face the reality of Molly's illness and the situation at his home, he might well lose Ann, too.

When questioned further about his confrontation with Ann the evening before, he seemed unable to understand why Ann felt so angry about her mother. Further discussion focused on the way Ann's roles and responsibilities in the family had changed during the past few months. As he slowly identified these changes for the therapist, he began to obtain an intellectual understanding of parent-child role reversal and its effect upon the child, particularly on one as young as Ann.

Gradually he began to recognize Ann's confrontation for what it was; it was a cry for his understanding of what was happening to her. She was overwhelmed by her inability to meet the ever-increasing dependency needs of her mother without some help from him. Unable to communicate her own dependency needs to either him or her mother, she saw escape from the entire situation as her only solution.

It was suggested to Frank that one of his first priorities was to find someone else to assume major responsibility for Molly's care and supervision. Until this happened, he could expect further confrontations with Ann and should not be surprised if Ann carried out her threat to leave home.

As an interim measure, Frank decided to take a few weeks of his long overdue vacation and stay at home to help out until he could find someone to provide full-time help with Molly's care.

During the second session Frank appeared much more optimistic as he described his past week at home. He said that he and Ann had talked together "for hours" the evening after his first session at the clinic. He reflected that it had been difficult at first for either of them to come face to face with their feelings. "But," he added, "it was such a relief when we did. Until then, neither of us had realized just how far apart we had become and how much we needed to stick together to work things out."

During the past week Frank also had contacted the local Alzheimer's disease group. By prearrangement two members visited his home to meet with him, Ann, and Molly. He recalled his surprise at how easily Molly had appeared to accept the "strangers'" visit and the apparent ease with which they included her in the conversation. As a result of the visit, appropriate resources were identified for assistance in Molly's care. After several interviews with applicants for a housekeeper's position, and with Molly's agreement, they finally hired a woman who seemed best able to cope with Molly's needs. The woman had moved in 2 days before this session and, he reported, "Molly hasn't scared her off yet." However, he would continue to remain at home for another week to help Molly adjust to any new changes in her daily activities.

Frank and Ann also had attended a meeting of the local Alzheimer's group. It surprised them both to find several other young people of Ann's age present. When asked to describe his feelings about the meeting, he said that both he and Ann had gone to the meeting "not expecting much—maybe coffee, cake, and sympathy—but that's all." Instead, they found a group of people who, he said, seemed to know exactly what his family had been going through. He learned that many of his experiences were not unique, but common to all of them. "For the first time," he said, "I was able to get some answers that were useful to us. Maybe no one could tell us *why* she got this disease, but this group of people could give me some good suggestions of how to help all of us deal with it." Most important for both him and Ann, as they left the meeting, was their feeling of no longer being alone with their problems and that now a support group was available to them as problems arose.

ANTICIPATORY PLANNING

Before the end of the session the therapist and Frank reviewed and assessed the adjustment that he had made and his insights into his own feelings about Molly and the effects of her illness on his future. They also discussed his understanding of

CASE STUDY: FRANK

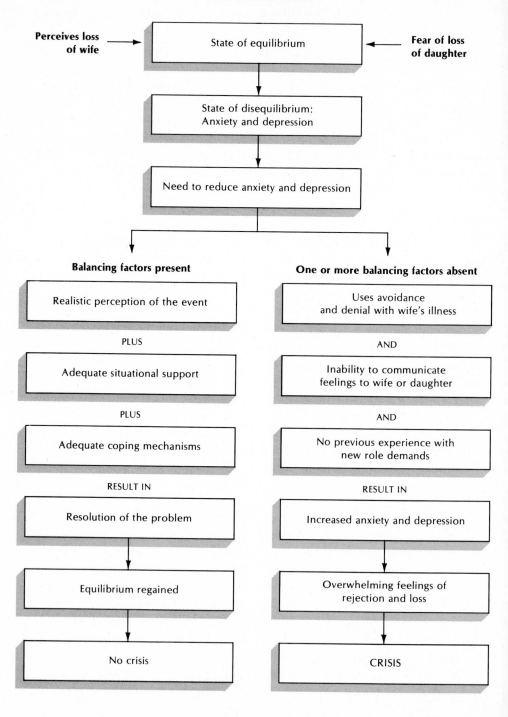

the effect that the process of role-reversal with her mother was having on Ann. It was strongly suggested that he encourage Ann's continued attendance at the Alzheimer's group meetings. The purpose was to provide her with ongoing peer support as she dealt with her changing relationship with her mother.

He was commended for taking direct action during the past week and obtaining appropriate resources to help with his ongoing situation at home. Such action strongly suggested that he no longer was coping solely through denial and avoidance but was making a conscious effort to perceive the situation realistically.

Frank was encouraged to continue to be more direct in his communications with Ann, letting her know that he was recognizing that she had needs, too. Before termination, he was reassured that he could return for help with any future crises, should the need arise.

SUMMATION OF THE PARADIGM

Frank had used denial and avoidance as methods for coping with his feelings toward Molly's illness and eventual death. His behavior was seen by Ann as a rejection of her efforts to communicate to him the realities of her mother's deteriorating condition and its effect upon her own unmet dependency needs. Failing to recognize the extent to which the process of role reversal with her mother had affected Ann's life, Frank perceived her threat to leave home as yet another rejection and threatened loss of someone close to him. Lacking any previous coping experience with his new role demands, his anxiety and depression increased to an intolerable level; Frank was in a state of crisis.

Intervention focused on helping him to identify and understand his unrecognized feelings toward Molly, to obtain an intellectual understanding of the effects of role-reversal on Ann, and to obtain appropriate situational support for the family because they, individually and as a unit, would undoubtedly be confronted with more stress-provoking situations in the progress of Molly's illness.

Chronic psychiatric patient—theoretical concepts

Crisis intervention has gained recognition as a viable therapy modality to assist individuals through acute traumatic life situations. As large psychiatric facilities, slowly or rapidly according to individual state laws, are beginning to shorten the length of hospitalization, the chronic psychiatric patient is returning to his community where continuity of care must be maintained. The questions to be asked and answered are: (1) Does crisis intervention work successfully with chronic psychiatric patients? (2) If not, what other methods must be used to keep this patient functioning in his community?

With a chronic psychiatric patient, as with any patient, identification of the precipitating event, the symptoms the patient is exhibiting, his perception of the event, his available situational supports, and his usual coping mechanisms are crucial factors in resolving his crisis.

Situational supports are those persons in the environment whom the therapist can find to lend support to the individual. A patient may be living with his family or friends; are they concerned enough—and do they care enough—to give him help? The patient's situational supports can serve as "assistants" to the therapist and the patient. They are with him daily and are encouraged to have frequent communication with the therapist. Usually situational supports are included in some part of the therapy sessions. This provides them with the knowledge and information they need to help the *identified* patient.

If the patient is living in a board-and-care facility, the therapist must determine if any of its members are concerned and willing to work with the therapist to help the individual through the stressful period. This involves visiting the facility and conducting collateral or group therapy with the patient and other members to get and keep them involved in helping to resolve the crisis.

Occasionally the patient has *no* situational supports. He may be a social isolate; he may have no family and may have acquaintances but no real friends with whom he can talk about his problems. Usually an individual such as this has many difficulties in interpersonal relationships at work and school and socially. It is then the therapist's role to provide situational support while the patient is in therapy.

Our experiences have verified for us that crisis intervention can be an effective therapy modality with chronic psychiatric patients. If a psychiatric patient with a history of repeated hospitalizations returns to the community and her family, her reentry creates many stresses. While much has been accomplished to remove the stigma of mental illness, people are still wary and hypervigilant when they learn that a "former mental patient" has returned home to her community.

In her absence the family and community have, consciously or unconsciously, eliminated her from their usual life patterns and activities. They then have to readjust to her presence and include her in activities and decision making. If for any reason she does not conform to their expectations, they want her removed so that they can continue their lives without the possibility of disruptive behavior.

The first area to explore is to determine who is in crisis: the patient or her family. In many cases the family is overreacting because of its anxiety and is seeking some means of getting the *identified* patient back into the hospital. The patient is usually brought to the center by a family member because her original maladaptive symptoms have begun to reemerge. Questioning the patient or her family about medication she received from the hospital and determining if she is taking it as prescribed are essential. If the patient is unable to communicate with the therapist about what has happened or what has changed in her life, the family is questioned about what might have precipitated her return to her former psychotic behavior.

A cause-and-effect relationship usually exists between a change, or anticipated change, in the routine patterns of life-style or family constellation and the beginnings of abnormal overt behavior in the identified patient. Often families forget or ignore telling a former psychiatric patient when they are contemplating a change because "he wouldn't understand." Such changes could include moving or changing jobs. This is perceived by the patient as exclusion or rejection by the family and creates stress that he is unable to cope with; thus he retreats to his previous psychotic behavior. Such cases are frequent and can be dealt with through the theoretical framework of crisis intervention methodology.

Rubinstein (1972) stated that family-focused crisis intervention usually brings about the resolution of the patient's crisis without resorting to hospitalization. In a later article in 1974 he advocated that family crisis intervention can also be a viable alternative to rehospitalization. Here the emphasis is placed on the period immediately after the patient's release from the hospital. He suggested that conjoint family therapy begin in the hospital before the patient's release and then continue in an outpatient clinic after his release. This approach has also served to develop the concept that a family can and should share responsibility for the patient's treatment.

In Decker's 1972 study, two groups of young adults were followed for 2½ years after their first psychiatric hospitalization. The first group was immediately hospitalized and received traditional modes of treatment, and the second group was hospitalized after the institution of a crisis-intervention program. The results of the study indicated that crisis intervention reduced long-term hospital dependency without producing alternate forms of psychological or social dependency and also reduced the number of rehospitalizations.

The following brief case study illustrates how a therapist can work with a chronic psychiatric patient in a community mental health center using the crisis model.

Case study   *Chronic psychiatric patient in the community*

ASSESSMENT OF THE INDIVIDUAL AND THE PROBLEM

Jim, a man in his late thirties, was brought to a crisis center by his sister because, as she stated, "he was beginning to act crazy again." Jim had many prior hospitalizations, with a diagnosis of paranoid schizophrenia. The only thing Jim would say was, "I *don't* want to go back to the hospital." He was told that our role was to help him stay out of the hospital if we possibly could. A medical consultation was arranged to determine if he needed to have his medication increased or possibly changed.

Information was then obtained from his sister to determine what had happened (the precipitating event) when his symptoms had started and, specifically, what she meant by his "acting crazy again." His sister stated that he was "talking to the television set, muttering things that made no sense, staring into space, prowling around the apartment at night," and that "this behavior started about 3 days ago.'' When questioned about anything that was different in their lives before the start of his disruptive behavior, she denied any change. When asked about any changes that were contemplated in the near future, she replied that she was planning to be married in 2 months but that Jim did not know about it because she had not told him yet. When asked why she had not told him, she reluctantly answered that she wanted to wait until all of the arrangements had been made. She was asked if there was any way Jim could have found out about her plans. She remembered that she had discussed them on the telephone with a girlfriend the week before.

She was asked what her plans for Jim were after she married. She said that her boyfriend had agreed, rather reluctantly, to let Jim live with them.

Since her boyfriend was reluctant about having Jim live with them, other alternatives were explored. She said that they had cousins living in a nearby suburb but that she did not know if they would want Jim to live with them.

PLANNING THE INTERVENTION

It was suggested that Jim's sister call her cousins, tell them of her plans to get married and her concerns about Jim, and in general find out their feelings about him living with them. The call was placed, and she told them her plans and concerns. Fortunately their response was a positive one. They had recently bought a fairly large apartment building and were having difficulty getting reliable help to take care of the yard work and minor repairs. They felt that Jim would be able to manage this, and they would let him live in a small apartment above the garage.

INTERVENTION

Jim was asked to come back into the office so that his sister could tell him of her plans to marry and the arrangements she had made for him with their cousins. He listened but had difficulty comprehending the information. He just kept saying, ''I *don't* want to go back to the hospital.''

He was asked if he had heard his sister talking about her wedding plans. He admitted that he had and that he knew her boyfriend would not want him around—''they would probably put him back in the hospital.'' As the session ended he still had not internalized the information he had heard. He was asked to continue in therapy for 5 more weeks and to take his medication as prescribed. He agreed to do so.

By the end of the sixth week he had visited his cousins, seen the apartment where he would be living, and had discussed his new ''job.'' His disruptive behavior had ceased, and he was again functioning at his precrisis level.

ANTICIPATORY PLANNING

Since Jim had had many previous hospitalizations and did not want to be rehospitalized, time was spent in discussing how this could be avoided in the future. He

CASE STUDY: JIM

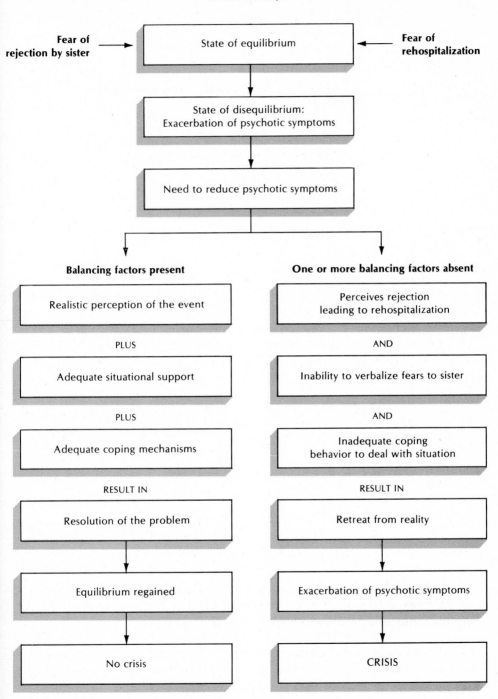

**Fear of
rejection by sister** → State of equilibrium ← **Fear of
rehospitalization**

State of disequilibrium:
Exacerbation of psychotic symptoms

Need to reduce psychotic symptoms

Balancing factors present

Realistic perception of the event

PLUS

Adequate situational support

PLUS

Adequate coping mechanisms

RESULT IN

Resolution of the problem

Equilibrium regained

No crisis

One or more balancing factors absent

Perceives rejection
leading to rehospitalization

AND

Inability to verbalize fears to sister

AND

Inadequate coping
behavior to deal with situation

RESULT IN

Retreat from reality

Exacerbation of psychotic symptoms

CRISIS

was given the name, address, and telephone number of a crisis center in his new community and told to visit them when he moved. He was assured that the center could supervise his medication and be available if he needed someone to talk to if he felt he again needed help.

SUMMATION OF PARADIGM

Jim's sister neglected to tell him about her impending marriage, which he perceived as rejection. Because of his numerous hospitalizations, he feared that his sister would have him rehospitalized "to get rid of him." He was unable to verbalize his fears, retreated from reality, and experienced an exacerbation of his psychotic symptoms.

The therapist adhered to the crisis model by focusing the therapy sessions on the patient's immediate problems, *not* on his chronic psychopathology.

Wife abuse—theoretical concepts

Throughout history women have been subjected to the whims and brutality of their husbands. In the United States the statistics reflect no epidemic of domestic violence, only a recent effort to collect often inexact figures which are startling even when allowances are made for error. Nearly 6 million wives will be abused by their husbands in any 1 year; some 2000 to 4000 women are beaten to death annually. The police spend one third of their time responding to domestic violence calls. Battery is the single major cause of injury to women, more significant than automobile accidents, rapes, or muggings.

In the United States wife beating is no longer widely accepted as an inevitable and private matter. This change in attitude, while far from complete, has come about in the past 10 to 15 years as part of the transformation of ideas about the roles and rights of women in society. Legal structures and social service networks, prompted by grass-roots women's organizations, have begun to redefine spouse abuse as a violation of the victim's civil rights and a criminal act of assault subject to the same punishments as other acts of violence (O'Reilly, 1983).

Marital abuse has been called "the silent crime." Bringing it out into the open by talking about it is the first step toward a solution. But for most people, including the victim and the abuser, the almost reflexlike response to the subject is to deny its existence.

Battering involves a pattern of escalating abuse in a situation from which the victim feels she cannot escape. Because they are usually physically stronger than their wives, men are less likely to be battered. Often a battered woman has grown up with violence and accepts it as a pitiful form of caring, or at least as something inevitable in a relationship. She may feel that the world is a dangerous place and that she needs a protector, even a man who beats her. Ashamed, terrified that any resistance will provoke greater violence, isolated from her family and friends, often without any means of support other than her husband, many a battered woman sinks into despairing submission from which the only escape is eventual widowhood, her own murder (or her husband's), or suicide.

Doctors, social workers, and psychiatrists have frequently been less helpful than the police. Straus (1981), in a study of family violence, concluded that the medical profession and social agencies are an essential part of the battered syndrome. They often treat the women like they are "crazy"; physicians fail to note signs of abuse, label battered women psychotic or hypochondriacal, prescribe tranquilizers, and tell them to go home. They make battered women doubt their own sanity by sending them to a family therapist for psychotherapy.

What kind of man would hit a woman? Not only hit her, but blacken her eyes, break the bones in her face, beat her breasts, kick her abdomen, and menace her with a gun? There is a very good chance that he was beaten as a child. Perhaps because of his early trauma, he is often emotionally stunted. An interesting analogy exists between a male batterer and a 2- or 3-year-old child; their tantrums are very similar. Like a narcissistic child, the batterer bites when he's throwing a tantrum.

The wife beater probably drinks; but he doesn't beat because he drinks—he drinks to beat. Unemployment does not cause battering, but hard times make it worse. The typical spouse beater is unable to cope with the traditional notion of masculinity, or the male role, which requires men to be stoic. It requires men not to need intimacy, to be in control, to be the "big wheel," and when there is a problem to "give 'em hell." The difficulty is that nine out of ten men fail at that list, at least in their own judgment. The batterer is often afflicted with extreme insecurity. The man's wife is the emotional glue that holds him together, and, as a consequence, he is desperately afraid of losing her. The husband is trying to make her be closer to him by controlling her physically, but he doesn't realize that he is driving her away (O'Reilly, 1983).

Batterers can be very calculating in how they deal with their wives and with the authorities once they are caught. They are frequently charming to a fault. They can play therapy off against the court system and not have to be responsible.

The first self-help group for abusive men was formed in Boston in 1977. There are now about 50. Very few men go to such centers on their own. Either their partner has left or is threatening to, or they are attending under court order. By and large, they do not believe they have done anything wrong, sometimes insisting they they are not batterers at all. Those who own up to being violent frequently believe their partners are at fault.

Historically, batterers have fallen between the cracks, being considered neither crazy nor criminal, at least by the standards of the day. A man beats up his wife because he can. He usually does not beat up his boss or male acquaintances; the consequences—loss of job, a charge of criminal assault, an old-fashioned black eye—

are simply too great. Now the consequences are rising for violence against one's wife. Shelters for abused women have created a safety net for wives who previously would have been afraid to take their husbands to court. Newspapers, judges, hospitals, neighbors, even a growing number of once exasperated police officers, are beginning to understand the dimensions of the problem. More important, states and municipalities are enacting laws that give women a realistic chance of getting protection and redress through the courts.

Ten years ago there were no real, specific laws providing remedies for women. If a woman wanted protection using the courts, she would have to get it as part of a domestic relations proceeding, that is, separation or divorce.

At that time police could not make an arrest without actually witnessing violence or seeing compelling physical evidence of abuse. Nowadays such requirements are being eased (Appleton, 1980).

The tightening of laws against wife beating has resulted in higher conviction rates. Still, only a fraction of abusive husbands are even reported to the authorities, much less arrested and convicted. For the glib, angry men who pummel their wives, a brush with the law sometimes has a sobering effect. In general, arrests work because they show the man that such behavior is inappropriate. They also show the woman that somebody will help her.

The crackdown represents an important shift in how the nation views wife abuse. No longer does a woman have to go it alone in a legal system that is stacked against her; no longer does she have to deny the suggestion, either stated or implied, that she got what she deserved. Now the courts and the community are swinging to her side, and the bullying husband is beginning to pay the price.

Case study   *Wife abuse*

ASSESSMENT OF THE INDIVIDUAL AND THE PROBLEM

Suzan, a 39-year-old housewife and mother of two daughters, (Karen, aged 15, and Leslie, aged 12) was admitted to a large metropolitan hospital. Her husband, Ron, aged 43, drove her to the emergency room and stated that she had "fallen down the stairs in their home." When asked by the resident the name of their family physician, Ron casually shrugged his shoulders and said, "We don't have one." The resident asked permission to call in an internist and an orthopedic specialist because he felt Suzan was badly injured.

The resident ordered x-rays for Suzan "from head to toe" and then contacted an internist and orthopedist and told them he suspected a possible case of wife beating. Both physicians stated they would be at the hospital within 30 minutes to see the x-rays and Suzan. Suzan went through the series of x-rays and was admitted to the hospital.

The internist, Dr. W., and the orthopedist, Dr. V., arrived at the x-ray department and looked at the x-rays with a sense of shock and disbelief. Suzan's current injuries included two black eyes, two fractures in the pelvic girdle, and two fractured ribs. The x-rays also revealed past injuries: four fractured ribs, fractured left wrist and left arm in two places, and fractures of the right ankle.

The two physicians went to Suzan's room, introduced themselves, and asked Suzan if they could sit down. Suzan's blackened eyes were almost swollen shut but both physicians could see the fear in her eyes as she looked past them to see if her husband was with them. Dr. W. ordered no visitors for Suzan, including family, unless they had the permission of one of the doctors. Suzan appeared to relax slightly.

During the taking of her medical history, Suzan stated that she had *no* previous injuries. Dr. W. then casually asked Suzan how she had sustained her present injuries. Suzan responded quickly, "I tripped and fell down the stairs at home."

Dr. V. told her about her current injuries, stating that they were quite extensive for a fall down a flight of stairs. Dr. V. then told Suzan that she would have to stay in the hospital from four to six weeks for the fractures in her pelvic girdle to heal. Suzan gasped and repeated, "Four to six weeks! What about my daughters— they need me!" Dr. V. asked, "Don't you have family that could stay with them?" Suzan replied, "My mother would love to come out and take care of them, but Ron doesn't get along with her."

The doctors explained the extent of Suzan's injuries to Ron, and then Dr. W. told him that Suzan's mother would be called to take care of their daughters. Dr. W. called Suzan's mother, who, when told of her daughter's injuries, commented that Ron had probably beat her again. Her mother made arrangements to be at the hospital the next morning.

Dr. W. then faced Suzan with her mother's accusation that Ron had beat her in the past; Suzan denied this. After discussing the case Dr. W. and Dr. V. decided to call in a psychotherapist with experience in dealing with battered wives.

PLANNING THE THERAPEUTIC INTERVENTION

The clinical psychologist called in to assist felt that he would have to work with Suzan's mother and her two daughters to break through Suzan's denial. The first step would be to confront Suzan with the x-rays that clearly showed the previous injuries and to demand an explanation. He would use Suzan's mother's statement that Ron had "beaten her many times before" as leverage against Suzan's denial. He would plan to see the daughters alone to see if they would admit that their father had abused their mother in the past as well as in the most recent accident. The second step would be to get Suzan to realize that other women had been battered by their spouses and that it was not her fault that she had been beaten. She had to be made to view the events in a realistic manner. The third step was to get situational support for Suzan and have her talk with other wives who had been battered and hear how they had coped with their situations. The fourth step would be to tell Suzan about the facilities that were available for battered wives and the therapeutic groups her husband could attend with other men who had battered their wives.

INTERVENTION

The next morning Suzan was introduced to the psychotherapist and told that one of his areas of expertise was working with battered wives. The therapist showed Suzan all her old fractures on the x-rays and asked her when and how she had received them and told Suzan he would ask her mother and her daughters if she did not answer. Then the therapist sat back in his chair and waited in silence as Suzan began to cry. As Suzan continued to cry, occasionally he handed her more tissues but said nothing. Finally Suzan asked, "Aren't you going to say something?" The therapist replied, "No, it is time for you to answer my questions." (Since most individuals have difficulty coping with silence, it can be a very effective technique in psychotherapy—if the therapist can handle it.)

Suzan finally commented that none of the other doctors had ever asked her any questions, and the therapist asked her to start at the beginning. Suzan began by saying, "I know Ron loves me and I love him—you will see—I'll probably receive a dozen yellow roses today with a card asking me to forgive him. And I will—I always do. I probably deserve to be beaten—I am not a good wife or mother."

Suzan continued, "It really is my fault. Ron didn't want to get married, but I got careless and ended up pregnant. Ron wanted me to have an abortion, but I refused—I just couldn't. I am Catholic but Ron isn't, so we got married. Karen was born 7½ months after we were married. I loved him so much, and I really believed that he loved me." She said he was a good husband and a very good father. "I had no experience in taking care of a house, husband, or a baby. I didn't even know how to cook—thank heavens someone gave me a good cookbook when we got married. I still can't iron his shirts to suit him. I have truly been a failure. You see, I was an only child and my mother and father 'spoiled me rotten'—I never had to do anything around the house."

The first time Ron had hit her was after they had been married about 1½ years because she had burned the dinner. She said she had been taking care of Karen, who had a fever, and completely forgot the roast in the oven. When Ron came home, she was rocking Karen trying to get her to sleep. He walked into Karen's room and said very coldly, "Put the baby in her crib and come with me." Suzan put Karen down, and Ron grabbed her by the arm and pulled her into the kitchen. He had taken the roast out of the oven—it was burned to a crisp, and the kitchen was filled with smoke. Ron said, "Do you think money grows on trees?" and he slapped her. Then he just kept hitting her. She said, "I begged him not to, but he just kept punching me. Finally, he stopped, probably because he was tired, but that is when I received my first black eye. So you see, I did deserve it—it was my fault." The therapist told Suzan she did *not* deserve that beating and asked if the beatings continued. Suzan said that she "just couldn't seem to please him. He didn't like the way I ironed his shirts—that's when he broke my ribs. If I didn't season the food to his liking, another beating. Almost anything I did wrong ended up with his beating me. That's why we have never had just one doctor, he would take me to a different one or to a different emergency room every time." The therapist asked Suzan if Ron drank much. She said that he usually would have a couple of beers, maybe more occasionally. The therapist asked her if she could remember if he usually had been drinking when he beat her. She replied, "Yes, yes, I remember; every time he beat me he had been drinking—he wasn't drunk you understand. Even last night he had been drinking!" She asked, "Do you think his drinking makes him beat me?" The therapist answered, "Not really. Although he drinks to beat you, he doesn't beat you because he drinks."

The therapist asked about Ron's family. Suzan said that she really did not know them, and Ron wasn't very close to them. Apparently his father was a violent man who beat his three sons and his wife. She continued, saying that Ron's father was an alcoholic and that his mother had died five years ago. The therapist told Suzan that because his father had beaten him and his mother he considered this acceptable behavior between a husband and wife.

The therapist explained to Suzan that shelters had been established for battered women and their children and that therapy groups had been formed for men who battered their wives. The therapist then asked if he could have a woman who lived in one of the facilities come and talk to her. Suzan said that she would like very much to talk to someone who had been through what she had been through. The therapist told Suzan he would arrange it as soon as possible. He reminded her that she was safe in the hospital, but she must seriously think about whether she wanted to return home to more beatings or go to one of the facilities with her daughters.

As Suzan had predicted, Ron sent her roses and asked for her forgiveness. At the same time the flowers came Suzan's mother arrived at the hospital, and the therapist left so that Suzan and her mother could talk. When he returned they had decided that Suzan would divorce Ron and she and her daughters would move to Chicago and live with Suzan's parents. Suzan called Ron to come to the hospital so she could tell him of her decisions.

When Ron arrived Suzan very quickly told him that she wanted a divorce and that she and the girls would be moving. At first Ron was shocked and briefly tried to change her mind. Then he became angry with Suzan's mother, who he assumed was responsible for Suzan's unexpeced actions. At this point the therapist ushered Ron from the room and offered to talk with him later about his problems concerning his beating Suzan. Ron said he would call in a few days and then left the hospital.

ANTICIPATORY PLANNING

Ron never called, but the therapist continued to see Suzan every few days until she was discharged in the fifth week. She fairly blossomed under the loving care of

CASE STUDY: SUZAN

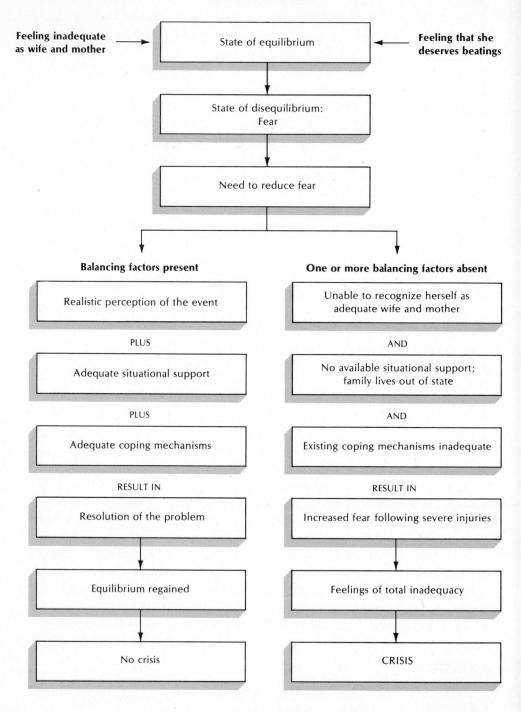

her mother. She filed for divorce, with no protest from Ron. Her daughters were delighted at the thought of moving to Chicago to live with their grandparents. They admitted they were terrified of their father and had been afraid of saying anything to anyone. They said he had moved out of the house because he could not stand being around their grandmother.

SUMMATION OF THE PARADIGM

Suzan was made to feel totally inadequate as a wife and mother. She had led a very sheltered life until her marriage and had no experience in keeping a home or caring for children. She felt that she deserved the beatings by her husband, and she was too embarrassed and ashamed to let anyone know that she was a battered wife. She had an unrealistic perception of the event. Her only situational supports were her family, who lived in another state. She had no adequate coping mechanisms. Her injuries from the last beating were so extensive that she was unable to deny her fear of her husband and thus entered a state of crisis.

Divorce—theoretical concepts

In Western society, divorce has become a common rather than a rare occurrence. Much has been written and hypothesized about the causes and effects of divorce on individuals and family members. According to the *Los Angeles Times,* April 2, 1980, the United States' divorce rate increased 96% in the last decade. This trend appears to be leveling off, according to the Bureau of the Census. In 1983 there were 1,179,000 divorces in the United States, or 75 divorces for every 1000 marriages. Since divorce rates are so high and many marriages are centers of friction and unhappiness, something must be lacking in the preparation for marriage. No event in life of equal importance is viewed with so little realism, and marriage seems to come about with little or no preparation.

Marriage and its demands on individuals can be stressful, and failure to sustain a marriage can precipitate a crisis. Rapoport (1963) delineates three subphases of marriage when stress is the most common: the engagement, honeymoon, and early marriage. Engaged couples confront major tasks on two levels—intrapersonal and interpersonal. The intrapersonal task implies a review of readiness for marriage on a conscious, preconscious, or unconscious level of psychological maturity. This readiness will be affected by the individual needs of the person and by her perceived subcultural norms. The interpersonal tasks are concerned with developing an interpersonal adjustment or accommodation that will be satisfactory in the marital relationship. The engagement period involves a process of separation from previous life patterns and of commitment of the couple to one another. The honeymoon period is a time for establishing a basic sense of harmony. The early marriage phase (the first 3 months) involves establishing a system of authority, decision-making patterns, and patterns of sexual relationships.

It is evident that individuals do not always accomplish these necessary tasks in the first few months of marriage. For some it may easily extend into the first few years of marriage. Additional stress factors may occur in this period to create even greater disequilibrium.

The largest proportion of divorces occurs in the early years of marriage among childless couples. The peak period of divorces is in the second year of marriage, after which the rate drops rapidly. A number of factors, other than those previously mentioned, are precipitating causes of divorce. Among these are urban background, early marriage (15 to 19 years of age), short courtship, short engagement, mixed racial or religious marriages, disapproval of friends and relatives, dissimilar backgrounds, and unhappy parental marriages.

Today there is greater acceptance of the possibility of divorce; because of this acceptance, divorced persons have lost some of the feelings of failure and guilt that were formerly associated with it. The higher divorce rate may reflect new values placed on marriage. Marriage is no longer accepted as an "endurance race" that is doggedly maintained "for the sake of the children." The current demands are for a "good marriage," one that meets the needs of the individuals involved. Even from the point of view of the children, who seemingly pay the highest price for marital failure, divorce in certain circumstances may create fewer psychological problems provided the children are not used as pawns by the separating parents.

The rate of remarriage after divorce is quite high, and in cases where both parties had been divorced two or more times the ratio climbs even higher. Greene (1968) assumes that divorce is a repetitive phenomenon. It is apparent that an unresolved neurotic pattern, carried over from one marriage to another, would tend to reinforce the individual's failure pattern in the subsequent marriage.

This case study (Morley and others, 1967) concerns a young woman, 23 years old, who sought help from a crisis center on the advice of her attorney because of an impending divorce. Neither Margie nor her husband had attained the psychological maturity or "readiness" necessary to enter marriage. Margie's impulsive marriages after brief courtships indicated her unrealistic expectations and attitudes toward marriage. Clues given in the assessment phase indicated that she believed herself a failure as a woman. These guilt feelings and lack of her usual situational supports precipitated a crisis. Intervention was planned to assist her to cope with her feelings of failure and guilt and to view her divorce in more realistic terms.

Case study   Divorce

ASSESSMENT OF THE INDIVIDUAL AND THE PROBLEM

Margie, an extremely attractive young woman in the process of divorce from her third husband, was referred to a crisis center for help because of severe depression and anxiety. This was manifested by insomnia, lack of appetitie, tremulousness, inability to concentrate, and frequent crying spells. These symptoms had begun 3 weeks earlier when she was notified of the date of the divorce proceedings. She had lost her job because she was unable to control her crying spells and had subsequently developed bursitis in her shoulder, which further limited her ability to work. Her symptoms had intensified so much in the past 3 days that she felt she was losing complete control over her emotions and needed help.

During the initial session, Margie stated that she did not want a divorce and that she still loved her husband, even though he did not love her. When questioned about the increased intensity of symptoms that had begun 3 days ago, she stated that at that time she had been informed by her attorney that the only way she could receive alimony would be to countersue for divorce.

In Margie's previous two divorces she had remained a passive participant; her husbands had sued her for divorce. She had accepted this and had not contested. Now, for the first time, due to her inability to work she was forced to become an active participant in a divorce she did not want. She stated frequently that "something must be wrong with me if I can't hold a husband," and later commented, "I don't feel this is a good marriage—but I hate to fail again." This ambivalence and her expressed guilt feelings were believed to be part of the crisis-precipitating event, as was the necessity of being forced to take an active part in a divorce she did not want.

As a result of the assessment, the therapist thought that, although Margie was depressed and expressed feelings of worthlessness, she was not suicidal and did not constitute a threat to others.

PLANNING OF THERAPEUTIC INTERVENTION

Margie had almost totally withdrawn from her social and family contacts. Her mother came occasionally to give her money for rent and bring her food. Beyond this social contact she remained isolated in the apartment she had previously shared with her husband, weeping at intervals, staring at her husband's picture, and unable to decide whether or not to contest the divorce.

Since she had not been forced into active decision making in her previous divorces, she had no coping experiences in this specific situation. When questioned about her previous methods of coping with stress, she stated that usually she had no problems because she remained involved in her work and its many social contacts, usually bowling and going to bars with friends. Her present inability to work eliminated these sources of social support, distractions from the problem, and her previous successful coping mechanisms could not be used.

The goal of intervention was established by the therapist to assist Margie to recognize and cope with her feelings of ambivalence and guilt. Unrecognized feelings about her marriage and the impending divorce were also to be explored.

INTERVENTION

In the next 3 weeks, through direct questioning and reflection of verbal and nonverbal clues to Margie, it became possible for her to view the present crisis and its effect on her in relationship to her previous marriages and divorces.

Margie wanted desperately to marry in order to become a housewife and mother. Her usual social contacts and previous patterns of meeting men (bowling alleys and bars) and her impulsive marriages (Las Vegas, three times) and reasons for marriage ("I thought I could help him—he needed me") were not meeting this need. The men she had met and married, and who later divorced her, were men who did not want to "settle down" with a wife and children. Instead, they wanted a fun-loving, attractive companion to show off to their friends. Margie always hoped that they would change after marriage. However, they remained unchanged and divorced Margie when she persistently suggested "starting a family." With each marriage and subsequent divorce her guilt feelings about her ability to be a good wife magnified. Since Margie could not use her previous coping mechanisms, the third divorce precipitated a crisis.

After the third session Margie's depression and symptoms had lessened as she recognized the possibility that the failure of her marriages may not have been in her "inability to be a good wife" but in the disparity between what she wanted and expected from a marriage and what the men she had married wanted and expected.

ANTICIPATORY PLANNING

Exploration with Margie about her usual modes of social contact and her impulsive marriages (usually after only 3 or 4 weeks' courtship) assisted her in viewing her current divorce in more realistic terms. This was an important phase in anticipatory planning.

By the fourth week Margie had made significant changes in her patterns of living. She moved from the apartment she had previously shared with her husband to a small house near her mother. She also signed the papers to contest the divorce and found a new job.

Margie was granted the divorce and was apparently able to view her past experience as a traumatic but valuable learning experience.

In discussion and review with Margie of her future plans, she was cautious but realistic. She was enjoying her new job and new friends, going to movies and occasionally dinner with girl friends. She stated that she was not accepting dates from men yet, "although I've been asked" and that if she married again, "it would not be in Las Vegas!"

Before termination Margie and the therapist reviewed and assessed the adjustments she had made in coping with the crisis, the insight she had gained into her own feelings, and her needs regarding future plans.

At termination Margie was reassured that she could obtain assistance in any future crisis that might occur.

CASE STUDY: MARGIE

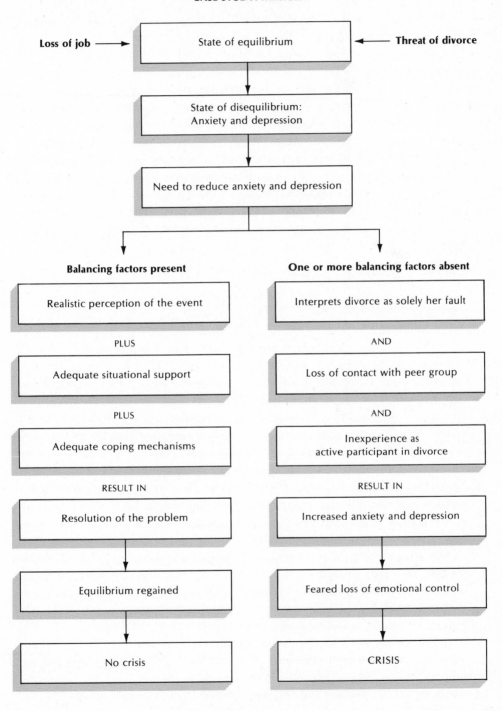

Loss of job ⟶ State of equilibrium ⟵ **Threat of divorce**

State of disequilibrium:
Anxiety and depression

Need to reduce anxiety and depression

Balancing factors present

Realistic perception of the event

PLUS

Adequate situational support

PLUS

Adequate coping mechanisms

RESULT IN

Resolution of the problem

Equilibrium regained

No crisis

One or more balancing factors absent

Interprets divorce as solely her fault

AND

Loss of contact with peer group

AND

Inexperience as
active participant in divorce

RESULT IN

Increased anxiety and depression

Feared loss of emotional control

CRISIS

SUMMATION OF THE PARADIGM

Margie's inability to cope with a third divorce was precipitated by the lack of her usual situational supports, that is, her involvement and social contacts at work. This was also the first time Margie was forced into the role of an active participant in the divorce process, and she had no previous coping skills. Her inability to work as a result of illness further isolated her from her usual contacts, and she began to introspect about her previous divorces and saw herself as a failure as a woman. As her doubts increased, her feelings of guilt and failure magnified until she feared complete loss of emotional control.

The intervention ws focused on encouraging Margie to bring her feelings of failure and guilt into the open. By direct questioning and reflecting the information back to Margie it became possible for her to view her current divorce and its effect on her in more realistic terms. She was given support by the therapist as she began to explore what she wanted and expected from marriage in the future.

Cocaine: substance abuse—theoretical concepts

Cocaine is a vegetable alkaloid derived from leaves of the coca plant. It is often referred to as Coke, C, snow, happy dust, and white girl. Cocaine is fast becoming the all-American drug. No longer is it a sinful secret of the moneyed elite or an exclusive glitter of decadence in raffish society circles. Today, in part because it is such an emblem of wealth and status, cocaine is the drug of choice for millions of solid, conventional, and upwardly mobile citizens—lawyers, businessmen, students, bureaucrats, politicians, secretaries, bankers, real estate brokers, and waitresses.

Superficially, cocaine appears to be a beguiling and relatively risk-free drug—so its devotees innocently claim. But cocaine can be a very dangerous drug. Although in very small and occasional doses cocaine is no more harmful than equally moderate doses of alcohol or marijuana, the euphoric lift, the feeling of being confident and on top of things that comes from a few brief "snorts," is often followed by a letdown, and regular use can induce depression, edginess, and weight loss. As usage increases, so does the danger of paranoia, hallucinations, and a total physical collapse. And usage does tend to increase.

Cocaine is classified as a narcotic, as are opium, heroin, and morphine. The last three are "downers," which quiet the body and dull the senses, whereas cocaine is an "upper," a stimulant, similar to amphetamines. It increases the heartbeat, raises the blood pressure and body temperature, and curbs the appetite. Unlike such downers as heroin and Quaaludes, cocaine is physically nonaddictive. It can, however, damage the liver, cause malnutrition, and increase the risk of heart attacks. Coming down from a high may cause such deep gloom that the only remedy is more cocaine. Bigger doses often follow, and soon the urge may become a total obsession. This pattern can lead to a psychological dependence, the effects of which are not all that different from physical addiction. There is growing clinical evidence that when cocaine is taken in the most potent and dangerous forms—injected in solution or chemically converted and smoked in a process called freebasing—it may become addictive.

A cocaine high is an intensely vivid, sensation-enhancing experience; there is no evidence, as claimed, that it is an aphrodisiac. There is evidence that the sustained use of cocaine can cause sexual dysfunction and impotence. Even casual sniffing can lead to more potent and potentially damaging ways of using cocaine and other drugs. Many cocaine users take sedative pills such as Quaaludes to calm them down after the high and to take the edge off their yearning for more cocaine. A few smoke marijuana for the same purpose or mix their cocaine with heroin in a process called speedballing or boy-girl. The latter produces a tug-of-war in which the exhilaration of cocaine is undercut by the heroin.

A few middle-class users who dabble with heroin in conjunction with cocaine smoke it rather than inject it; they believe this prevents addiction. This is false; heroin, however used, is a fiercely addictive drug. Treatment centers are receiving an influx of well-dressed, well-to-do men and women who have gravely underestimated heroin's effects. One of cocaine's biggest dangers is that it diverts people from normal pursuits; it can entrap and redirect people's activities into an almost exclusive preoccupation with the drug.

Little likelihood exists that the cocaine blizzard will soon abate. A drug habit born of a desire to escape the bad news in life is not likely to be discouraged by the bad news about the drug itself. Middle-class Americans will continue to succumb to the powder's crystalline dazzle. Few are yet aware or willing to concede that, at the very least, taking cocaine is dangerous to their psychological health (Demarest, 1981).

Today's drug was yesterday's drug as well; we are now experiencing the third or fourth cocaine epidemic. Historically, it dates back 5000 years. Its real claims to fame occurred in the nineteenth century. Angelo Mariani, a Corsican chemist, may have come the closest to "turning the world on" by inventing an elixir with coca and alcohol. Numerous medical giants including Freud, Koller, Corning, Halsted, Crile, and Cushing praised the merits of the discovery of the age; its benefit to mankind would be incalculable. Its opponents labeled it the third scourge of mankind (after alcohol and morphine). The *New York Times* stated that it wrecks its victim more swiftly and surely than opium. Coca-Cola went "clean," replacing coca with caffeine. In the Harrison Tax Act (1914) cocaine was erroneously classified as a narcotic, and since then debate has continued about its abuse and addictive potential.

In the United States between 1975 and 1980 the number of individuals seeking treatment for cocaine abuse increased fivefold, the number of emergency room admissions fourfold, and the number of deaths fourfold. At least 1 million are now profoundly dependent on cocaine, a new corps more numerous than heroin addicts. About 10% of high school seniors are regular users. Cocaine has become a $25 billion business, ranking it in sales among the top 10 U.S. companies. No longer is it the recreational drug of the affluent; 20% of blue collar workers engage in frequent cocaine misuse. Men outnumber women by a 2:1 ratio. The emerging profile appears to be a white, college-educated man in his 30s with an annual income of $25,000. Recent bumper crops in South America will alter the supply-demand ratio to lower the price and augment the already massively escalating epidemic.

Cocaine is readily absorbed from all mucous membranes, although concomitant local vasoconstriction limits its rate of absorption. Despite this fact, absorption may easily exceed the rate of detoxification and excretion, leading to high toxicity. Cocaine undergoes rapid biotransformation in the body. Its two main metabolites, ecgonine and benzoylecgonine, are excreted in the urine in amounts equivalent to one fourth to one half the original dose within 24 to 36 hours. Depending on urine acidity, 10% to 20% of cocaine is excreted unchanged. Addicts attempt to enhance excretion to avoid detection by consuming large volumes of cranberry juice or ingesting megadoses of vitamin C. Physicians treat in similar fashion with intravenous ammonium chloride. After 100 mg of intravenous cocaine, a plasma peak occurs at 5 minutes and the distributional half-life is 20 to 40 minutes. The most popular routes for abuse purposes are intranasal (snorting), intravenous (running), and free-basing inhalation (smoking) (Hankes, 1984).

Cocaine is a beguiling drug that does not result in hangovers, lung cancer, or holes in the arm. Instead, a user takes a snort and for the next 20 to 30 minutes there is an increase in drive, sparkle, and energy without a feeling of being drugged. Reported subjective effects include mood elevation to the point of euphoria, decrease in hunger, increases in energy and sociability, indifference to pain, and significant decrease in fatigue. Users experience a feeling of great muscular strength and increased mental capacity leading to an overestimation of their capabilities. The powerful experience of the cocaine high can lead the user into a pattern of regular and escalating use. The most commonly reported side effects of regular use include anxiety, dysphoria, suspiciousness, disruption in eating and sleeping habits, weight loss, fatigue, irritability, concentration difficulties, and perceptual problems. Increasing use may lead to hyperexcitability, marked agitation, paranoia, hypertension, and tachycardia. As the individual becomes more and more "strung out," alcohol, other sedatives, or narcotics are often taken to combat the overstimulation. Paranoid psychoses are manifested by a variety of symptoms such as visual distortion and hallucinations ("snow lights," geometric patterns), tactile hallucinations (sensation of insects on, in, or under the skin—cocaine "bugs"), delusions (being chased by the police—"bull horrors"), and violent behavior. Cocaine interacts with the catecholamine neurotransmitters, norepinephrine and dopamine, and alters normal interneuronal communication. It augments the effects of these catecholamines, probably by blocking (or prolonging) reuptake at the synaptic junction, leaving an excess of these neurotransmitters to restimulate receptors. Dopamine is a precursor of norepinephrine and is found in the corpus striatum—part of the network governing motor functions—and in that portion of the hypothalamus regulating thirst and hunger. Norepinephrine is the prime neurotransmitter of the ascending reticular activating system (RAS), regulating mechanisms of external attention and arousal. It acts as a vital transmitter as well in the hypothalamus, which regulates body temperature, sleep, and sexual arousal and, in general, mediates emotional depression. It also mediates neural activation in the median forebrain bundle of the hypothalamus, which is believed to serve as an individual's "pleasure center."

When we look at a drug taken, but not prescribed, for a mood or behavioral change, we consider the following: first, the potential for overdose; second, the potential for acute toxicity; third, physical derangements; fourth, its effects on mental status; and fifth, behavioral modification. That is, how much does it incapacitate a person or hinder his or her ability to function in an environment that was not a preexisting problem? Acute consequences include hyperpyrexia; hypertension with possible cerebrovascular accident (CVA), arrhythmia, or myocardial infarct; accidents because of impaired judgment and timing; and the dangers that lurk around some less than desirable purchase zones. Seizures are common and often progress to status epilepticus. Chronic complications depend on purity, route of administration, sterility, and frequency of use. Users confuse cleanliness with sterility. One of the frequent chronic medical complications is not strictly medical but dental. Cocaine is a powerful local anesthetic and users neglect their teeth, often presenting with missing fillings, holes in teeth, loose teeth, impaction with inflammation, and even periodontal abscesses. A detailed oral examination is mandatory. Malnutrition is common because food intake is ignored. Most patients are thin, rarely obese, and some are emaciated; 73% have at least 1 major vitamin deficiency, usually pyridoxine followed by thiamine and then ascorbic acid. Intranasal users develop rhinorrhea, nasal septal necrosis and perforation, hoarseness, aspiration pneumonia, and frontal sinusitis. Routine chest and frontal sinus x-ray examinations are suggested. Freebasing often results in burns from explosion of the volatile ether used in preparation of the base. Chronic smoking patients should be evaluated with pulmonary function tests. Intravenous users are subject to infections of the skin, lung, heart valves, brain, and eye with multiple unusual bacteria and fungi. Some 86% of intravenous coke users have antibody evidence of prior exposure to hepatitis B. Talc and silicone adulterants produce granuloma formation in the lungs, liver, brain, and eye. Cocaine is metabolized by the liver and excreted by the kidney; any preexisting dysfunction will exacerbate most conditions previously discussed.

Patients will often "tank up" just before admission, that is, use very large doses in anticipation of cold turkey withdrawal. This increases the toxicity potential, and some centers are reluctant to admit on weekends and nights unless medical supervision is available. The lethal dose of cocaine is about 1.2 gm, but severe toxicity has occurred with an average dose of 20 mg. Tolerance and route of administration play an important role in the lethal dose. Sudden death from cocaine is so sudden that the only medical person to see the patient is often the coroner. Death occurs from status epilepticus, respiratory paralysis, myocardial infarction or irritability, and rarely anaphylaxis. It does not appear that antiepileptic medications will reduce or block cocaine-related seizures. The combined chronic lack of sleep and throat anesthesia may interact to cause a deep "crash" (sleep), which is accompanied by airway obstruction (suffocation) induced by a flaccid jaw or failure to remove secretions (drowning). The number of deaths involving cocaine with other drugs also has rapidly increased but not as much as cocaine-related homicide victims. Death can and does occur in young people who drink and use cocaine. The cocaine keeps the person awake enough to continue drinking and try to drive home; the cocaine wears off before the alcohol and the high blood alcohol level oversedates, causing a fatal accident. Often only the blood alcohol level is analyzed, falsely attributing the death to alcohol alone. Concomitant use of narcotics in an attempt to boost the cocaine high, or to self-medicate its side effects, often results in disaster. Finally, another factor involved in cocaine-related deaths is cocaine-related suicides. These dependent individuals feel hopeless and helpless. Suicide may be seen as the only solution to deteriorating health and personal-domestic-financial situations. However, fear of disability or disease from various sources will not deter use, since most users discount these medical reports or doubt that any disability or disease will happen to them (Hankes, 1984).

The life-style that civilized people generally accept as normal involves major efforts to obtain and enjoy food, water, shelter, friendship, and a sexual partner. Brain researchers assume that a major function of the brain's reinforcement centers is to make it possible for the individual to strive to achieve these goals despite the fact that their availability is limited. Cocaine's main danger is its bypassing of the normal reinforcement process. In doing this, it reprograms or reprioritizes the person so that getting cocaine is supreme and all normal drives are subverted. People and their cocaine problems can be separated on the basis of access. Pharmacists and doctors who have tried cocaine or who have access to pharmaceutical cocaine have a special kind of problem. People who have a lot of disposable income (such as athletes and entertainers) have a different problem—unlimited access; they can easily end up addicted. Cocaine is a drug of disposable income—what you have the drug will soon dispose of. The remainder of the population of users may be temporarily saved from this fate by lack of resources or access. But if the price drops or availability changes, all bets are off.

Many physicians and users debate whether cocaine is addicting, the underlying premise being that if it is not addicting, it is not dangerous. The state of the art definition of addiction encompasses three concepts: compulsive use, loss of control in the face of the drug, and continued use despite adverse consequences. Using this definition, cocaine is obviously very, very addicting. It lends itself to reinforcement. Toxic manifestations do not even curtail use. Taking cocaine stimulates taking cocaine. Drug-craving and drug-seeking behavior are notable with cocaine, clearly indicating a high level of psychological dependence. It is this effect, coupled with cocaine's property to reinforce its own abuse, that leads to disaster. Regular users, especially high dose snorters, freebasers, and injectors, generally want to maintain the elation. Cocaine's price and pharmacology do not lend themselves to a self-regulated maintenance program. So if price and access can be conquered, users may "base" continuously for days or inject intravenously every 10 minutes. For some, the anxiety, suspiciousness, and hypervigilance become overwhelming. Even as the user comes down and recalls the paranoid experience, he will generally start up again with the notion that this time he will stop short of insanity. Success-oriented people who rarely use drugs may discover cocaine and in less than 2 or 3 years find themselves hopelessly involved in illicit activities or facing incarceration. Consistent use can result in a severe depressive reaction, which may be due to depletion of norepinephrine stores. This may lead to another temporary "cure" perpetuating the habit. Others with mild depression will self-medicate with cocaine. They quickly learn that they are nothing and that the drug is everything. Any subsequent success is misattributed to the drug, and these abusers come to believe that normal functioning without the drug is nearly impossible (Garwin and Kepler, 1984).

Acute cocaine reaction. Medical intervention must be without hesitation and directed to support of cardiovascular and respiratory functions. Needed are a source of positive pressure ventilation, supplemental oxygen, proper endotracheal equipment, suction, a stretcher that will allow the Trendelenburg position, intravenous infusion lines, continuous ECG monitor, and proper medications. All drugs should be titrated to clinical need. For signs of advancing central nervous system stimulation, 2.5 to 5.0 mg diazepam may be given intravenously and repeated as many as 4 times at 5-minute intervals. If impending disaster is perceived, the ultrashort-acting barbiturate, thiopental, 50 to 100 mg, along with the depolarizing muscle relaxant, succinylcholine, 40 to 100 mg, may be given for immediate control of the airway and ablation of convulsive movement. Should tachycardia, hypertension, or ventricular ectopy appear, 1 mg propranolol by intravenous bolus may be given. This may be repeated 6 times at 1-minute intervals. Titrate to a diastolic pressure of about 90, and an apical/radial pulse around or less than 100. Lidocaine may be employed to suppress ventricular ectopy in a dosage of 50 to 100 mg intravenous bolus; keep intravenous lines open in order to administer 2 to 4 mg lidocaine per minute, as needed. Core temperature should be monitored with a cooling blanket, fans, and cold sponging available. Metabolic acidosis should be treated with bicarbonate. In administering drugs, remember the dangerously high levels of catecholamines. Central nervous system and cardiovascular events must be scrupulously watched.

Chronic cocaine toxicity. A commonly seen clinical phenomenon is a patient 3 to 14 days into a binge who exhibits signs of late State I (premonitory to the collapse of Stages II and III). These individuals show hyperkinetic behavior, tachycardia, hypertension, tachypnea, dyspnea, tics, jerks, tremors, stereotypical movements, distorted perception, and, possibly, violent protective behavior, which is delusional. Such patients are at prime risk for cardiac arrhythmia, cerebrovascular accident and high output congestive heart failure. Such cases of adrenergic or dopaminergic storm have been found to respond dramatically to the lytic effects of propanolol. Again, careful monitoring is mandatory. Give propanolol either in slow intravenous increments of 1 mg at 1-minute intervals up to a total of 6 mg or orally in a dosage of 40 to 80 mg at 4- to 6-hour intervals for a period of up to 1 week with a pulse of 90 or less the goal. Give sips of 5% glucose solution or perhaps cranberry juice rich in benzoic acid. Acidify urine with IV ammonium chloride at 75 mg/kg four times daily, with a maximum dose of 6 gm per day. Administer diazepam at bedtime. Using the IV method, the hyperkinetic state will be reversed within 3 to 5 minutes and within 20 to 40 minutes following oral medication. The use of phenothiazines and haloperidol have been specifically avoided because of their propensity to lower seizure threshold. The tricyclic antidepressants are avoided because of the danger of the appearance of true life-threatening arrhythmias in an already sensitized patient.

Withdrawal. The actual existence of physiological dependency and a related cocaine abstinence syndrome is widely debated; yet a relatively consistent withdrawal syndrome is observed following cessation of chronic use. It consists of irritability, alternating anxiety and depression, boredom, perceptual problems, inability to concentrate, hypersomnia, fatigue, and intense drug craving. Medical detoxification should be accomplished in an inpatient medically supervised setting. Premature departures against medical advice occur most frequently at 24 and 96 hours. These are the times when drug craving is most intense, paranoid ideation increases, and intolerance to rigid treatment unit regulations surfaces. The science of "ART" should be employed: "A"—Acceptance as a caring, understanding intermediary is essential; "R"—Reduction of stimuli; rest and reassurance will diminish most disruptive behavior; "T"—"Talkdown" technique with sincere concern and gentle manipulation will abort hostile actions. Initial restrictions should include no pass-phone-visitor privileges. After 2 days daytime naps are not allowed. The night personnel often need extra staffing to handle the increased hallway traffic then. L-tryptophan, 2 gm before meals three times daily, and 4 gm at bedtime with a carbohydrate snack is an effective aid to sleep. Tyrosine is being studied as an adjunctive measure. Vigorous structured physical activity plays an important role also.

Diazepam appears to be the ideal sedative for the over-amped cocaine user. Oral dosage of 10 to 20 mg every 6 to 8 hours is quite effective.

Postdetoxification. Does cocaine addiction require a specific therapeutic program? This is an unsettled question. More often than not, the traditional 28-day inpatient alcoholism program is the only available resource. Administrators of such programs frequently do not want to handle cocaine abusers because they believe cocaine abuse is a completely different problem. Although it is true that it is overly simplistic to lump all addictions under the umbrella of "chemical dependency," the striking similarities between cocaine addiction and alcoholism merit treating both in similar fashion. Both are culturally accepted, and although cocaine is illegal, its use generally does not occur within the same milieu as the other illicit drugs, especially the narcotics. These considerations as well as the existence of any polydrug abuse should be noted when structuring and tailoring a treatment plan specifically for cocaine addiction. In the meantime, traditional inpatient alcoholism programs appear to have the most to offer the cocaine addict. Didactic education, individual and group counseling, cognitive restructuring based on reality therapy, family therapy, and ongoing participation in posttreatment self-help groups are essential ingredients of an effective treatment program.

Cocaine addiction is viewed by "addictionologists" as a primary disease of multifactorial etiology. The addiction is not merely a symptom of underlying psychopathology. This is a critical distinction. For therapy to be successful, treatment must focus on the toxic consequences of cocaine. The goal must be a cocaine-free recovery. To accomplish this, the treatment team helps the patient find positive and constructive alternatives to deal with the drug hunger, emphasizing that any attempt to return to the drug is a relapse. Once an addictive disease is established, the person cannot return to any recreational use; total abstinence is required (Laurie, 1971).

Case study   *Cocaine abuse*

ASSESSMENT OF THE INDIVIDUAL AND THE PROBLEM

Late one Thursday afternoon, Steve D., an open-heart surgeon, called his friend, who was a psychotherapist. He was quite concerned that no one hear their conversation; he wanted to talk to his friend but not at the hospital where other staff members might see him. They made arrangements for him to meet with her at her home early that evening.

The therapist recalled that Dr. D. had a very distinguished background; his father, grandfather, and great-grandfather had been highly respected physicians; he was a Phi Beta Kappa from a well-known and distinguished eastern school, had graduated magna cum laude, had married an intelligent and attractive woman, had three lovely children, had finished at the top of his class, and had done his residency with a famous cardiologist-surgeon. Everyone, including peers, nursing staff, and patients, respected and liked him. In other words, he had everything going for him.

When Dr. D. arrived at his friend's home, she immediately noticed that he was tense and trembling. Then he lit a ciagarette, which she had never seen him do before; he had always disapproved of smoking. He seemed hesitant about telling the therapist what was wrong. She reminded him that she could not help him if she did not know what the problem was, and he obviously had a problem.

Steve began by telling her that he had been indefinitely suspended from the hospital staff. His explanation started with his internship when the hours were long and the physical and emotional demands were constant. He started using cocaine then, "not every day or night—just when I was so tired I didn't think I could keep my eyes open from fatigue and complete exhaustion." The therapist was shocked and saddened by his confession, but she made no outward sign of her feelings and told him to continue his story. The residency had been very difficult; Steve had felt that nothing he did pleased the surgeon. However, when the residency was completed, the surgeon wrote a "glowing report," which stated that Steve had a "brilliant career" ahead of him and that he had been the surgeon's most outstanding resident. Steve told the therapist he had used cocaine while he was a resident, maybe a little more than when he was an intern but still not every day.

The therapist asked how he was using it and he replied, "I was just snorting it—then." She asked about the present, and he said, "Now I am smoking it—freebasing—and injecting it." He also said that he was not combining heroin with it when he injected it, because he was "not that crazy." He had been freebasing for about 2½ years and injecting a little over a year.

She asked Steve who found out about his cocaine use and when. He started pacing up and down and asked for a drink. Since he admitted smoking some coke right before coming to see her, the therapist refused his request. She became very firm with him and offered him a choice of answering her questions right then or leaving. After only a moment's hesitation, the doctor started talking. He had scheduled a triple bypass on a patient for the previous Monday morning. He explained that he never injected himself for three days before surgery, but he did freebase. He made it a point to be scrubbed early, before anyone else was around, and gowned so no one could see his arms (with tracks from injecting the cocaine). He said everything was going well in surgery on this particular morning until he accidentally cut his finger with a scalpel. He added that he had been a little shaky that morning for some reason (probably because of his heavy use of cocaine). One of his partners took his place to continue the surgery, and he went out to rescrub. Unfortunately, Dr. A., the chief of staff, was in the scrub room when Steve entered. Steve stripped his gloves and gown off and started to rescrub at a basin as far from

Dr. A. as possible. Dr. A. asked him why he was rescrubbing, and Steve explained that he had cut his finger. Dr. A. asked to see his finger. Steve quickly held up his hand and said it was nothing. However, the other doctor apparently saw the tracks on Steve's arm and quietly but firmly asked him to hold out both his arms. Steve did as he was asked, and Dr. A. looked at his arms and told him to stay where he was. Dr. A. then called for a resident to replace Steve in surgery and told Steve to cancel all his appointments for the rest of the week and wait for Dr. A. in his office. Dr. A. arrived at his office and asked Steve what he had been shooting up on, how long, and why. After Steve related his story, Dr. A. told him he had no excuse for doing it—they were all dealing with human lives and could not afford to make even one mistake. Dr. A. called an emergency staff meeting of the ethics committee for an hour later. He made it clear that he was doing nothing to help Steve, who was to "try to explain" his behavior to the committee members.

Steve stopped talking at this point and had to be prodded into continuing. He said the committee meeting was "horrible," that the persons attending "stared at me as if they had never seen me before." All they had asked him was how much he was using and where he got his supply (by writing prescriptions for nonexistent patients). They informed him that he would have to enter a substance abuse facility and stay there until he was determined "clean" by the discharge clinic staff. He was automatically suspended from hospital privileges immediately. If he did not report to a facility by the end of the week, they would notify the Board of Medical Quality Assurance and his license to practice medicine would be revoked. The therapist asked him if he were going to do as the committee had told him or not by the next day. He replied. "I don't know. That's why I had to talk to you—can't you work with me and get me over the need to use coke?" She answered firmly, "Absolutely not—it can't be done!" She explained that the amount he used, the methods, and the length of time all made outpatient psychotherapy inappropriate and dangerous. She told him he could die trying to get "clean" himself.

At that point Steve said, "It would be better if I were dead." His friend pointed out to him that he would be leaving his wife and children a terrible legacy. She told him that he could continue to be a famous surgeon, but that it would not be easy. She then asked if he had discussed the matter with his wife, Jennifer, and he said no.

The therapist sent Steve home to talk to his wife and told him to bring her back with him that night. While he was gone, she would make some plans for him. He agreed to do as she said.

PLANNING THE THERAPEUTIC INTERVENTION

The first step would be to talk with Steve and Jennifer together to determine if his wife would stand by the decision that he enter a substance abuse facility. The next step would be to contact the best facility the therapist knew to see if a private

CASE STUDY: STEVE

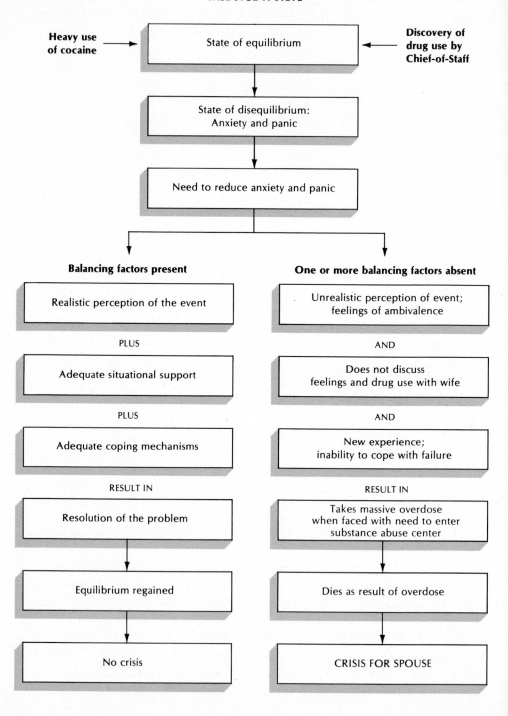

room was available for Steve. She also needed to know if he could be admitted that night. The facility under consideration was approximately 100 to 125 miles away. The therapist did not think Steve would willingly accept a facility in the city.

INTERVENTION

The psychotherapist called the substance abuse facility and related her story to the director, Mr. B., a friend of hers. Mr. B. informed her that he definitely had a room and suggested that Steve might want to use an assumed name while there. He agreed that Steve and Jennifer should come that night; he would make the train reservations and would pick them up.

Steve returned to the therapist's home with his wife. Jennifer was shaken by what her husband had told her, but she said they were very willing to do anything that the therapist suggested to help her husband. The therapist told them to make arrangements immediately to go to the facility that night. She told Steve that she would talk to the chief of staff and inform him of Steve's decision. Before leaving, Jennifer requested therapy after she returned from the facility; she did not understand how her husband could have become involved in using cocaine.

After they left, the therapist called Dr. A. and told him what had happened that evening. He asked her what she felt the chances were for Steve to come out of his addiction really "clean," with no desire to go back on cocaine. She responded that if he could get through the first week, he *might* make it. The length of time he had been using it and the methods he used made a more optimistic response impossible. However, the therapist felt they had done all they could for him.

During the night the therapist received a call from the director of the facility. He informed her that Steve had died on the train; he had apparently "tanked up" and died in his sleep. Jennifer had been admitted to the hospital in a state of shock.

ANTICIPATORY PLANNING

Since nothing could be done for Steve, anticipatory planning would involve helping his wife and children through the grief and mourning process. They would have to rebuild their lives without him.

SUMMATION OF THE PARADIGM

Dr. Steve D. was accustomed to success, to being "the best at everything he tried." His use of cocaine, which became heavy and dangerous, was discovered by his chief-of-staff. Suddenly he was faced with entering a substance abuse facility or having his license revoked. He agreed to enter a facility but was ambivalent because of his heavy use. He did not use his available situational support, his wife. He took a massive overdose and died on the way to the facility. This left his wife in a state of crisis.

Suicide—theoretical concepts

Each year suicide accounts for more than 13.3 deaths per 100,000 population in the United States, which makes it a leading cause of death. It ranks second as a cause of death for adolescents and college students. Although this death rate has remained relatively stable during the past decade, suicide attempts, suicide threats, drug overdoses, and other forms of self-destructive behavior have increased dramatically. At large general hospitals a night rarely goes by in any emergency room without at least one admission for attempted suicide.

The most common form of attempted suicide is the ingestion of a sedative or hypnotic drug. Suicide attempts by other methods, such as hanging, wrist cutting or other body mutilation, gas inhalation, gunshot wounds, and jumping from high places, are less frequent.

In addition to actual suicide attempts, other persons are referred or brought to hospitals or mental health centers because they have threatened suicide or because they have demonstrated some form of self-destructive behavior, such as running into highway traffic or threatening to jump from a bridge or freeway overpass.

Regardless of how the suicidal behavior is manifested, the basic question remains, "Why suicide?" There is no single answer to this question. The complex motivations, weaknesses, and strengths that determine all types of human behavior apply also to suicide. Consequently there are many roads that individuals may take in reaching a decision to commit suicide. Usually the process is long, and often it is complicated by other physical and emotional symptoms of distress. Despite the multiplicity of causes and patterns, suicidal behavior can usually be related to three primary motivations: loss of communication, ambivalence about life and death, and the effects of suicidal behavior on significant others.

Communication

Usually, suicidal reactions are associated with feelings of hopelessness and helplessness and are often related to the separation or loss of a significant or valued relationship. Suicidal behavior can best be understood as an expression of intense feelings when other forms of expression have failed. The expression of feelings can range from sad cries for help to desperate statements of despair. A suicidal person is driven to this act because he feels unable to cope with a problem and believes that others are not responding to his need. The suicidal behavior becomes expressed verbally or by actions. Either directly or indirectly, the communication is frequently aimed at a specific person—the significant other. Recognizing the intent of the disguised message and understanding its real content becomes a problem for the recipient when the message is indirectly communicated.

Ambivalence

Only a small number of people who threaten or attempt suicide actually succeed. The general explanation for an incomplete or partially effective suicidal act is that the individual is filled with contradictory feelings about living and dying. This state is termed "ambivalence." One should realize that ambivalence is a universal human trait. We all have it at times, and it is not a weakness. Everyone feels ambivalence over decisions at one time or another, in choosing a career, a spouse, or a place to live. The choice of a place and time to die is no exception. In making the decision of whether to live or die one would expect to find even more than the normal amount of ambivalence. This psychological characteristic accounts for the sometimes puzzling fact that a person will take a lethal or near-lethal action and then counterbalance it with some provision for rescue. The very fact that every person is divided within himself over decisions provides the chance for successful intervention with a suicidal patient. By making use of the patient's wish to live, his "cry for help," suicide may be averted. The myth that "if a person talks about suicide, he won't do it" is actually that—a myth. Every statement or ideation of the wish to die should be taken seriously and explored with the individual.

Effects on others

Suicidal behavior can be further understood in terms of its effect on those receiving the communication. A suicidal attempt may arouse feelings of sympathy, anxiety, anger, or hostility on the part of the individual's family or friends and therefore serve to manipulate relationships. The therapist may also experience similar feelings unless he or she can anticipate and counteract these reactions. The therapist must resist the desire to be omnipotent. No one is truly omnipotent, just as no one can solve all the problems and meet all the demands of every patient. This is especially true when dealing with intensely dependent patients who often attribute tremendous powers to the potential rescuer.

Many suicidal situations will arouse feelings of anxiety and self-doubt in the therapist about her own ability to handle them. Although a moderate level of anxiety is appropriate, too much may seriously hamper the effort to help, especially if it is transmitted to the patient, who is depending on someone to help him solve his problems. Already feeling helpless and lost, the suicidal person who perceives excessive anxiety may lose hope of being helped and may bluntly state so. As in any form of intervention, the therapist develops confidence in her ability with training and experience.

Suicidal potential

Before considering the factors that influence the probability of suicide, the therapist should consider her own attitudes toward suicide and death because they definitely affect how she will function with patients. Death is a process and is a part of life and living. From the moment one is born, movement toward death begins. Unfortunately, Western cultures have surrounded death with many powerful taboos. The feelings that these taboos can arouse may very well interfere in the therapist's interactions with her patients. She must be sensitive to her own thoughts about death and suicide, and regardless of personal attitudes, she must avoid any moralistic judgments about what has happened. The professional point of view must be that death is to be prevented, if possible. A therapist will often be placed in the position of actually debating life and death questions with upset people. Although she must recognize the existence and merits of other viewpoints, her role is to represent life and to assist distressed, helpless people.

From the first conversation with a suicidal individual, a therapist immediately assumes some responsibility for preventing the suicide. In working out some plan for prevention, the therapist must first determine the individual's suicidal potential, that is, the degree of probability that the person will try to kill himself in the immediate or near future. In some individuals the suicidal potential will be minimal, whereas in others it will be immediate and great. The therapist must decide the degree of risk for each patient.

The prediction of suicide is by no means an exact science. Even the most experienced therapist can be misled in assessing a problem. However, certain criteria allow suicidal potential to be evaluated with some assurance. Assessment of suicidal potential depends on obtaining detailed information about the patient in each of the following categories.

Age and sex. Statistics indicate that women attempt suicide more often than men but that men commit suicide more often than women. Currently, this trend is changing as women are beginning to feel the same stresses in their changing social roles as men feel. They are also beginning to use more lethal methods in their suicide attempts. It is also known that the rate for completed suicide rises with increasing age. Consequently, an older man presents the greatest threat of actual suicide and a young woman, the least. Within this framework age and sex offer a general, though by no means clear-cut, basis for evaluating suicidal potential. One must remember that young women and young men do kill themselves, even though their original aim was to manipulate other people. Each case requires individual appraisal.

Suicidal plan. How an individual plans to take his life is one of the most significant criteria in assessing suicidal potential. The therapist must consider the following three elements:

1. Is it a relatively lethal method? An individual who intends to commit suicide with a gun, by jumping from a tall building or bridge, or by hanging is a far greater risk than someone who plans to take pills or cut her wrists. Since the person who plans either of the latter two methods is amenable to treatment or resuscitation, these methods are less lethal than the irrevocable consequences of putting a gun to one's head.

2. Does the individual have the means available? It must be determined if the method of suicide the individual has considered is in fact available to her. An actual threat to use a gun, if the person has one, is obviously more serious than the same threat without a gun.

3. Is the suicide plan specific? Can the individual say exactly when she plans to do it (for example, after the children are asleep)? If she has spent time thinking out details and specific preparations for her death, her suicidal risk is greatly increased. Changing a will, writing notes, collecting pills, buying a gun, and setting a time and place for suicide suggest a high risk. When a patient's plan is obviously confused or unrealistic, one should consider the possibility of an underlying psychiatric problem. A psychotic person with the idea of suicide is a particularly high risk because she may make a bizarre attempt based on her distorted thoughts. The therapist should always find out if the patient has a past history of any emotional disorder and whether she has ever been hospitalized or received other mental health care.

Stress. The therapist needs to find out about any stressful event that may have precipitated the suicidal behavior. The most common precipitating stresses are losses: the death of a loved one; divorce or separation; loss of a job, money, prestige, or status; loss of health through illness, surgery, or accident; and loss of esteem or prestige because of possible prosecution or criminal involvement. Not all stresses are the result of bereavement. Sometimes increased anxiety and tension are a result of success, such as a promotion with increased responsibilities. Always investigate any sudden change in the individual's life situation.

Learning to evaluate stress from the individual's point of view rather than from society's point of view is necessary. What may be minimal stress for the therapist could be perceived by the patient as severe stress. The relationship between stress and symptoms is useful in evaluating prognosis.

Symptoms. The most common and most important suicidal symptoms relate to depression. Typical symptoms of severe depression include loss of appetite, weight loss, inability to sleep, loss of interest, social withdrawal, apathy and despondency, severe feelings of hopelessness and helplessness, and a general attitude of physical and emotional exhaustion. Other persons may exhibit agitation through such symptoms as tension, anxiety, guilt, shame, poor impulse control, or feelings of rage, anger, hostility, or revenge. Alcoholics, homosexuals, and all substance abusers tend to be high suicidal risks.

The patient who is both agitated and depressed is particularly at high risk. Unable to tolerate the pressure of his feelings, the individual in a state of agitated depression shows marked tension, fearfulness, restlessness, and pressure of speech. He eventually reaches a point where he must act in some direction to relieve his feelings. Often he chooses suicide.

Suicidal symptoms may also occur with psychotic states. The patient may have delusions, hallucinations, distorted sensory impressions, loss of contact with reality, disorientation, or highly unusual ideas and experiences. As a baseline for assessing psychotic behavior, the therapist should use his own sense of what is real and appropriate.

Resources. The patient's environmental resources are often crucial in helping the therapist decide how to manage the immediate problem. Who are his situational supports? The therapist must find out who can be used to support him through this traumatic time: family, relatives, close friends, employers, physicians, or clergymen. To whom does he feel close? If the patient is already under the care of a therapist, the new therapist should try to contact him.

The choice of various resources is sometimes affected by the fact that the patient and the family may try to keep the suicidal situation a secret, even to the point of denying its existence. As a general rule, this attempt at secrecy and denial must be counteracted by dealing with the suicidal situation openly and frankly. It is usually better, both for the therapist and the patient, if the responsibility for a suicidal patient is shared by as many people as possible. This combined effort provides the patient with a feeling that he lacks: that others are interested in him, care for him, and are ready to help him.

When there are no apparent sources of help or support, the therapist may be the person's only situational support, his one link to survival. This is also true if available resources have been exhausted or family and friends have turned away from the individual. In most cases, however, people will respond to the situation and provide help and support if given the opportunity.

Life-style. How has the person functioned in the past under stress? First, has his style of life been stable or unstable? Second, is the suicidal behavior acute or chronic?

The stable individual will describe a consistent work record, sound marital and family relationship, and no history of previous suicidal behavior. The unstable individual may have had severe character disorders, borderline psychotic behavior, and repeated difficulties with major situations, such as interpersonal relationships or employment.

A suicidal person responding to acute stress, such as the death or loss of someone he loves, bad news, or loss of a job, which has pushed him into an unwanted and unfamiliar status, presents a special concern. The risk of early suicide among this group is high; however, the opportunity for successful therapeutic intervention is greater. If the suicidal danger can be averted for a relatively short period of time, individuals tend to emerge without great danger of recurrence.

By contrast, individuals with a history of repeated attempts of self-destruction may be helped through one emergency, but the suicidal danger can be expected to return at a later date. In general, if an individual has made serious attempts in the past, his current suicidal situation should be considered more dangerous. Although individuals with chronic suicidal behavior benefit temporarily from intervention, the emphasis should fall more on continuity of care and the maintenance of relationships.

Acute suicidal behavior may be found in either a stable or an unstable personality; however, chronic suicidal behavior occurs only in an unstable person. In dealing with a stable person in a suicidal situation, the therapist should be highly responsive and active. With an unstable person, the therapist needs to be slower and more thoughtful, reminding the patient that he has withstood similar stresses in the past. The main goals will be to help him through this period and assist him in reconstituting an interpersonal relationship with a stable person or resource.

Communication. The communication aspects of suicidal behavior have great importance in the evaluation and assessment process. The most important question is whether or not communication still exists between the suicidal individual and her significant others. When communication with the suicidal patient is completely severed, it indicates that she has lost hope in any possibility of rescue.

The form of communication may be either verbal or nonverbal, and its content may be direct or indirect. The suicidal person who communicates nonverbally and indirectly makes it difficult for the recipient of the communication to recognize or understand the suicidal intent of these communications. Also, this type of communication in itself implies a lack of clarity in the interchange between the suicidal person and others. At the same time, it raises a danger that the individual may "act out" suicidal impulses. The primary goal is to open up and clarify communication among everyone involved in the situation.

The patient's communication may be directed toward one or more significant persons within her environment. She may express hostility, accuse or blame others, or may demand openly or subtly that others change their behavior and feelings. Her communication may express feelings of guilt, inadequacy, and worthlessness or indicate strong anxiety and tension.

Significant other. When the communication is directed to a specific person, the reaction of the recipient becomes an important factor in evaluating suicidal danger. One must decide if the significant other can be an important resource for rescue, if she is best regarded as nonhelpful, or if she might even be injurious to the patient.

The nonhelpful significant other either rejects the patient or denies the suicidal behavior itself by withdrawing, both psychologically and physically, from continued communication. Sometimes this other person resents the patient's increased demands, insistence on gratification of dependency needs, or the demands to change her own behavior. In other situations, the significant other may act helpless, indecisive, or ambivalent, indicating that she does not know what the next step is and has given up. A reaction of hopelessness gives the suicidal individual a feeling that aid is not available from a previously dependable source. This can increase the patient's own hopelessness.

By contrast, a helpful reaction from the significant other is one in which the other person recognizes the communication, is aware of the problem, and seeks help for the individual. This indicates to the patient that her communications are being heard and that someone is doing something to provide help.

ASSESSMENT OF THE INDIVIDUAL AND THE PROBLEM

Carol was referred to a crisis center for help by a physician in the emergency room of a nearby small suburban hospital. The night before, she had attempted suicide by severely slashing her left wrist repeatedly with a large kitchen knife, and she had severed a tendon as a result.

When she was first seen by the therapist at the center, her left wrist and arm were heavily bandaged. She appeared tense, disheveled, very pale, and tremulous. She described her symptoms as insomnia, poor appetite, recent inability to concentrate, and overwhelming feelings of hopelessness and helplessness.

Carol was a 30-year-old single woman who lived alone. She had come to a large midwestern city about 4 years ago, immediately after graduating with a master's degree in business administration from an eastern university. Within a few weeks she had obtained a management trainee position with a large manufacturing distributor company. In the next 3 years she had been advanced rapidly to her current position as manager of the main branch office. She stated that she was considered by her co-workers to be highly qualified for the position. She denied any on-the-job problems other than "the usual things that anyone in my position has to expect to deal with on a day-to-day basis." As a result of her rapid rise in the company, however, she had not allowed herself much leisure time to develop any close social relationships with either sex.

About a year ago Carol met John, a 40-year-old widower who had a position similar to hers with another company. His office was on the same floor as hers. Within a few weeks they were spending almost all of their leisure time together, though still maintaining separate apartments.

Carol's symptoms began about 2 weeks ago when John was offered a promotion to a new job in his company, which he accepted without mentioning it to her first. It meant that he would be transferred to another office about 30 miles away in the suburbs. She stated that she did feel upset "for just a few minutes" after he told her of his decision; "I guess that was just because he hadn't even mentioned anything about it to me first."

They went out that evening for dinner and dancing to celebrate the occasion. Before dinner was even over John had to bring her home because she "suddenly became dizzy, nauseated, and chilled" with what she described as "all of the worst symptoms of stomach flu."

Carol remained at home in bed for the next 3 days, not allowing John to visit her because she felt she was contagious. After she returned to work she continued to feel very lethargic, had difficulty concentrating, could not regain her appetite, "and felt quite depressed and tearful for no reason at all."

Convincing herself that she had not yet fully recovered from the "flu," she cancelled several dates with John so that she could get more rest. She described him as being very understanding about this, even encouraging her to try to get some time off from work to take a short trip by herself and really rest and relax.

During this same time, John had begun to spend increasing amounts of his time at his new office. Their coffee-break meetings at work became very infrequent. Within the next week he expected to be moved completely.

The night before Carol came to the crisis center she had come home from work expecting to meet John there for dinner; instead she found a note under her door written by her neighbor. It said that John had telephoned him earlier in the day and left word for her that he had "suddenly been called out of town—wasn't sure when he would be back, but would get in touch with her later."

She told the therapist, "Suddenly I felt empty . . . that everything was over between us. It was just too much for me to handle. He was never going to see me again and was too damned chicken to tell me so to my face! I went numb all over—I just wanted to die." She paused a few minutes, head down and sobbing, then took a deep breath and went on, "I really don't remember doing it, but the next thing I was aware of was the telephone ringing. When I reached out to answer it, I suddenly realized I had a butcher knife in my right hand and my left wrist was cut and bleeding terribly! I dropped the knife on the floor and grabbed the phone. It was John calling me from the airport to tell me why he had to go out of town so suddenly—his father was critically ill."

Through sobs she told him what she had just done to herself. He told her to take a kitchen towel and wrap it tightly around her wrist. After she had done that, he told her to unlock the front door and wait there, that he would get help to her.

He immediately called her neighbors, who went to her apartment and found her with blood-soaked towels around her wrist and sitting on the floor beside the door. They took her to the hospital, and John continued on his trip. After being treated in the emergency room, Carol went home to spend the night with her neighbors. They drove her to the crisis center the next morning.

During her initial session Carol told the therapist that she had no close relatives. Her father and mother had died within a few months of each other during her last year in college. Soon after she had fallen in love with another graduate student, and at his suggestion they had moved into an apartment together. She had believed that they would marry as soon as they had both graduated and had jobs.

Just before graduation, however, her boyfriend had come home and informed her that he had accepted a postdoctoral fellowship in France and would be leaving within the month. They went out for dinner "to celebrate" that night because, she said, "I couldn't help but be happy for him—it was quite an honor—I just couldn't tell him how hurt I felt."

The next morning after he had left for classes she stated that she "suddenly realized I would never see him again after graduation—that he had never intended to marry me—and I was helpless to do anything about it." She took some masking tape and sealed the kitchen window shut, closed the door and put towels along the bottom, and turned on all of the stove gas jets.

About an hour later a neighbor smelled the gas fumes and called the fire department. The firemen broke into the apartment, found her lying unconscious on the floor, and rushed her to the hospital. She was in a coma for 2 days and remained in the hospital for a week. Her boyfriend came only once to see her. When she returned to the apartment, she found that he had moved out, leaving her a note saying that he had gone home to see his family before taking off for France. He never contacted her again. A month later Carol moved to the Midwest.

For the first few months after meeting John, Carol was very ambivalent about her feelings toward him. She frequently felt very anxious and fearful that she was "setting myself up for another rejection." Even when John proposed marriage, she found herself unable to consider it seriously and told him that they should wait a while longer "to be sure that they both wanted it." Continuing, she stated, "Until about 2 days ago I had never felt so secure in my life—I'd begun to seriously consider proposing to him! Then, suddenly, the bottom began to fall out of everything."

When John accepted the new job without telling her first, Carol saw this as the beginning of another rejection by someone highly significant in her life. As her anxiety increased, she withdrew from communication with John "because of her flu." John's well-intentioned agreement to cancel several dates so that she could get more rest further cut off her opportunities to communicate her feelings to him. His suggestion that she take a trip alone compounded her already strong fear of imminent rejection by him.

Finding the neighbor's note under the door was, for her, "the last straw," final proof that he was leaving her, "just like my boyfriend did in college."

Unable to cope with overwhelming feelings of loss and anger toward herself for "letting it happen to me again," she impulsively attempted to commit suicide.

PLANNING OF THERAPEUTIC INTERVENTION

Carol's two suicide attempts, except for the method used, were quite similar. Both were precipitated by the threat of the loss of someone highly significant in her life; both were impulsive, maladaptive attempts to cope with intense feelings of depression, hopelessness, and helplessness; and both demonstrated an inability to communicate her feelings in stressful situations.

When asked by the therapist how she usually coped with anxiety in the past Carol said that she would keep herself so busy at work that she did not have much time to worry about personal problems. This had been her method of coping with anxiety at school, too, until her first suicide attempt. Since she had been too ill to work full time the past 2 weeks, her previous successful coping mechanisms could not be effectively used.

The goal of intervention was to help Carol gain an intellectual understanding of the relationship between her crisis and her inability to communicate her intense feelings of depression and anxiety caused by the threat of the loss of John.

INTERVENTION

Before the end of the first session the therapist's assessment was that Carol was no longer acutely suicidal. However, because of her continuing feelings of depression, a medical consultation was arranged and an antidepressant prescribed. A verbal contact was agreed on; Carol was to call the therapist if she felt suicidal again. Carol agreed to the suggestion that she have a friend move into her apartment to help her out until her arm was less painful. Before leaving she assured the therapist that she would call him immediately if she again began to feel overwhelmed by anxiety before her next appointment.

When Carol returned for her next session, she was markedly less depressed. She told the therapist that John had called her soon after she came home from the center the week before. Although he had expressed great concern for her, she had been unable to tell him exactly why she had attempted suicide. "I just couldn't tell him that I thought he had left me for good—he'd think that I was trying to blame him—after all, I've been telling him for months that we both should keep our independence!" However, she said she felt much more reassured of his love for her. John expected to be back in about 2 more weeks.

During this and the next few sessions the therapist explored with Carol why she found it difficult to communicate her feelings to someone so significant in her life. Carol was reluctant at first to admit that this was a problem that could have contributed to her recent crisis. She saw herself as someone who was completely self-sufficient and denied any dependency needs on John. As a child she had been expected to control her emotions, to appear "ladylike" and composed at all times. Efforts on her part to communicate her feelings as she passed through the normal maturational crises of childhood and adolescence were met with rejecting behavior from those most significant in her life—her parents. Slowly she began to gain insight into the ways in which she had learned maladaptive methods to cope with stress, such as withdrawing from contact with others whenever she felt threatened by a stressful situation; by somatizing her anxiety rather than admit it was more than she could handle. By the end of the third session she reported that she had been able to communicate her feelings to John more openly and honestly than she had ever done in the past. She appeared to be surprised and pleased that John had responded so positively to her. When asked what she would have done if he had not responded this way, she paused thoughtfully, then answered. "It was a risk I

CASE STUDY: CAROL

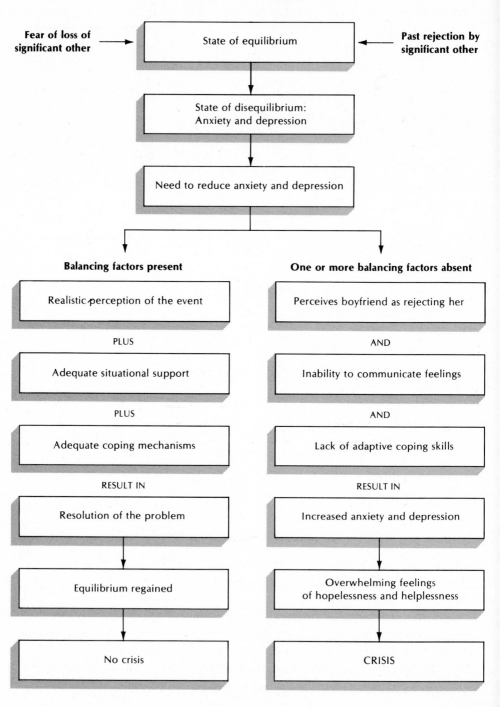

had to take. I just had to find out for sure if I could handle it this time." She added that although she had been very anxious while talking to him, she at no time felt as though she could not go on living if things had turned out differently.

By the end of the fourth session John had returned to the city, and Carol had returned to her job full time. She no longer felt depressed, and her wrist was slowly regaining its functioning. They were seeing each other frequently despite the distance between their offices, and Carol now said that she felt much more comfortable talking things out with him.

ANTICIPATORY PLANNING

Because Carol had attempted suicide once before under much the same crisis-precipitating stressful situation, she continued in therapy for the full 6 weeks. The purpose was to ensure that she could depend on situational support from the therapist while adjusting to the fact that she would no longer be seeing John every day. She was encouraged to telephone the therapist at any time she began to feel a recurrence of her earlier symptoms and felt unable to communicate these feelings to John.

Because she now seemed to have a better understanding of the relationship between her suicide attempts and the precipitating events, she said that she felt more secure in being able to cope with stressful situations in a more positive manner.

SUMMATION OF PARADIGM

Carol's distorted perception of rejection by John was compounded by her previous experience in losing someone highly significant in her life. Unable to directly communicate her feelings to John, her anxiety and depression increased. Lacking adequate coping mechanisms and situational support, she became overwhelmed with feelings of hopelessness and helplessness. Anticipating another rejection, Carol, entering a state of crisis, impulsively attempted suicide. Intervention was focused on getting her to understand why she was unable to communicate and cope with her intense feelings of inadequacy in interpersonal relations.

Death and the grief process—theoretical concepts

Death is a certainty. This universal phenomenon is ominous because it is inescapable. Since every human being will at some time be subject to death, it seems that death is most significant. Much is unknown of the process of death, and human beings are noted for their fear of the unknown. It might be said that this is a basic fear, and throughout the ages human beings have sought self-preservation. Advances in medical science and allied areas support this contention.

The critical question is not the sham dichotomy of life and death but the way in which each person relates to the knowledge that death is certain. This fear may be the prototype of human anxiety. Throughout history, death has posed an external mystery that is the core of religious and philosophical systems of thought. Anxiety relates to the fact that each person is powerless; he or she may postpone death, may lessen its physical pain, may rationalize it away or deny its very existence, but there is no escape from it, and so the fight for self-preservation is inevitably lost.

The attitudes of the persons involved in the situation are basic to the process of dying. Concepts, philosophies, and attitudes about death evolve from centuries of conflicting ideas and thought.

Traditionally the attitude of a society toward death has been a function of its religious beliefs. Religion denies the finality of death and affirms the continuation of the human personality either in its psychophysical totality or as a soul. The medical and social sciences, by challenging these traditional beliefs, have indirectly caused alienation and a serious mental health problem.

Family reaction to the death of a member develops in stages varying in time. The death of a loved one must produce an active expression of feeling in the normal course of events. Omission of such a reaction is to be considered as much a variation from the normal as is an excess in time and intensity. Unmanifested grief will be found expressed in some way or another; each new loss can cause grief for the current loss as well as reactivate the grieving process of previous episodes.

Lindemann (1944) states that following the loss there are three phases of mourning.

Phase I: Shock and disbelief. There is a focus on the original object with symptoms of somatic distress occurring in waves, lasting from 20 minutes to an hour at a time, a feeling of tightness in the throat, choking with shortness of breath, need for sighing, an empty feeling in the abdomen, and lack of muscular power. There is commonly a slight sense of unreality, a feeling of increased emotional distance from other people, and an intense preoccupation with the image of the deceased.

There is a strong preoccupation with feelings of guilt, and the bereaved searches the time before death for evidence of failure to do right by the lost one, accusing himself of negligence and exaggerating minor omissions.

Phase II: Developing awareness. Disorganization of personality occurs in this phase, accompanied by pain and despair because of the persistent and insatiable nature of yearning for the lost object. There is weeping and a feeling of helplessness and possible identification with the deceased.

Phase III: Resolving the loss. Resolution of the loss completes the work of mourning. A reorganization takes place with emancipation from the image of the lost object, and new object relationships are formed.

Engel (1964) states that the clearest evidence that mourning or grieving is successfully completed as is the ability to remember *completely* and *realistically* the pleasures *and* disappointments of the lost relationship.

In this phase one must also consider pathological mourning, in which there is an inability to express overtly these urges to recover the lost object. When all reactions are repressed, they will influence behavior in a strange and distorted way; for example, a schizophrenic person's reaction to the death of a significant individual may be laughter. There may be a delayed reaction or an excessive reaction; or the grief reaction may take the form of a straight agitated depression with accompanying tension, agitation, insomnia, feelings of worthlessness, bitter self-accusation, and obvious need for punishment. Individuals reacting in this way may be dangerously suicidal.

Proper management of grief reactions may prevent prolonged and serious alterations in an individual's social adjustment. The essential task is that of sharing and understanding the individual's grief work. Comfort alone does not provide adequate assistance. He has to accept the pain of the bereavement. He has to review his relationships with the deceased. He will have to express his sorrow and sense of loss. He must accept the destruction of a part of his personality before he can organize it afresh toward a new object or goal. Although they are unwelcome, such phases are a necessary part of life (Lindemann, 1944).

The following case study concerns a retired widower who is threatened by a second loss before completing "grief work" from the recent death of his wife. Initial assessment of the crisis situation provided clues in the determination that he was probably in the last phase of mourning and became overwhelmed by the threat of losing another highly cathected object, his son. The goal of intervention was to assist Mr. P. in reentering his social world and in gaining an intellectual understanding of the grief process as it related to his symptoms.

Case study   *Death and the grief process*

ASSESSMENT OF THE INDIVIDUAL AND THE PROBLEM

Mr. P., 67 years old and recently widowed, came to a crisis center for help on the advice of his family physician because of severe depression and anxiety. He described his symptoms as loss of appetite, inability to concentrate, restlessness, insomnia, and loss of energy. These symptoms had been first manifested a month earlier, following the death of his wife. He thought that they had been subsiding, but they suddenly increased to an intolerable level and he feared loss of emotional control. He denied any suicidal ideas, stating, "I don't want to die, it's just that I've lost all interest in life and no longer care what happens to me."

During the initial visit, Mr. P. was at first unable to determine any specific event that might have caused the sudden and acute rise in his symptoms. His wife's death was not unexpected, and he had felt "well prepared" for a future life without her. He viewed himself as realistic in his attitudes and planning before she died and as having experienced a "normal amount of grief" afterward.

After a mandatory retirement when he was 65 years old, he had devoted most of his time to helping to care for his wife, a semi-invalid with severe coronary disease. "I think I was really glad when I retired, because I'd had so little time for myself in those last few years, working all day and then going home and trying to catch up with things I had to do there." Having little time for social activities with his business friends, he had felt little sense of their loss when he left his job.

He had one son, married and living nearby. The son and his wife had had close relationships with Mr. and Mrs. P., helping them out with their household activities and with the care of Mrs. P. Mr. P. had made tentative plans to move into an apartment after his wife's death, feeling fully able to care for his own needs. However, just after she died his son and daughter-in-law brought up the idea of their moving into his home with him. It was a large home, much larger than their rented one, and they would pay him monthly amounts toward eventually buying it from him. He said that he was quite pleased with the idea, preferring to remain in his home but unable to justify to himself any reason for staying there alone. They had moved in 2 weeks ago, and he had felt an immediate lessening in his grief reaction to his wife's death.

A week ago his son had received an unexpected offer of a better job in another state. Mr. P. related that he felt very proud of the offer to his son, strongly urging him to accept it. The decision had to be made within the month. Since he had previously begun plans to live alone, he had not felt too concerned for himself if his son and daughter-in-law did decide to leave.

That same night he had suddenly awakened, feeling nauseous, tense, anxious, and very depressed, and sleep had become increasingly difficult as these symptoms had increased in the past few days. Although he no longer experienced nausea, he had a loss of appetite, insomnia, and a feeling of total exhaustion. He summed up his feelings by saying, "Maybe I'm not as happy about my son leaving as I told him I was."

The therapist thought that Mr. P.'s recovery from the grief at the loss of his wife had evolved through the stage of shock and disbelief. He had anticipated her death realistically and had accepted it as inevitable. He had begun to overcome his feelings of guilt and sense of failure, as well as his persistent longing for a lost object (his wife). Mr. P. was probably in the last phase of mourning, that of emancipation from the image of the lost object and the initial formation of new object relationships. At this stage, before final resolution of his grief, he was unexpectedly threatened with loss of another highly cathected object, his son.

PLANNING OF THERAPEUTIC INTERVENTION

Mr. P. had few social contacts because of his total involvement with the care of his wife during the past few years. His son and daughter-in-law had been providing situational support before and during his period of mourning, and this support was now in jeopardy. He had unrecognized ambivalence with regard to the job offer made to his son. Although intellectualizing plans to move into an apartment by himself, he lacked skills that would be necessary to repeople his social world. The anxiety generated by his unresolved grief and his ambivalence about his personal future was then compounded by the unexpected threat of a new loss.

When asked how he had coped with stress in the past, he said that he had always been able to keep busy caring for his wife and the housework. He had also been able to talk things over with his son. He now felt unable to talk to his son about his present feelings "for fear he might think he'd have to give up the job offer and stay here with me."

The goal of intervention was to help Mr. P. gain an intellectual understanding of his crisis in order to recognize the relationship between the threatened loss of his son and his present severe discomfort. His unrecognized ambivalence between his needs for independence as opposed to dependency would be explored.

INTERVENTION

During the next 2 weeks it became possible for him to see the present crisis and its accompanying symptoms in relation to his reactions to the loss of his wife and the threatened loss of his son.

During Mrs. P.'s illness he had narrowed his own life-style to conform to hers. In failing to acknowledge his lack of the interpersonal skills necessary to maintain a social life of his own, he justified his action as "what would be expected of any husband in a similar situation." Mrs. P. had been the dominant member of the marriage. Even when bedridden, she had guided the decision making that he thought was independent on his part. The additional support and assistance by his son and daughter-in-law only served to increase his dependency on others for decision making.

At times during the past few years he had thoughts of "all the things we could have done if I'd retired when my wife had not been so ill." He had deflected these thoughts into overt sympathy for her rather than for himself and what he was missing. As her death became imminent and inevitable, his wife began to make plans with him for his future. She told him to sell the home and to move into an apartment, even selecting which furniture he should keep and which he should give away.

When she died, he was finally faced with the reality of his inability to cope with the changes. Crisis at this time was circumvented by the offer of his son to move into his home. He was able to continue in much the same life pattern that had previously existed for him, with the son and daughter-in-law assuming the leadership role. With their strong situational support the work of grief had not become overwhelming.

The sudden threat of their loss had precipitated the crisis. Unrecognized feelings of inadequacy and dependency had come into painful focus. He feared both the physical loss of his son and the loss of his son's love if the job were turned down "because he'd think I couldn't take care of myself if he left me here alone."

By the third session, through discussion and clarification with the therapist,

Mr. P. was able to recognize his ambivalent feelings and relate them to his own needs for dependency. He saw the disparity between his concept of what he thought others expected of him and what he could actually achieve alone. His acceptance of this enabled him to reestablish meaningful communication with his son and to gain his support in making more realistic plans.

ANTICIPATORY PLANNING

Mr. P.'s exploration of his feelings related to his loss and subsequent grief helped him to gain an intellectual understanding of the process of working through the period of mourning. His recognition of his symptoms as part of the process helped to reduce his anxiety and enabled him to better perceive the reality of the situation and to utilize his existing coping skills. Realization was gained that he himself was withdrawing from available situational support because of his concept that his role was to be "an independent person." He was able to accept the fact that this might not be true and, as a result, he felt better about communicating his fears to his son and enlisting his assistance in planning.

By the third week his son had made the decision to accept the position and move out of the state in another month. Through joint efforts they located an apartment-hotel for Mr. P., where he would have the independence to "come and go as I'd always planned for in my retirement." Since the hotel preferred its guests to be in the retirement-age group, there were programs established for the guests' interests and social needs.

Mr. P. moved into the hotel 3 weeks before his son left town. The period of transition was facilitated with minimal rise in his anxiety. There was a gradual removal of his son's situational support, which was being replaced by the support gained in new social contacts. Although he felt grief when his son and daughter-in-law left town, Mr. P. could recognize and relate his symptoms to the event and so was able to cope with them.

In discussion and review of his future plans Mr. P. was optimistic about his ability to live independently within the framework of his new environment. He was slowly entering new activities and making new friends, although he admitted "being a bit rusty about how to do it."

Before termination of therapy, Mr. P. and the therapist reviewed the adjustments that he had made, as well as his new insights into his own feelings. He thought that the crisis situation, although being very painful to him at the time, had provided him with a "good idea of how to face up to things in the future." His future plans were also reviewed, and he was reassured by the therapist that he could always return for future help should the occasion arise.

SUMMATION OF THE PARADIGM

Mr. P. had failed to recognize any relationship between his feelings of increased anxiety and the death of his wife. His inexperience with independent decision mak-

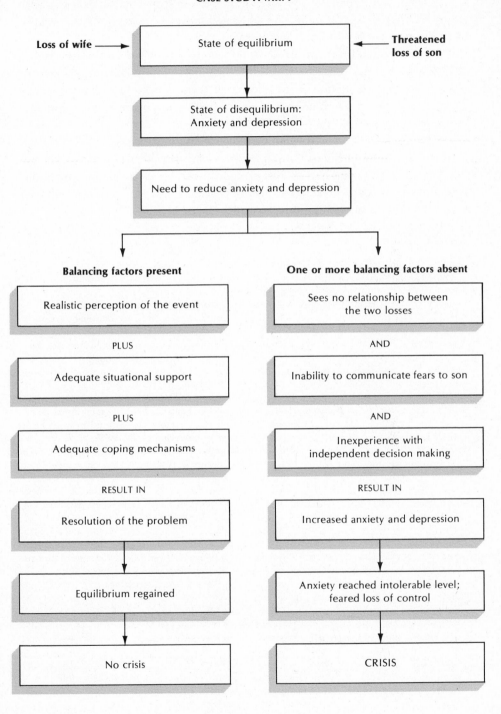

CASE STUDY: MR. P

Loss of wife ⟶ State of equilibrium ⟵ **Threatened loss of son**

State of disequilibrium:
Anxiety and depression

Need to reduce anxiety and depression

Balancing factors present

Realistic perception of the event

PLUS

Adequate situational support

PLUS

Adequate coping mechanisms

RESULT IN

Resolution of the problem

Equilibrium regained

No crisis

One or more balancing factors absent

Sees no relationship between
the two losses

AND

Inability to communicate fears to son

AND

Inexperience with
independent decision making

RESULT IN

Increased anxiety and depression

Anxiety reached intolerable level;
feared loss of control

CRISIS

ing made him inadequate to cope with the stressful event alone. Intervention with strong situational support by his son and daughter-in-law assisted him to begin to work through the grief process and averted a crisis.

The unexpected threat of his son and daughter-in-law's departure and his inability to communicate his fears resulted in their loss to him as situational supports. These factors were compounded by uncompleted grief work and a failure to see any connection between his recurrence of severe anxiety and his reaction to a second loss.

In the assessment phase the therapist kept focus on the areas of stress to determine the adequacy of his past coping skills with bereavement. Intervention was directed toward assisting him to explore and ventilate his feelings of dependency. Anticipatory planning was directed toward providing him with situation supports when his son moved from town.

References

Aguilera, D.C.: Review of psychiatric nursing, St. Louis, 1977, The C.V. Mosby Co.

Allport, G.W.: Pattern and growth in personality, New York, 1961, Holt, Rinehart & Winston.

Amir, M.: Patterns in forcible rape, Chicago, 1971, University of Chicago Press.

Appleton, W.: The battered woman syndrome, Ann. Emerg. Med. 9(2):84, 1980.

Bandura, A.: Aggression: a social learning analysis, Englewood Cliffs, N.J., 1973, Prentice-Hall, Inc.

Bard, J., and Zacher, M.: Assaultiveness and alcohol use in family disputes, Criminology 12:283, 1974.

Bernstein, R.: Are we still stereotyping the unmarried mother? Soc. Work 5:22, 1960.

Bowlby, J.: Separation anxiety, Int. J. Psychoanal. 41:89, 1960.

Brown, H.F., Burditt, V.B., and Lidell, W.W.: The crisis of relocation. In Parad, H.J., editor: Crisis intervention, New York, 1965, Family Service Association of America.

Bryant, H.: Seattle prosecutors crack down on wife beaters, Seattle Post-Intelligencer, p. A3, July 30, 1978.

Burgess, A.W., and Holmstrom, L.L.: The rape victim in the emergency ward, Am. J. Nurs. 73(10):1741, 1973.

Burgess, A.W., and Holmstrom, L.L.: Rape trauma syndrome, Am. J. Psychiatry 131:982, Sept. 1974.

Caplan, G.: An approach to community mental health, New York, 1961, Grune & Stratton, Inc.

Caplan, G.: Principles of preventive psychiatry, New York, 1964, Basic Books, Inc., Publishers.

Carlson, B.: Battered women and their assailants, Soc. Work 22:455, 1977.

Chanda, S.K., Sharma, V.K., and Banergee, S.P.: Andreoceptor sensitivity following psychotropic drug treatment. In Usdin, E., editor: Catecholamines: basic and clinical frontiers, New York, 1979, Pergamon Press.

Chown, S.M., editor: Human aging, New York, 1972, Penguin Books, Inc.

Claridge, G.: Drugs and human behavior, Middlesex, England, 1972, Penguin Books, Ltd.

Cohen, I., editor: The battered woman, Emergency Medicine 11:24, 1979.

Comstock, B.S., and McDermott, M.: Group-therapy for patients who attempt suicide, Int. J. Group Psychother. 25(1):44, 1975.

Croog, S.H., Levine, S., and Lurie, Z.: The heart patient and the recovery process, Soc. Sci. Med. 2:111, 1968.

de Smit, N.W.: Crisis intervention and crisis centers: their possible relevance for community psychiatry and mental health care, Psychiatr. Neurol. Neurochir. 75(4):299, 1972.

Decker, J.B., and Stubblebine, J.M.: Crisis intervention and prevention of psychiatric disability: a follow-up study, Am. J. Psychiatry 129(6):725, 1972.

Demarest, M.: Cocaine: middle class high, Time, July 6, 1981.

Drake, V.K.: Battered women: a health case problem in disguise, Image 14(2):40, 1982.

Engel, G.L.: Grief and grieving. Am. J. Nurs. 64:93, Sept. 1964.

Faberow, N., and Shneidman, E., editors: The cry for help, New York, 1961, McGraw-Hill Book Co.

Foss, S.: Experts agree spouse abuse part of American way, The Oregonian, p. C1, Feb. 9, 1978.

Frederick, C.J.: Organizing and funding suicide prevention and crisis services, Hosp. Community Psychiatry 23(11):346, 1972.

Garwin, F., and Kepler, H.: Cocaine abuse treatment, Arch. Gen. Psychiatry 41:903, 1984.

Gelles, R.J.: The violent home, Beverly Hills, Calif., 1972, Sage Publications.

Giarretto, H.: Humanistic treatment of father-daughter incest. In Helfer, R.E., and Kempe, C.H., editors: Child abuse and neglect: the family and the community, Cambridge, Mass., 1976, Ballinger Publishing Co.

Gil, D.C.: Violence against children, Cambridge, Mass., 1970, Harvard University Press.

Gil, D.C.: Unravelling child abuse, Am. J. Orthopsychiatry 45:352, 1975.

Glass, A.T.: Observations upon the epidemiology of mental illness in troops during warfare, Symposium on Preventive and Social Psychiatry sponsored by Walter Reed Army Institute of Research, Walter Reed Medical Center, and National research Council, April 15-17, Washington, D.C., 1957, U.S. Government Printing Office.

Glatt, M.M.: A guide to addiction and its treatment, New York, 1974, John Wiley & Sons, Inc.

Gouirand, Y., and Soubrier, J.P.: Possibilities of psychotherapeutic intervention in suicide attempters and those who are suicidal, Perspect. Psychiatriques 3(47):153, 1974.

Grayford, J.J.: Wife battery: a preliminary survey of 100 cases, Br. Med. J. 169:194, 1975.

Greene, B.L.: Sequential marriage: repetition or change. In Rosenbaum, S., and Alger, I., editors: The marriage relationship, New York, 1968, Basic Books, Inc., Publishers.

Grinspoon, L., and Bakalar, J.B.: Drug dependence: non-narcotic agents. In Kaplan, H.I., Freedman, A.M., and Sadock, B.J., editors: Comprehensive textbook of psychiatry, ed. 3, Baltimore, 1980, Williams & Wilkins Co.

Halperin, M.: Helping maltreated children: school and community involvement, St. Louis, 1979, The C.V. Mosby Co.

Hankes, L.: Cocaine: today's drug, J. Fla. Med. Assoc. 71(4):235, 1984.

Hankoff, L.D., and others: Crisis intervention in the emergency room, Am. J. Psychiatry 131:47, 1974.

Helfer, R.E., and Kempe, C.H., editors: Child abuse and neglect: the family and the community, Cambridge, Mass., 1976, Ballinger Publishing Co.

Heller, S., and Kornfeld, D.: Delerium and related problems. In Reiser, M., editor: America's handbook of psychiatry, vol. 4, New York, 1975, Basic Books, Inc., Publishers.

Hellerstein, H., and Goldstone, E.: Rehabilitation of patients with heart disease, Postgrad. Med. 15:265, 1954.

Hinkle, L.E., Jr.: Social factors and coronary heart disease, Soc. Sci. Med. 2:107, 1968.

Hollender, M.H.: The psychology of medical practice, Philadelphia, 1958, W.B. Saunders Co.

Holmstrom, L.L., and Burgess, A.W.: Assessing trauma in the rape victim, Am. J. Nurs. 75(8):1288, 1975.

Hubbard, L.: The Alzheimer's puzzle: putting the pieces together, Modern Maturity, Aug.-Sept. 1984.

Jacobson, G.F.: Emergency services in community mental health: problems and promise, Am. J. Public Health 64(2):124, 1974.

Justice, B., and Justice, R.: The abusing family, New York, 1976, Human Sciences Press, Inc.

Justice, B., and Justice, R.: The broken taboo, New York, 1979, Human Sciences Press, Inc.

Kameron, S., and Kahn, A.: Social services in the United States, Philadelphia, 1976, Temple University Press.

Kaplan, D.M., and Mason, E.A.: Maternal reactions to premature birth viewed as an acute emotional disorder. In Parad, H.J., editor: Crisis intervention, New York, 1965, Family Service Association of America.

Kempe, C.H.: The battered child syndrome, J.A.M.A. 181:17, 1962.

Kempe, C.H., and Helfer, R.: Helping the battered child and his family, Philadelphia, 1972, J.B. Lippincott Co.

King, S.H.: Perceptions of illness and medical practice, New York, 1962, Russell Sage Foundation.

Kleber, H.D., and Garwin, F.H.: Cocaine abuse: current and experimental treatments, National Institute on Drug Abuse Research Monograph Series, 1984.

Kubie, L.S., cited by Kaufman, J.G., and Becker, M.D.: Rehabilitation of the patient with myocardial infarction, Geriatrics **10:**355, 1955.

Kübler-Ross, E.: On death and dying, New York, 1969, Macmillian Inc.

Kübler-Ross, E.: Questions and answers on death and dying, New York, 1974, Collier Books.

Labell, L.S.: Wife abuse: A sociological study of battered women and their mates, Victimology **4:**258, 1979.

Landsgraf, S.: Battered women, Renton (Wash.) Record-Chronicle, p. 2, July 2, 1978.

Laurie, P.: Drugs; medical, psychological and social facts, ed. 2, Middlesex, England, 1971, Pelican, C. Nicholls & Co. Ltd.

Lee, P.R., and Bryner, S.: Introduction to a symposium on rehabilitation in cardiovascular disease, Am. J. Cardiol. **7:**315, 1961.

Levinger, G.: Sources of marital dissatisfactions among applicants for divorce, Am. J. Orthopsychiatry **36:**803, 1966.

Lindemann, E.: Symptomatology and management of acute grief, Am. J. Psychiatry **101:**141, Sept. 1944.

Linton, R.: Culture and mental disorders, Springfield, Ill., 1956, Charles C Thomas, Publisher.

Lipowski, J.: A new look at organic brain syndrome, Am. J. Psychiatry **137:**674, 1980.

Lystad, M.A.: Violence at home: literature review, Am. J. Orthopsychiatry **45:**328, 1975.

Mace, N.L., and Rabins, P.V.: The 36-hour day, Baltimore, 1981, The Johns Hopkins University Press.

Mason, E.A.: Method of predicting crisis outcome for mothers of premature babies, Public Health Rep. **78:**1031, Dec. 1963.

McDonald, J.M.: Rape: offenders and their victims, Springfield, Ill., 1971, Charles C Thomas, Publisher.

McGee, R K., and others: The delivery of suicide and crisis intervention services. In Resnik, H.: Suicide prevention in the 70's, Rockville, Md., 1973, National Institute of Mental Health.

McIver, J.: Psychiatric aspects of cardiovascular diseases in industry. In Warshaw, L.J., editor: The heart in industry, New York, 1960, Harper & Row, Publishers.

Moore, H.E.: Tornadoes over Texas: a study of Waco and San Angelo in disaster, Austin, 1958, University of Texas Press.

Morley, W.E., Messick, J.M., and Aguilera, D.C.: Crisis: paradigms of intervention, J. Psychiatr. Nurs. **5:**540, Nov.-Dec. 1967.

O'Reilly, J.: Battered wives, Time, pp. 23, Sept. 5, 1983.

Parsons, F.: The social system, New York, 1951, The Free Press.

Pert, A., and others. In Post, R.M., and others: Effect of chronic cocaine on behavior and cyclic AMP in cerebrospinal fluid of rhesus monkeys, Commun. Psychopharmacol. **3:**143, 1979.

Prescott S., and Letko, C.: Battered women: a social psychological perspective. In Roy, M., editor: Battered women: a psychosociological study of domestic violence, New York, 1977, Van Nostrand Reinhold Co., Inc.

Rapoport, L.: The state of crisis: some theoretical considerations, Soc. Service Rev. **36:**211, 1962.

Rapoport, R.: Normal crises, family structure, and mental health, Fam. Process **2:**68, 1963.

Rehabilitation of patients with cardiovascular diseases, WHO Tech. Rep. Ser., 1966.

Reisberg, B.: A guide to Alzheimer's disease, New York, 1981, The Free Press.

Reiser, M.F.: Emotional aspects of cardiac disease, Am. J. Psychiatry **107:**781, 1951.

Resnik, H.L.P., and Hathorne, B.C.: Summary of recommendations of the task force on suicide prevention. In Resnik, H.: Suicide prevention in the 70's, Rockville, Md., 1973, National Institute of Mental Health.

Rosenbaum, A., and O'Leary, K.D.: Marital violence: characteristics of abusive couple, J. Consult. Clin. Psychol. **49:**63, 1981.

Rounsaville, B.: Theories in marital violence: evidence from a study of battered women, Victimology **3:**11, 1978.

Roy, M.: A current survey of 150 cases. In Roy, M., editor: Battered women: a psychosociological study of domestic violence, New York, 1977, Van Nostrand Reinhold Co., Inc.

Rubenstein, D.: Rehospitalization versus family crisis intervention, Am. J. Psychiatry **129**(6):715, 1972.

Rubenstein, D.: Family crisis intervention as an alternative to rehospitalization, Curr. Psychiatric Ther. **14:**191, 1974.

Rubinelli, J.: Incest: it's time we faced reality, J. Psychiatr. Nurs. **18**(4):17, 1980.

Salholz, E., and others: Beware of child molesters, Newsweek, p. 45, Aug. 9, 1982.

Selkin, J.: Rape, Psychol. Today, Jan. 1975, pp. 71-76.

Seltzer, B., and Frazier, S.: Organic mental disorders. In Nicholi, A., editor: The Harvard guide to modern psychiatry, Cambridge, Mass., 1978, Harvard University Press.

Sihier, L.: Does violence breed violence? Study of the child abuse syndrome, Am. J. Psychiatry **126**:404, 1969.

Singh., A.N., and Brown, J.H.: Suicide prevention: review and evaluation, Can. Psychiatr. Assoc. J. **18**(2):117, 1973.

Smitson, W.: Focus on service, Ment. Hyg. **56**(4):22, 1972.

Steinmetz, S.K., and Straus, M.A.: Family as cradle of violence, Society **10**:50, 1973.

Steinmetz, S.K., and Straus, M.A.: Social myth and social system in the study of intrafamily violence. In Steinmetz, S.K., and Straus, M.A., editors: Violence in the family, New York, 1974, Harper & Row, Publishers, Inc.

Stewart, M.A., and deBlois, C.S.: Wife abuse among families attending a child psychiatry clinic, J. Am. Acad. Child Psychiatry **20**:845, 1981.

Storaska, F.: How to say no to a rapist and survive, New York, 1976, Warner Books, Inc.

Straus, M.: Behind closed doors: violence in the American family, Garden City, New York, 1981, Anchor Books.

U.S. Congress, Child abuse prevention and treatment act, Public Law 93-247. 93rd Congress, 1974.

U.S. Department of Health and Human Services: Executive summary: national study of the incidence and severity of child abuse and neglect, DHHS Publ. No. (OHDS) 81-30329, Washington, D.C., 1982, U.S. Government Printing Office.

Vernick, J.: The use of the life space interview on a medical ward, Soc. Casework **44**:465, 1963.

Wales, E.: Crisis intervention in clinical training, Professional Psychology **3**(4):357, 1972.

Walker, L.: The battered woman, New York, 1979, Harper & Row, Publishers, Inc.

Walker-Hooper, A.: Domestic violence: assessing the problem. In Warner, C.G., editor: Conflict intervention in social and domestic violence, Bowie, Md., 1981, Robert J. Brady Co.

Woods, J.H., and Downs, D.A.: The psychopharmacology of cocaine. In Drug use in America: problem in perspective, Appendix, vol. 1: Patterns and consequences of drug use, Washington, D.C., 1973, National Commission on Marijuana and Drug Abuse.

Zinberg, N.E., and Robertson, J.A.: Drugs and the public, New York, 1972, Simon & Schuster, Inc.

Additional readings

Binder, R.L.: Difficulties in follow-up of rape victims, Am. J. Psychother. **35**(4):534, 1981.

Bowlby, J.: Attachment and loss, vol. 1, New York, 1980, Basic Books, Inc., Publishers.

Brown, V.B.: The community in crisis, N. Direction Ment. Health Serv. **6**:45, 1980.

Burns, D.: Feeling good, New York, 1981, The New American Library, Inc.

Calhoun, L.G., and others: Reactions to the family of the suicide, Am. J. Community Psychol. **7**:571, May 1979.

Capodanno, A., and Targum, S.: Assessment of suicide risk: some limitations in the prediction of infrequent events, J. Psychosocial Nurs. **21**(5):11, 1983.

Cassems, G., and others: Amphetamine withdrawal: effects on threshold of intracranial reinforcement, Psychopharmacology **73**:318, 1981.

Claus, K.E., and Bailey, J.T.: Living with stress and promoting well-being, St. Louis, 1980, The C.V. Mosby Co.

Cobbin, D.M., and others: Urinary MHPG levels and tricyclic antidepressant drug selection: a preliminary communication on improved drug selection in clinical practice, Arch. Gen. Psychiatry **36**:1111, 1979.

Colpaert, F.C., Niemegeers, C.J., and Janssen, P.A.: Discriminative stimulus properties of cocaine: neuropharmacological characteristics as derived from stimulus generalization experiments, Pharmacol. Biochem. Behav. **10**:535, 1979.

Courtois, C.A.: Victims of rape and incest, Couns. Psychologist **8**(1):38, 1979.

Cousins, N.: Anatomy of an illness, New York, 1979, W.W. Norton & Co., Inc.

Dohrenevend, B.P., and Egri, G.: Recent stressful events and episodes of schizophrenia, Schizophrenia Bulletin **7**(1):12, 1981.

Ellis, E.M., and others: An assessment of long-term reaction to rape, J. Abnorm. Psychol. **90**(3):263, 1981.

Fischman, M.W., and others: Cardiovascular and subjective effects of intravenous cocaine administration in humans, Arch. Gen. Psychiatry **33**:983, 1976.

Fitzpatrick, J.: Suicidology and suicide prevention: historical perspectives from the nursing literature, J. Psychosoc. Nurs. **21**:5, May 1983.

Friederick, C.J.: Current trends in suicidal behavior in the United States, Am. J. Psychother. **32**:172, 1979.

Garfield, C.A.: Stress and survival: the emotional realities for life-threatening illness, St. Louis, 1979, The C.V. Mosby Co.

Gaston, S.K.: Death and midlife crisis, J. Psychiatr. Nurs. 18(1):31, 1980.

Goldberg, S.: Premature birth: consequences for parent-infant relationship, Am. Scientist 67(2): 214, 1979.

Goodwin, F.K., Post, R.M., and Sack, R.L.: Clinical evidence for neurochemical adaptation to psychotropic drugs. In Mandell, A.J., editor: Neurobiological mechanisms of adaptation and behavior, New York, 1975, Raven Press.

Grodon, V.: Themes and cohesiveness observed in a depressed women's support group, Issues in Ment. Health 4:115, 1982.

Guttentag, Marcia, and others, editors: The mental health of women, New York, 1980, Academic Press.

Hansell, N.: Services for schizophrenics: a lifelong approach to treatment, Hosp. Community Psychiatry 29(2):105, 1978.

Hargreaves, A.G.: Coping with disaster, Am. J. Nurs. 80(4):683, 1980.

Hoeffler, K.H.: Social, psychological, and situational factors in child abuse, Palo Alto, Calif., 1982, R&E Research Associates, Inc.

Hohenshil, T.H.: Counseling handicapped persons and their families, Personnel Guidance J. 58:213, April 1979.

Horowitz, M.J., and Kaltreider, N.B.: Brief treatment for posttraumatic stress disorder, N. Directions Ment. Health Serv. 6:67, 1980.

Jacobson, D.S.: Crisis intervention with stepfamilies, N. Directions Ment. Health Serv. 6:35, 1980.

Kalish, R.A.: Death, grief, and caring relationships, Monterey, Calif., 1981, Brooks/Cole Publishing Co.

Kerr, M.: Emotional factors in physical illness, The Family 7:59, 1980.

Kieth, L.S., and Mosher, L.R., editors: N.I.M.H. Special Report: schizophrenia, Washington, D.C., 1980, U.S. Department of Human Services.

Klerman, G.: The age of melancholy? Psychol. Today 12(11):36, 1979.

Kline, N.: From sad to glad, New York, 1981, Ballantine Books.

Kokkinidis, L., and Zacharko, R.: Response sensitization and depression following long-term amphetamine treatment in a self-stimulation paradigm, Psychopharmacology. 68:73, 1980.

Kosman, M.E., and Unna, K.R.: Effects of chronic administration of the amphetamines and other stimulants on behavior, Clin. Pharmacol. Ther. 9:240, 1968.

Kraus, J.B., and Slavinsky, A.: The chronic psychiatric patient and the community, Oxford, England, 1982, Blackwell Scientific Publications, Ltd.

Kubler-Ross, E.: To live until we say goodbye, Englewood Cliffs, N.J., 1978, Prentice-Hall, Inc.

Labell, L.S.: Wife abuse: a sociological study of battered women and their mates, Victimology 4(2):258, 1979.

Lambert, V.A., and Lambert, C.E.: The impact of physical illness and related mental health concepts, Englewood Cliffs, N.J., 1979, Prentice-Hall, Inc.

Langsley, D.G.: Crisis intervention and the avoidance of hospitalization, N. Directions Ment. Health Serv. 6:81, 1980.

Leith, N.J., and Barrett, R.J.: Amphetamine and the reward system: evidence for tolerance and post-drug depression, Psychopharmacology 46:19, 1976.

Leith, N.J., and Barrett, R.J.: Self-stimulation and amphetamine: tolerance to *d* and *l* isomers and cross tolerance to cocaine and methylphenidate, Psychopharmacology 74:23, 1981.

Lindemann, E.: Beyond grief: studies in crisis intervention, New York, 1979, Jason Aronson, Inc.

Moss, D.M.: Near-fatal experience: crisis intervention and the anniversary reaction, Pastoral Psychol. 18:75, Feb. 1979.

Murphy, S.: Learned helplessness: from concept to comprehension, Perspect. in Psychiatr. Care 20(1):27, 1982.

Norris, J., and Feldman-Summers, S.: Factors related to the psychosocial impacts of rape on the victim, J. Abnorm. Psychol. 90(6):562, 1981.

Pao, P.: Shizophrenic Disorders: theory and treatment from a psychodynamic point of view, New York, 1979, International Universities Press.

Papa, L.: Responses to life events as predictors of suicidal behavior, Nurs. Res. 29(6):362, 1980.

Perry, G.F., and others: Clinical study of mianserin, imipramine and placebo in depression: blood level and MHPG correlations, Br. J. Clin. Pharmacol. 5:35S, 1978.

Ruben, H.L.: Managing suicidal behavior, J.A.M.A. 241(3):282, 1979.

Rush, J.A.: Short term psychotherapies for depression, New York, 1982, The Guilford Press.

Schildkraut, J.J., and others: Amphetamine withdrawal: depression and MHPG excretion, Lancet **2:**485, 1971.

Shapiro, S.A.: Contemporary theories of shizophrenia, New York, 1981, McGraw-Hill Book Co.

Shrier, D.K.: Rape: myths, misconceptions, facts and interventions, J. Med. Soc. N.J. **78**(10): 668, 1981.

Simpson, D.: Depressed rates of self-stimulation following chronic amphetamine in the rat: evaluation of these depressed rates by desmethylimipramine, Paper presented at the meeting of the Eastern Psychological Association, Washington, D.C., April 19, 1974.

Simpson, D.M., and Annau, Z.: Behavioral withdrawal following several psychoactive drugs, Pharmacol. Biochem. Behav. **7:**59, 1977.

Skelton, S.C., and Nix, L.: Development of a divorce adjustment group program in a social service agency, Soc. Casework **60:**309, May 1979.

Spector, Rachel E.: Cultural diversity in health and illness, New York, 1979, Appleton-Century-Crofts.

Strauss, J., and Carpenter, W.: Schizophrenia, New York, 1981, Plenum Medical Books.

Strob, Richard L.: Alzheimer's disease: current perspectives, J. Clin. Psychiatry, **41**(4):110, 1980.

Tierney, K.J., and Baisden, B.: Crisis intervention programs for disaster victims: a source book and manual for smaller communities, Publication No. (ADM) 79-675, Washington, D.C., 1979, Department of Health, Education, and Welfare.

Watson, R., Hartmann, E., and Schildkraut, J.J.: Amphetamine withdrawal: affective state, sleep patterns and MHPG excretion, Am. J. Psychiatry **129:**263, 1972.

Werner-Beland, J. A., editor: Grief responses to long-term illness and disability, Reston, Va., 1980, Reston Publishing Co.

Wise, R.A.: Direct action of cocaine on the brain mechanisms of complex behavior. In Jeri, F.R., editor: Cocaine 1980, Lima, Peru, 1980, Pacific Press.

Wolanin, M.O., and Phillips, L.R., editors: Confusion: prevention and care, St. Louis, 1981, The C.V. Mosby Co.

Wu, R.R.: Stressors at birth, Fam. Community Health **2**(4):1, 1980.

chapter 7

Maturational crises

A person's life-style is continually subject to change by the ongoing processes of maturational development, shifting situations within the environment, or a combination of both. Potential crisis areas occur during the periods of great social, physical, and psychological change experienced by all human beings in the normal growth process. These changes could occur during concomitant biological and social role transitions such as birth, puberty, young adulthood, marriage, illness or death of a family member, the climacteric, and old age.

Maturational crises have been described as normal processes of growth and development. They usually evolve over an extended period of time, such as the transition into adolescence, and they frequently require that the individual make many characterological changes. There may be an awareness of increased feelings of disequilibrium, but intellectual understanding of any correlation with normal developmental change may be inadequate.

The hazardous situations that occur in daily life may serve to compound normal maturational crises. When a person requests help at these times, it is necessary to determine what part of the presenting symptomatology is the result of transitional maturational stages and what, in turn, is the result of a stressful event in his current social orbit.

The theoretical concepts used in this chapter are derived primarily from Erikson's (1950, 1959, 1963) psychosocial maturational tasks (trust, autonomy, initiation, industry, identity, intimacy, generativity, and integrity); Piaget's (1963) ontogenetic development of intellectual abilities (sensorimotor—birth to 2 years; preoperational thought—2 to 7 years; concrete operations—7 to 11 years; and formal operations—11 to 14 years); and Cameron's (1963) personality development, which is based on a synthesis of recent theories of general psychology and dynamic psychopathology.

For the sake of clarity maturational crises discussed here are presented in the more generally familiar phases: infancy and early childhood, preschool, prepuberty, adolescence, young adulthood, adulthood, late adulthood, and old age.

The case studies and paradigms presented here illustrate some common maturational crises. It must be emphasized that seldom are hazardous events and maturational crises this clearly defined.

190

Infancy and early childhood—theoretical concepts

The first year of life is one of almost total helplessness and dependency. The infant must learn to trust the maternal figure and become able to allow her out of his sight without fear or rage. He must also be able to develop confidence in the sameness and continuity of his environment and to internalize it through his developing tactile, auditory, olfactory, and visual senses. Deprivation in any one or a combination of these senses could lead to maladaptive response patterns affecting his biopsychosocial development.

During this stage the symbiotic relationship that develops between the infant and the maternal figure forms a foundation for the behavioral patterns of later personality development. This relationship goes beyond the symbiosis of mutual dependency for biological survival; in the psychosocial development of the infant it implies that the mother is willing and ready to assume responsibility for the infant, who in turn accepts her care passively without reciprocating.

During infancy the mouth is the primary organ of gratification and exploration; feeding becomes an important aspect of meeting needs. This is controlled by someone else, usually the mother, and her consistency in meeting her infant's needs for oral gratification is the beginning of his development of trust in his environment.

As a result of the varied experiences that he and his mother share, the infant develops confidence that his needs will be met. Through her own dependability, the mother structures these situations so that there is a basis for a mutual sense of confidence. For example, if the infant is fed regularly at times when he has come to expect a feeding, his sense of trust is encouraged. But, should the feedings become sporadic, he will become uncertain and anxious about his environment, and a sense of mistrust will begin to appear. His resulting fretful, anxious behavior may inspire further inadequate mothering. Another essential component of the healthy symbiotic relationship is the comfort brought by the mother; if discomfort is inflicted, any continued trust can be destroyed.

Environmental consistency and stimulation are important for cognitive and effective growth. The infant usually becomes aware of his mother as a person by 9 months; however, absence of *mothering* can provoke symptoms of insecurity at 4 weeks, such as crying and rocking, withdrawal, depression, and even death.

Piaget (1963) describes the infant's development of intelligent behavior in this stage as *sensorimotor*. During the first year the reflex patterns she was born with are repeated and strengthened with practice. As a newborn, the infant is capable of grasping, sucking, auditory and visual pursuit, and other stereotyped behavior patterns. These can be activated by nonspecific stimuli in the environment; after being activated a number of times the response becomes spontaneous without further external stimulation. For example, at birth the infant is able to suck at the breast; continued practice improves her coordination and facility until this ability becomes well adapted to the goal of taking nourishment.

These primary reflex actions become coordinated into new actions. For example, the hand accidentally comes in contact with the mouth and initiates sucking movements that may lead to more coordinated actions and to thumbsucking as an established form of behavior. Later actions become oriented toward objects in the environment that stimulate seeing and hearing, and intentional behavior emerges as the infant seeks to repeat these actions. She learns to begin meaningful actions in sequence and to explore new objects within reach, thus developing goal-oriented activity. In this way physical activity patterns develop into mental activity patterns of response.

By the end of the first year the stage of purposeful behavior is reached, and exploration of further boundaries of the environment is begun. Motor actions have gradually become internalized as thought patterns. During this period the trend is toward a higher level of sensory experiences and related mental activities. By the end of the second year there is a functional understanding of play, imitation, causality, objects, space, and time. By the age of 2 years a child can truly imitate such behavior as eating, sleeping, washing himself, and walking.

If the child does not develop the beginnings of trust, in later life there may be a sense of chronic mistrust, dependency, depressive trends, withdrawal, and shallow interpersonal relationships.

During the second year the child begins a struggle for autonomy. He shifts from dependency on others toward independent actions of his own. As his musculature matures, it is necessary for him to develop the ability of coordination such as "holding on" and "letting go." Since these are highly opposing patterns, conflict may occur; one example is the conflict arising over bowel and bladder control. A power struggle may develop between the child and his parents, since elimination is completely under his control, and approval or disapproval become strong influences because of his parents' attitudes toward eliminative habits. The child is expected to abandon his needs for self-gratification and substitute ones that meet the demands of his parents, representing the later demands of society.

Cognitive development in this stage includes the first symbolic substitutions, words and gross speech. The child begins to manipulate objects and will look for hidden items. He recognizes differences between "I" and "me," "mine," and "you" and "yours." He also begins to manipulate others by words such as "no," and the origins of concrete literal thinking are developed; this is the period of *preoperational thought* that continues to the age of 7 years (Piaget, 1963). One of its characteristics is egocentrism, in which the child is unable to take the viewpoint of another person; at the end of this period, egocentrism is replaced by social interaction. The child has now formed concepts in primitive images, thing to thing. He cannot cope intellectually with problems concerning time, causality, space, or other abstract concepts, although he understands what each is by itself in concrete situations. His perceptions dominate his judgments, and he operates on what can be seen directly.

The psychosocial task during this stage is to develop self-esteem through limited self-control. The achievement of bowel and bladder control within the prescribed cultural expectations allows also for self-control without loss of self-esteem.

This is an important time for establishing a ratio between love and hate, cooperation and willfulness, and freedom of self-expression and its suppression. Failure during this stage is manifested in childhood by feelings of shame and doubt, fear of exposure, and ritualized activity; in later adulthood the failure to achieve "autonomy" is seen in the individual who is a "compulsive character," with an irrational need for conformity and a concomitant irrational need for approval.

Preschool—theoretical concepts

Erikson (1950, 1959, 1963) believes that in the preschool stage the child has the task of developing *initiative*. She will discover what kind of person she is going to be, she learns to move around freely and has an unlimited radius of goals, her language skills broaden, and she will ask many questions. Her skill in using words is not matched by her skill in understanding them, and she is thus faced with the dangers of misinterpretation and misunderstanding. Language and locomotion allow her to expand her imagination over such a broad spectrum that she can easily frighten herself with dreams and thoughts.

The prerequisites for masculine and feminine initiative are developed. Infantile sexual curiosity and preoccupation with sexual matters arise. Oedipal wishes can occur as a result of increased imagination, and terrifying fantasies and a sense of guilt over these fantasies may develop.

Initiative becomes governed by a firmly established conscience. The child feels shame not only when she is found out but also when she fears being found out; guilt is felt for thoughts as well as deeds, and in this stage anxiety is controlled by play, by fantasy, and by pride in the attainment of new skills.

The child is ready to learn quickly and to share and to work with others toward a given goal; she begins to identify with people other than her parents and will develop a feeling of equality of worth with others despite differences in functions and age.

At 4½ to 5 years of age the shift from infantile to juvenile body build is rapid, and the beginning of hand-eye coordination as well as an intellectual growth spurt occurs. The social base of gender role is firmly laid down by the end of the fifth year. If this stage is successfully accomplished, the child develops the fantasy of "I who can become"; but if the child is excessively guilt-ridden, her fantasy is "I who shouldn't dream of it." The desired self-concept at the end of this stage is "I have the worth to try even if I am small."

Failure or trauma at this time leads to confusion of psychosexual role, rigidity and guilt in interpersonal relations, and loss of initiative in the exploration of new skills.

Prepuberty—theoretical concepts

Prepuberty years are characterized as the learning stage; that is, "I am what I learn" (Erikson, 1959). The child wants to be shown how to do things both alone and with others; he develops a sense of industry in which he becomes dissatisfied if he does not have the feeling of being useful or a sense of his ability to make things and make them well, even perfectly. He now learns to win recognition by *producing things*. He feels pleasure when his attention and diligence produce a completed work.

Slow but steady growth occurs as maturation of the central nervous system continues. In terms of psychosexual development pressure is reduced in the exploration of sensuality and the gender role while other skills are developed and exploited.

The cognitive phase of development includes the mastery of skills in manipulating objects and the concepts of his culture. Thinking enters the period of *concrete operations* (Piaget, 1963), and the ability to solve concrete problems with this ability increases, so that toward the end of this period the child is able to abstract problems. The solution of real problems is accomplished with mental operations that the child was previously unable to perform. By puberty the child exhibits simple deductive reasoning ability and has learned the rules and the basic technology of his culture, thus reinforcing his sense of belonging in his environment.

Self-esteem is derived from the sense of adequacy and the beginning of "best" friendships and sharing with peers. This also marks the beginning of friendships and loves outside the family, as he begins to learn the complexities, pleasures, and difficulties of adjusting himself and his drives, aggressive and erotic, to those of his peers. By learning and adjusting he begins to take his place as a member of their group and social life. In making this adjustment he seeks the company of his own sex and forms groups and secret societies. The gangs and groups, especially the boys, fight each other in games, baseball, and cops and robbers, working off much hostility and aggression in a socially approved manner.

Feelings of inadequacy and inferiority may begin if the child does not develop a sense of adequacy. Family life may not have prepared him for school, or the school itself may fail to help him in developing the necessary skills for competency. As a result, he may feel that he will never be good at anything he attempts.

In general, children are better able to cope with stress when normal familial supports are available. Any real or imagined threat of separation from a nuclear family member could drastically reduce their abilities to cope with new or changing psychosocial demands. They are particularly vulnerable to such crisis-precipitating situations as the loss of a parent through death. Equally as stressful are recurring partial losses of a parent from the child's usual environment. Examples of the latter are repeated episodes of parental hospitalization or frequent, extended absences from home by one or both parents.

An increasingly common source of emotional distress for children of this age group is the entry, or reentry, of the "homemaker" parent into the work field. This major change in the parenting role demands reciprocal changes in the child's role. For some children, externally imposed demands to assume increased independence and responsibility for self may be more than the child is maturationally able to cope with. Not yet able to assume the level of expected independence, the child may actually perceive this as a form of rejection by the parent.

A common symbol of this role change is the home "latch key" that is bestowed upon the child, much like a rite of passage and with the accompaniment of new social rules and regulations. In general, such rules and regulations focus on protection of the child and the home, with the child given implicit, or explicit, responsibility for ensuring that neither is violated in the parent's absence.

The following case study is about Billy B., an 8-year-old boy for whom the latch key symbolized only rejection.

Case study *Prepuberty*

ASSESSMENT OF THE INDIVIDUAL AND THE PROBLEM

Billy B., 8 years old, was referred with his mother to the school counseling psychologist by his homeroom teacher. For the past few weeks, she reported, Billy had changed from his usual cheerful, outgoing, alert behavior to moodiness and apparent preoccupation. He was falling behind in his schoolwork and twice during the past week he had failed to return to his classes after the lunch hour. The first time that he had done this, the school had contacted his mother at her place of work. She told them that Billy had already telephoned her from home. He told her that his stomach was upset, so he had decided to go home and call her from there. She was planning to go right home when the call came from the school.

Yesterday, the counselor was told, Billy again failed to return to his classes after the lunch hour. This time he did not call his mother and he did not go home. After being notified by the school, his mother had telephoned home. She thought that Billy would be there, as before. Failing to get any answer, she went directly home from her work to begin looking for him around the neighborhood.

About an hour later, while making his routine security rounds, the apartment house custodian heard muffled sounds coming from a basement stairway and went to investigate. He found Billy crouched on the top steps, his head on his knees and sobbing. He was taken immediately to his mother. When questioned, he denied having been threatened by anyone or being injured, and he showed no signs of physical abuse. He refused to say why he had left school early again, or why he had not gone directly home.

Mrs. B. immediately called the school and told them that Billy had been located and was safe. She was asked, and agreed, to come to school the next day with Billy to meet with his homeroom teacher. At her request, during the meeting the following day a referral was made for Billy and her to meet with the counseling psychologist.

Billy was seen initially without his mother present. He was average in height and weight, appeared physically healthy, though pale, and spoke hesitantly. He sat slouched down in his chair, his eyes downcast, and appeared rather depressed. When asked why he had left school without permission twice that week, he muttered, "I don't know what everyone is so excited about—I can take care of myself—ask my mother—I can go home alone because I have the house key and can get in when my mother isn't home."

He stated that he'd always liked school, got A's and B's, and that he particularly enjoyed gym and outdoor sports, such as soccer and football. Until a week ago, he had attended an after-school boys' sport group with many of his friends. This, however, had been suddenly cancelled when the group director had resigned and moved to another city. He also said that his parents had been divorced when he was "a little kid" (4 years old) and that he now lived with his mother. He had frequently visited with his father, who lived nearby, until about 4 months ago. At that time his father had remarried and, a month later, his father's company had transferred him out of state.

After seeing Billy alone, the counselor talked to Mrs. B. to verify and to clarify this information and to assess her feelings about his problems and her ability to cope with them.

Mrs. B. was a tall, attractive, well-dressed woman who gave the impression that she was deeply concerned about the recent changes in Billy's behavior. She stated that Billy, an only child, had always been considered to be "well adjusted," got along well with his friends, and, until recently, could always be depended on to keep up with his schoolwork. She went on to say that she and the boy's father had been particularly concerned about what effect their divorce might have on him. They had met regularly with a family therapist during that period to help Billy through their separation and eventual divorce.

Mrs. B. had met her husband in college and they had married right after graduation. He was an electronics engineer and she had majored in business administration. During the 3 years before Billy was born, she had advanced to a well-paying position as administrative assistant to the director of a large advertising company. When she learned that she was pregnant, she arranged to take a 6-month leave of absence after his birth. However, as she described it to the counselor, Billy was not a healthy baby and seemed to have one medical problem after another for more than 2 years.

She described Billy's father as very possessive and domineering whenever it came to any decisions about Billy's care. "In fact," she said, "when the time came that I felt that I could safely leave Billy with a sitter and go back to work, it became clear to me that our marriage was in for a lot of rocky days ahead." After many days of arguing and eventual compromise, it was agreed that she would return to work on a part-time basis and this only if they were both satisfied that the baby-sitter was giving Billy the best of care. Furthermore, the father completely refused the idea of a day nursery, insisting that they get a sitter to come to their home, stating, "It's his home as much as it is ours, and he is entitled to be here—not in some stranger's house where I can't check up on things whenever I want."

By the time Billy was 3 years old, his mother reported, both parents realized that he was being emotionally "ping-ponged" between them and that her returning to work, even for a day, would always be a point of conflict with her husband. He had grown up in a very patriarchal family with his mother never daring to even dream of any other role than that of "Kinder, Kirche, und Kuche." It was difficult for him to consider any other role for his wife, now that they had a family.

On the other hand, Billy's mother had grown up in a family that encouraged equal rights for women. Her mother was a practicing attorney while rearing four children and her father had managed a produce company. She just could not understand why she and her husband were having so many conflicts with only *one* child.

By the time Billy was 4 years old they had separated and they were eventually divorced when he was 5. The final decree provided Mr. B. with ample visitation rights and they shared equally the responsibility for child support funds.

Until 4 months ago Billy's mother had been able to manage on part-time work and was able to be home each day when he returned from school. However, earlier this year Mr. B. had remarried and, when he transferred out of state 4 months ago, he was over 6 months delinquent in payments for his share of child support. Being, as she put it, "a very realistic person," Mrs. B. decided that she could no longer depend on Billy's father for regular payments in the future. Three months ago she went to her boss and asked if she could be reassigned to full-time work on an ongoing basis as soon as possible.

She stated that Billy had never expressed any particularly negative feelings about his father remarrying and moving away, only that he would miss seeing him as often as he had in the past. She had taken particular care in planning with Billy for her return to full-time work. She knew, for example, that she would not be able to be home before he got back from school at the end of the day, so they planned for him to join an afterschool supervised sport group. This was one that would pick him up at the school and return him to his home by supper-time each day. "By that time," she said, "I would be home and he wouldn't come home to an empty apartment." This, she felt, also took care of her worry about him playing unsupervised in the neighborhood without her there to "keep an eye on things."

Three weeks ago Mrs. B. had started her full-time work. She had always managed to get home before Billy returned from the sports group. It seemed to her that there were going to be no really major changes for either of them to adjust to. One week ago, however, the director of the sports group suddenly resigned without notice. A replacement had not been found yet, and the group had been temporarily cancelled. As the only interim choice that she could think of, Mrs. B. decided to give Billy his own key to the apartment.

Worried about all of the real and imagined things that might happen to him before she got home, she accompanied the key with many admonishments about coming directly home from school, checking in with the apartment manager when he got there, and being sure to keep the door locked until she got home. She said that Billy did not seem to object to this at all. In fact, he had purchased a key chain to hook on his belt just like the one that the building manager wore.

When the school called her the first time Billy cut classes and went home, she had counseled him to remain at school the next time he felt ill and she would pick him up there. She had told him that he must "never go home alone again without first telling her or someone at the school. I don't like the idea of your being alone and sick. You know I would worry about you." She had also reminded him that they had planned this together and that they both had certain responsibilities to each other in working out this new living schedule. "Neither of us had much choice in this, you know," she told the counselor. "I'm making the best of things that I know how, and Billy is just going to have to cooperate. I just don't know why he is acting this way now."

PLANNING THERAPEUTIC INTERVENTION

The sudden, rapid changes in Billy's life during the past few months had forced him into assuming a degree of independence and self-responsibility beyond his maturational level of skills. Not yet accepting the loss of his father and perceiving it as a rejection of himself, he was forced to full dependence on his mother for any sense of security and all decision making. The timely entrance into the after-school sports group had provided him with opportunities to express his feeling of anger and hostility about the situation through the competitive, aggressive sports activities with his peers. Unfortunately, the group was cancelled about the same time his mother started her new job, and he lost his normal outlet for expressing such feelings. Not only did he lose situational support of his peers when he most needed it, he had the further situational loss of his mother from her familiar roles. He could no longer depend on her being at home when he might need her during the day. His anxiety increased as he perceived this to be another sign of rejection from a parent figure. Billy had no coping mechanisms in his repertoire with which to handle these feelings of added anxiety and depression. At the particular time when he needed to use his usually successful coping behaviors, the opportunity was not available because of the demand by his mother that he "come home directly after school—you can't play in the neighborhood after school with your friends."

It was believed that Mrs. B. needed assistance in gaining a realistic, intellectual understanding of the situation as it related to Billy's current behaviors. Increasingly anxious about the added responsibility that had been placed upon her during the past few months, she was possibly projecting her own feelings of insecurity into overprotective behaviors toward Billy, that is, "it is Billy, not *I,* who should not be out alone and unprotected. Something terrible might happen to *him* when there is no longer a strong, dependable person nearby to help keep an eye on things."

Billy would need to explore his perceptions and feelings about the psychosocial losses of both parents from the usual family roles that they had occupied in his life. He needed to be helped to express his feelings constructively and to make a positive adaptation to the new role demands made of him.

INTERVENTION

During the first session the counselor focused on identifying with Mrs. B. the many critical changes that had occurred in Billy's life during the past few months and their impact on his level of maturational skills' development. The goal was to provide her with insight into how Billy might be perceiving such events at his level of comprehension and concrete thinking. Although he was old enough to be fully aware of the events happening, he was still too young to deal with them abstractly. For example, when his father had remarried and then had moved away soon after, Billy most likely had perceived these actions as signs of complete rejection by his father and blamed himself in some way. In his mind he may have wondered, "Why else would my father marry someone else and then move away, abandoning both me and my mother?"

It was also suggested to Mrs. B. that her comments at the time such as, "If I don't go back to full-time work, we won't have a roof over our heads or food to eat," were probably taken quite literally by Billy. So, also, was her later admonishment to him always to come straight home from school, implying that he was one more source of problems for her.

In the next two sessions, through the use of direct questioning and reflection of verbal and nonverbal clues with Mrs. B., it became possible for her to express her own feelings about the recent chain of events in her life and to begin to relate them to Billy's behavioral changes. It was suggested that she try to find some alternative supervised peer-group activities for Billy after school. The purpose was to reinstate, for him, the opportunity for some normal, acceptable outlets for the angry, hostile feelings that he must be still having from the recent losses in his life.

The counselor met with Billy at the beginning of each session to discuss with him how he was doing in school classes and what things he was doing to occupy his time after school before his mother got home from work. Billy's feelings of rejection and insecurity were dealt with during this time.

The remaining time was spent with Mrs. B. She was encouraged to continue to

CASE STUDY: BILLY

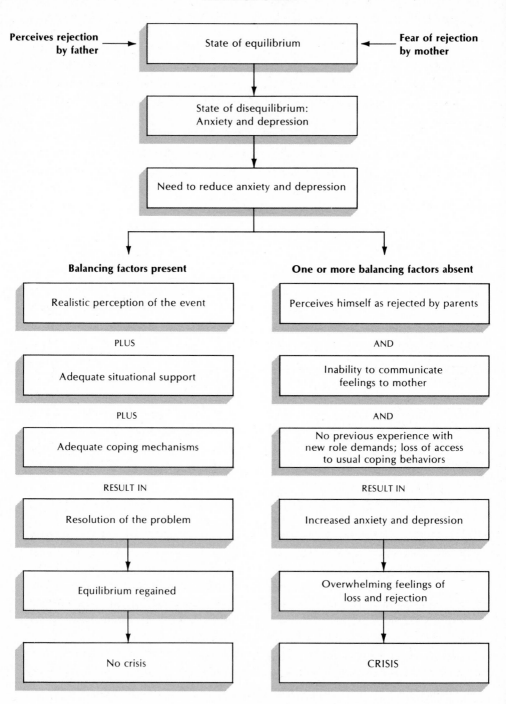

**Perceives rejection
by father** →   State of equilibrium   ← **Fear of rejection
by mother**

State of disequilibrium:
Anxiety and depression

Need to reduce anxiety and depression

Balancing factors present

Realistic perception of the event

PLUS

Adequate situational support

PLUS

Adequate coping mechanisms

RESULT IN

Resolution of the problem

Equilibrium regained

No crisis

One or more balancing factors absent

Perceives himself as rejected by parents

AND

Inability to communicate
feelings to mother

AND

No previous experience with
new role demands; loss of access
to usual coping behaviors

RESULT IN

Increased anxiety and depression

Overwhelming feelings of
loss and rejection

CRISIS

provide Billy was as much independence as feasible, yet not expect him to assume any more than he could comfortably cope with at this time. The importance of providing Billy with every opportunity to learn new social skills and to develop strong feelings of competency and self-adequacy was emphasized. The fact that closing off his access to usual after-school activities with his peers would greatly limit his chances for new learning experiences was discussed. It might also precipitate his return to the same maladaptive coping behaviors that he had been demonstrating during the past few weeks.

Mrs. B. was not able to locate another supervised activity group for her son to attend after school. However, she did make arrangements with a retired gentleman who lived in the same apartment house to "keep an eye" on Billy and to be a contact for him when he came home and played in the neighborhood with his friends after school.

ANTICIPATORY PLANNING

An important focus of anticipatory planning was to review with Mrs. B. the maturational changes that she could expect to see developing in Billy over the next few years. The need for her to continue to allow him normal opportunities for growth and development was stressed. The fact that Billy was now a member of a single-parent family should not create any particular peer group problems, since this situation was increasingly common among children his age. However, potential stressful situations were identified with her and discussed in terms of how she might approach coping with them as they arose, both for herself and in her dealings with Billy.

Billy was encouraged to be more direct in questions to his mother and in letting her know when he felt confused or angry about things that were happening to him. He understood that he could stop in and talk to the counselor whenever the need arose, but that he would also be expected to keep in close touch with his mother about his feelings in the future.

SUMMATION OF THE PARADIGM

Billy had perceived his father's remarriage and move out of state as a rejection of himself. Unable to express his feelings to his mother, he coped by acting out his anger and hostility in competitive, aggressive sports activities with his peers. Despite Mrs. B.'s assumptions to the contrary, planning with Billy for her return to full-time work had served to reactivate his fears of another rejection. No longer having his sports activities available to him as before, his anxiety increased. Lacking any other available coping skills, he became overwhelmed.

Intervention focused on helping Billy explore his feelings of loss and rejection. Time was spent with his mother, helping her understand the level of maturational skills and the need to better recognize when her demands of him, or expectations, might exceed his abilities to meet them.

Adolescence—theoretical concepts

The adolescent has a strong need to find and confirm her identity. Rapid body growth equals that of early childhood, but it is compounded by the addition of physical-genital maturity. Faced with the physiological revolution within herself, the adolescent is also concerned with consolidating her social roles. She is preoccupied with the difference between what she appears to be in the eyes of others and what she believes herself to be. In searching for a new sense of continuity, some adolescents must refight crises left unresolved in previous years.

Changes that occur while secondary sex characteristics emerge make the adolescent self-conscious and uncomfortable with herself and with her friends. Body image changes and the adolescent constantly seeks validation that these physiological changes are "normal" because she feels different and is dissatisfied with how she thinks she looks. If sudden spurts of growth occur, she concludes she will be too tall; conversely, if growth does not occur as expected, she thinks she will be too short, or too thin, or too fat. In this period of fluctuation, half-child and half-adult, the adolescent reacts with childish rebellion one day and with adult maturity the next.

The adolescent is as unpredictable to herself as she is to parents and other adults. On the one hand she seeks freedom and rebels against authority, on the other she does not trust her own sense of emerging maturity and covertly seeks guidelines from adults. In her struggle for an identity she turns to her peers and adopts their mode of dress, mannerisms, vocabulary, and code of behavior, often to the distress of adult society. The adolescent desperately needs to belong, to feel accepted, loved, and wanted.

This is the age for cliques and gangs. The "in group" can be extremely clannish and intolerant of those who do not belong. Banding together against the adult world, its members seek to internalize their identity, but because of different and often rebellious behavior they are frequently incorrectly labeled as "delinquent."

Having achieved a sense of security and acceptance from peers, the adolescent begins to seek heterosexual involvement. This occurs first at group-oriented social events, such as dances, parties, and football games. As comfort and confidence increase, the adolescent progresses to more meaningful and deeper emotional involvements in one-to-one heterosexual relationships. Because of conflict between sexual drives, desires, and the established norms of society, this stage can be extremely stressful, and again the adolescent is faced with indecision and confusion.

Occupational identity also becomes a concern at this time. There are continual queries by parents and school authorities about career plans for the future. Uncertainties are compounded when a definite choice cannot be made because of an inability to fully identify with the adult world of work. Having only observed or participated in fragments of work situations, the adolescent finds it difficult to commit herself to the reality of full-time employment and its inherent responsibilities. It is easier and more realistic to state what is *not* wanted rather than what is wanted as a career.

Piaget (1963) refers to the cognitive development at this stage as *formal operations,* the period in which the capacity for abstract thinking and complex deductive reasoning becomes possible. At this time the goal is "independence," and in mid-adolescence acceptance of the idea that it is possible to love and at the same time to be angry with someone is one problem that should be solved. If this stage is successfully negotiated, the individual develops a capacity for self-responsibility; failure may lead to a sense of inadequacy in controlling and competing.

Because of the number and wide variety of stimuli and rapid changes to which she is exposed, the adolescent is in a hazardous situation. A crisis situation may be compounded by the normal amount of flux characteristic of adolescent development (Cameron, 1963; Erikson, 1950, 1959, 1963; Piaget, 1963; Zachry, 1940).

The following case study illustrates some of the conflicts that adolescents face while trying to find their identity, to strive for independence, and to win acceptance from their peer group. It also points out the need for understanding and patience on the part of parents as their adolescents grow up.

Case study   *Adolescence*

ASSESSMENT OF THE INDIVIDUAL AND THE PROBLEM

Mary V., a 14-year-old high school sophomore, was referred to a crisis center with her parents by a school nurse. During the past few weeks she had shown signs of increased anxiety, cried easily, and had lost interest in school activities. That morning, for no apparent reason, she had suddenly left the classroom in tears. The teacher followed and found her crouched in a nearby utility closet, crying uncontrollably. Mary seemed unable to give a reason for her loss of control and was very anxious. When her mother came in response to a call from the school nurse, they agreed to follow her advice and seek family therapy.

During the first session the therapist saw Mary and her parents together in order to assess their interaction and communication patterns and to determine Mary's problems.

Mrs. V. was quiet and left most of the conversation up to her husband and Mary. When she attempted to add anything to what was being said, she was quickly silenced by Mr. V.'s hard, cold stare or by Mary exclaiming in an exasperated tone, "Oh, Mother!" Mr. V. spoke in a controlled, stilted manner, saying that he had no idea what was wrong with Mary, and Mrs. V. responded hesitantly that it must be something at school.

Mary was particularly well developed for her age, a fact that was apparent despite the rather shapeless shift she was wearing. She might have been very attractive if she had paid more attention to her posture and general appearance.

When questioned, Mary said that she had not been sleeping well for weeks, had no appetite, and could not concentrate on her schoolwork. She did not know why she felt this way, and her uncontrolled outburst of tears frightened and embarrassed her. She was also afraid of what she might do next, adding that her crying that morning was probably because she had not slept well for the past 2 nights. At first she tried to brush this off as final exam jitters.

She evaded answering repeated questions about sudden changes in her life in the past few days. When the therapist asked if she would be comfortable talking alone, without her parents, she gave her father a quick glance and replied that she would. Mr. and Mrs. V. were asked if they objected to Mary talking to the therapist alone. Both agreed that it might be a good idea and went to the waiting room.

For a time Mary continued to respond evasively. It was obvious that she had strongly mixed feelings about how to relate to the male therapist. Should it be "woman to man" or "child to adult?" Throughout this and the following sessions she alternated between her child-adult roles. The therapist recognized the role ambivalence of adolescence and adjusted his role relationship, using whichever was most effective in focusing on the problem areas and making Mary more comfortable.

Mary eventually relaxed and began to talk freely about her relationship with her family, her activities at school, and some of the feelings that were troubling her. She said that she had two older brothers. The younger of the two, Kirk, was 16 years old and a senior in high school. She felt closer to him because "he understands and I can talk to him." Mary said that she had "as good a childhood" as the rest of her friends. However, she did think that her father kept a closer eye on her activities than did the parents of most of her friends. He still called her his "baby" and "my little girl" and lately had begun to place more restrictions on her friendships and activities than usual.

She admitted that during the past year she had gone through a sudden spurt of body growth and development. She was keenly aware of these differences in her appearance and sensed the changing attitudes of her father and her friends. She felt her father was worried about her growing "up and out so fast." He was the one who insisted that she wear the almost shapeless shifts. She said she knew "It wasn't really because I outgrow things so fast right now—he thinks I look too sexy for my age!"

About 3 weeks ago she had been invited to the junior-senior prom by a friend of her brother Kirk. She liked the boy and wanted to go but was not sure Kirk would approve, because he would be at the prom too. Another problem was getting her parents' permission to go and to buy the necessary formal clothes. She had looked at dresses and knew exactly the one she wanted but knew her father would not let her have it.

Mary was asked if she felt able to tell her parents these things that were bothering her if the therapist were present to give her support. She thought that she could if he would "sort of prepare them first" and explain how important it was for her to go dressed like the rest of her girl friends. He suggested that Mary discuss the situation with Kirk to see how he felt about her going to the prom with his friend, and she agreed to do this before the next session. The therapist assured her that he would spend the first part of the next session with her parents to discuss and explore their feelings about this.

PLANNING OF THERAPEUTIC INTERVENTION

It was thought that Mary needed support to assist her in convincing her parents that she be allowed to grow up. Mr. and Mrs. V. needed to gain an intellectual understanding of some of the problems that adolescent girls face as they search for an identity, seek independence, and feel the need to be like their peers. Mrs. V. would have to be encouraged to give support and guidance to Mary and help to resist Mr. V.'s attempts to keep Mary as the baby of the family.

INTERVENTION

At the next session the therapist went to the waiting room to get Mr. and Mrs. V. and saw that Mary had brought her brother Kirk with her. She asked if he could come in with them at the last half of the session when the family would be together. The therapist agreed, realizing that Mary had brought additional support and that apparently Kirk had approved of her going to the prom.

The first part of the session was spent discussing with the parents the general problems of most adolescents, as well as the reasons behind their often erratic and unusual behavior. Both parents seemed willing to accept this new knowledge, although Mr. V. said that he had not noticed any of this with the boys. Mrs. V. said, "No, but you treated them differently, you were glad they were becoming men." The therapist supported Mrs. V. and said that this was one of Mary's specific problems. He then repeated to the parents what Mary had said about the things that were bothering her. Both parents seemed slightly embarrassed, and Mr. V.'s voice and manner became quite angry as he tried to explain why he wanted to "protect" Mary, "She's so young, so innocent—someone may take advantage of her," and so on.

Discussion then focused on Mary's anxiety and the tension she was feeling because her father had made her feel different from her friends. Compromise between Mr. and Mrs. V. and Mary was explored when Mary and Kirk joined their parents

CASE STUDY: MARY

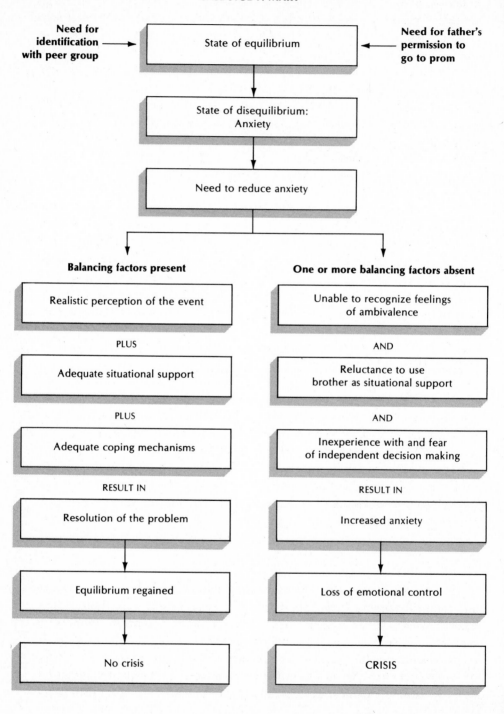

in the last half of the session. Mary was more verbal with Kirk present to support her, and Kirk told his father, "You are too old fashioned, Mary's a good kid; you don't have to worry about her; you make her dress like a 10-year-old," and so on. Mr. V. was silent for a while and then said, "You may be right, Kirk, I don't know." He then asked him, "Do you think I should let her go to the prom?" Kirk answered, "Yes, Dad, I'll be there; she can even double with me and my girl." Her father agreed, adding that Mrs. V. should go with her to pick out a "fairly decent dress." Mary began to cry, and Mr. V. in great consternation asked, "What's wrong now?" She replied, "Daddy, I'm so happy, don't you know women cry when they are happy too!"

ANTICIPATORY PLANNING

The next few sessions were spent in supporting the family members in their changing attitudes toward each other. Anticipatory planning was directed toward establishing open communication between the parents and Mary to avoid another buildup of tensions and misunderstandings. Mary was encouraged to use Kirk as a situational support in the future, since he and his father were not in conflict.

The V.'s were told they could return for help with future crises if necessary and were assured that they had accomplished a great deal toward mutual understanding.

SUMMATION OF THE PARADIGM

Mary suffered acute symptoms of anxiety because she had to ask her father for permission to go to a dance. She wanted to be a member of her peer group but felt uncomfortable because she was not allowed to dress as they did. She wanted independence but was inexperienced and afraid to make a decision that would oppose her father. Because the situation involved possible conflict with her brother, she did not feel comfortable in talking with him about her problem.

Intervention was based on exploring areas of difficulty with the family and assisting them to recognize, understand, and support Mary's adolescent behavior, her bid for independence, and her need to become a member of her peer group.

Young adulthood—theoretical concepts

Young adulthood is the time in which childhood and youth come to an end and adulthood begins. It involves studying for a specific career or seeking employment, as well as sociability with either sex. According to Cameron (1963), socioeconomic developments make it difficult to determine the transition from adolescence to adulthood. Originally this was determined by the young adult maintaining an independent job, having the capacity for marrying, and forming a new family unit. The young unemployed tend to live at home with their families in a dependent relationship that has some of the characteristics of adolescence and some of the independence of adulthood. The young adult can no longer look forward confidently to gainful employment; without technical or professional education he may have to be satisfied with unskilled temporary jobs. The more time he spends in technological or professional training, the longer he remains financially dependent on his family, and changes and uncertainties in modern socioeconomic situations may extend the period of dependence into the middle or late twenties. If the preceding stages of maturation have been successfully negotiated, the young adult will have confidence in himself and his ability for decision making and, as a result, will be able to establish and maintain a real intimacy with others.

Adult society demands that young adults not deviate from the established norm: they are expected to remain in school if studying for a career or be consistent and productive in a job while maintaining an active social life.

There is an exploration and exploitation, or the denial of cultural and familial heritage, and a clarification of self-identity and the social role. The psychosexual task is one of differentiating self from family without complete withdrawal from the family. Cognitive development should be at the level of deductive and inductive logic, with expansion and exploration of cognitive capacities and the beginning of creativity.

Unsuccessful transition at this stage or lack of inner resources may lead to confusion when decisions are made regarding future goals. There is an inability to establish a true and mutual psychological intimacy with another person; there is also a tendency toward self-isolation and the maintenance of only highly stereotyped and formal interpersonal relationships, characterized by a lack of spontaneity, warmth, and an honest exchange of emotional involvement.

In the next case study a young adult is faced with the problem of making a choice between conforming to society's norms for choosing a vocation and marriage or remaining self-absorbed in his own immature interests.

Case study   *Young adulthood*

ASSESSMENT OF THE INDIVIDUAL AND THE PROBLEM

Bob M., 18 years old, came for help at a crisis center stating he was "feeling bad." When the therapist asked him to be more specific, he said he was not sleeping, was nervous, and things seemed unreal to him. When asked who referred him to the center, he replied a friend who had been there when he had been in trouble.

Bob was small in stature, slim, with a shaggy black beard, neatly dressed in Levis, sport shirt, and cowboy boots. During the initial session Bob appeared overtly nervous and depressed. He sometimes spoke in short, rapid bursts, usually after a period of silence, but more often he spoke in a slow, hesitant manner. He would neither establish nor maintain eye contact with the therapist, continually looking down at the floor.

When asked about events occurring before the onset of his symptoms, Bob said that "during the past 10 days so many things have happened it's difficult to remember what happened first." He began to recite events. After working on his car for 6 months "it blew up" the first time he drove it. This was also the first time he had been able to drive in 6 months because his driver's license had been revoked for speeding. This precipitated a quarrel with his girlfriend, Lauri, because he had promised to take her out when his driver's license was reinstated and his car was fixed. He had recently received a promotion to foreman at work, but he was ambivalent—pleased with the promotion although uncertain of his readiness to accept the responsibility of a permanent job. Last, his best friend, a member of his motorcycle club, was out of town, and he felt that he had no one with whom to talk about his problems.

Further exploration with Bob revealed that his usual pattern of coping with stress was to ride his motorcycle with his friend "as fast and as far as we can go." They would stop someplace and "talk it out." He felt that this relieved his tension; things became clearer, and he could usually solve the problem.

Bob also expressed ambivalence in his relationship with Lauri. He loved her and wanted to marry her but was concerned because he thought that they had conflicting values; she was from a middle-class family with values that emphasized the importance of a steady job, conformity, and so forth, whereas he felt he belonged in the motorcycle club and liked their philosophy, or as he stated it, "to be free, take what you want, don't work." He was afraid that marriage to Lauri would inhibit his freedom and that to please her family he feared he would have to give up riding with his friends and working on his car and would have to trim his beard.

PLANNING OF THERAPEUTIC INTERVENTION

Because of the many problems presented it was necessary for the therapist to sift through extraneous data and concentrate on major areas of difficulty. She decided, at this time, to assume the role of available situational support until other support could be found. This would give Bob the opportunity to use his prior successful coping device of "talking it out." As tension decreased, other support would be provided for his attempts to solve his problems.

INTERVENTION

The goal of intervention was established by the therapist to assist Bob to recognize and cope with his feelings of ambivalence toward his job and Lauri and with the implications of making a choice. The areas of difficulty were determined to be a conflict of values and Bob's need to feel that he belonged to something or someone.

In the next two sessions, while the therapist acted as a situational support, Bob's symptoms diminished. He was able to discuss and explore his feelings about Lauri and his job; he also began discussing his fears of "giving up so much" if they married. Because Bob's relationship with Lauri appeared to be a major problem area, the therapist suggested that she be included in the sessions.

In the subsequent sessions, which Lauri did attend, they began discussing areas of mutual concern and conflict. Lauri said that she did not expect him to give up riding his motorcycle. "He can do it on weekends, and I'll go along." Bob became angry, saying that he did not want her along because she "was too nice for that crowd." He then admitted he was not certain he would continue with them anyway, *but* he wanted it understood that he could go riding with his friend occasionally if he wanted. Bob added that if they were married, he might not need them because he would have her (his need to belong).

When Bob spoke of her parents' comments about his shaggy beard, Lauri said that she liked his beard and that he was marrying her, not her family.

She insisted, however, that Bob spent too much time working on his car and not enough with her. Bob replied that the car was his hobby and said that he probably spent less time on his hobby than her father did on his golf.

In the concluding sessions Bob apparently resolved his conflicts and stated firmly that he thought he would be gaining more than he might lose if he married Lauri and kept his job. At the last session they made tentative plans to be married.

ANTICIPATORY PLANNING

The most important phase in anticipatory planning occurred when Bob agreed that Lauri be included in the therapy sessions. The necessity of choosing between present modes of behavior and gratifications and future expectations in his life led Bob to weigh the consequences involved. His decision to include Lauri in future planning indicated an orientation toward reality. In certain phases of life it is necessary to give up certain pleasures of youth that appear to be consistent with freedom. An orientation toward the future, where maturity of decisions reflects not only an inner freedom but also a sense of self-fulfillment and a recognition of one's own strength, is consistent with a strong ego-identity.

SUMMATION OF THE PARADIGM

Bob M. was forced to seek help because of increased symptoms of tension and anxiety. So many stressful events occurring in rapid succession had made it impossible for him to decide which problem should be solved first. His usual situational support, the friend from the motorcycle club, was out of town, and his normal method of coping with stress was unavailable.

Ambivalent feelings about his job situation and his girlfriend Lauri increased his feelings of tension; he became immobile and unable to make decisions or to solve his problems.

Intervention focused on providing Bob with the situational support of the therapist, and Lauri was included as an active participant in the later sessions. When

CASE STUDY: BOB M

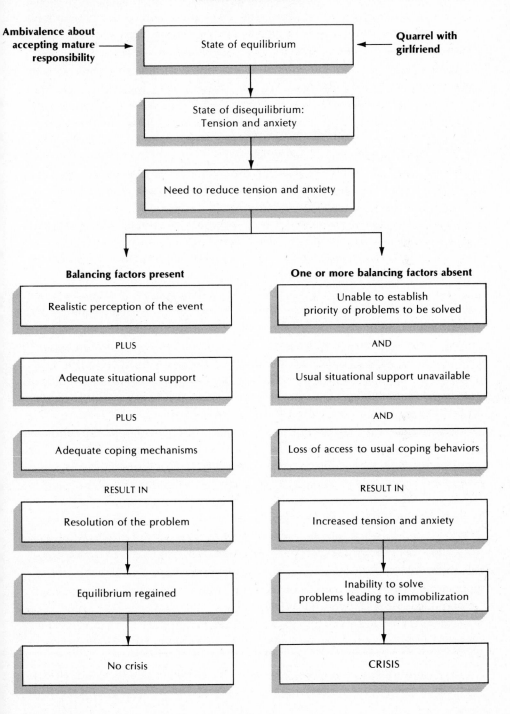

Bob was encouraged to ventilate his feelings, his anxiety decreased and he was able to perceive relationships between the stressful events and his crisis situation more realistically. Previous successful coping skills were reintroduced and proved adequate in assisting him to solve his problem. Major focus of the last sessions was anticipatory planning to help him cope with future areas of stress as he made the transition to increased maturity.

Adulthood—theoretical concepts

Adulthood is the usual period in life when the responsibilities of parenthood are assumed, involving the abilities of a man and woman to accept the strengths and weaknesses of one another and to combine their energies toward mutual goals. It is a crucial time for reconciliation with practical reality.

Maturity is always relative and is usually considered to develop in adulthood. Many adults who marry and have children never do achieve psychological maturity whereas others who choose not to marry may show a greater degree of mature responsibility than many of their married peers.

Adult normality, like maturity, is also relative. Normality requires that a person achieve and maintain a reasonably effective balance, both psychodynamically and interpersonally. The normal adult must be able to control and channel her emotional drives without losing her initiative and vigor. She should be able to cope with ordinary personal upheavals and the frustrations and disappointments in life with only temporary disequilibrium and be able to participate enthusiastically in adult work and adult play, as well as have the capacity to give and to experience adequate sexual gratifications in a stable relationship. She should be able to express a reasonable amount of aggression, anger, joy, and affection without undue effort or unnecessary guilt.

In actuality it is unreasonable to expect to find perfect normalcy in any adult. Absolute perfection of physique and physiology are rare rather than normal, and an adult with a perfect emotional equilibrium is equally as exceptional.

This case study concerns a young woman whose lack of psychosocial maturity created problems when she was faced with the responsibility of motherhood. Her husband's competence and pleasure in caring for their baby increased her feelings of inadequacy and rejection.

Case study   *Adulthood*

ASSESSMENT OF THE INDIVIDUAL AND THE PROBLEM

Myra and John, a young married couple, were referred by Myra's obstetrician to a crisis center because of her symptoms of depression. Myra said she was experiencing difficulty in sleeping, was constantly tired, and would begin to cry for no apparent reason.

Myra was an attractive but fragile blonde of 22 years whose looks and manners gave her the appearance of a 16-year-old. John, 28 years old, had a calm and mature demeanor. They had been married 1½ years and were the parents of a 3-month-old son, John, Jr.

John was an engineer with a large corporation. Myra had been a liberal arts major when they met and married. John was the oldest of four children and was from a stable family of modest circumstances; Myra, on the other hand, was an only child who had been indulged by wealthy parents.

When questioned by the therapist specifically about the onset of her symptoms, Myra stated that they had really begun after the baby was born, with crying spells and repeated assertions that she "wasn't a good mother" and that taking care of the baby made her nervous. She said she felt inadequate and that even John was better with the baby than she. John attempted to reassure her by telling her she was an excellent mother and that he realized she was nervous about caring for the baby. He suggested that he get someone to help her. Myra said she did not want anyone because it was her baby, and she could not understand why she felt as she did.

When questioned about her pregnancy and the birth of the child, she said there had been no complications and had added hesitantly that it had not been a planned pregnancy. When asked to explain further, she replied that she and John had decided to wait until they had been married about 3 years before starting a family. She went on to explain that she did not think she and John had enough time to enjoy their life together before the baby was born.

After she had recovered from the shock of knowing that she was pregnant, she became really thrilled at the thought of having a baby and enjoyed her pregnancy and shopping for the nursery. Toward the end of her pregnancy she had difficulty sleeping and was troubled by nightmares. She began to feel uncertain of her ability to be a good mother and was frightened because she had not been around babies before.

When she and John brought the baby home, they engaged a nurse for 2 weeks to take care of the child and to teach Myra baby care. She thought that basically she knew how, but it upset her if the baby did not stop crying when she picked him up. When he was at home, John usually took care of the baby, and his competency made her feel more inadequate. The precipitating event was thought to have occurred the week before when John had arrived home from work to find Myra walking the floor with the baby, who was crying loudly. Myra told him she had taken the baby to the pediatrician for an immunization shot that morning. After they returned home he had become irritable, crying continuously, and repeatedly refusing his bottle. When Myra said she did not know what to do, John told her the baby felt feverish. After they took the baby's temperature and discovered that it was

102 °F., John called the pediatrician, who recommended a medication to reduce the temperature and discomfort. John got the medication and gave it to the baby; he also gave the baby his bottle. The baby went to sleep, but Myra went to their bedroom crying and upset.

PLANNING OF THERAPEUTIC INTERVENTION

Myra's mixed feelings toward the baby would be explored in addition to her feelings of inadequacy in caring for him. She apparently resented the responsibility of the parental role, which she was not ready to assume. Unable to express her hostility and feelings of rejection toward the baby, she turned them inward on herself, with the resulting overt symptoms of depression. Bringing these feelings into the open would be a necessary goal. Myra also needed reassurance that her feelings of inadequacy were normal because of her lack of contact and experience with infants and also because most new parents felt this same inadequacy in varying degrees. John obviously was comfortable and knowledgeable in the situation as a result of his experience with a younger brother and sisters; he should be used as a strong situational support.

INTERVENTION

The therapist, believing that a mild antidepressant would help to relieve Myra's symptoms, arranged a medical consultation. It was not thought that she was a threat to herself or to others, and intervention was instituted.

Myra's mention in the initial session that she and John had not had enough time to enjoy each other before the baby was born was considered to be an initial reference to Myra's negative feelings regarding her pregnancy and the baby. In subsequent sessions, through the therapist's use of direct questioning and the reflection of verbal and nonverbal clues, Myra was able to express some of her feelings about their life as a family with a baby in contrast to her feelings when there had been just she and John.

Their previous life pattern revealed much social activity before the birth of the baby and almost none afterward. Myra said that although this had not really bothered her too much at first, recently she had felt as if the walls were closing in on her. John appeared surprised to hear this and asked why she had not mentioned it to him. Myra replied with some anger that it apparently did not seem to bother him, because it was obvious that he enjoyed playing with the baby after he came home from work. The possibility of reinstating some manner of social life for Myra and John was considered to be essential at this point. John told her that his mother would enjoy the chance to babysit with her new grandson and that he and Myra should plan some evenings out alone or with friends. Myra brightened considerably at this and seemed pleased at John's concern.

The therapist also explored their feelings about the responsibilities of parenthood and Myra's feelings of inadequacy in caring for the baby. Myra could commu-

CASE STUDY: MYRA

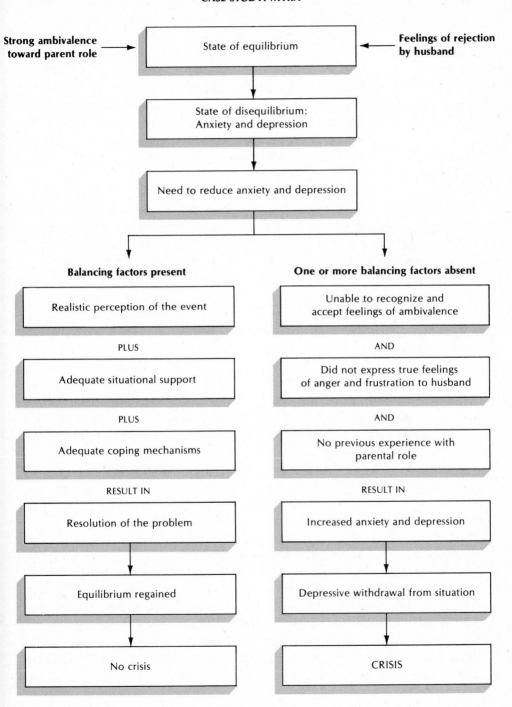

nicate to John and the therapist her feelings that the baby received more of John's attention than she and that she resented "playing second fiddle." John explained that he had originally assumed care of the baby so that she could get some rest and that he enjoyed being with her more than with the baby. He told her that he loved her and that she would always come first with him.

Myra was eventually able to see that she was being childish in resenting the baby and that she was competing for John's attention; as her social life expanded, her negative feelings toward the baby lessened and she said she was feeling more comfortable in caring for him. After the fourth session the medication was discontinued, and Myra's symptoms continued to decrease.

ANTICIPATORY PLANNING

Because of John's maturity it was thought important that he be aware of the possibility that Myra could occasionally have a recurrence of feelings of rejection. If the original symptoms returned, he would recognize them by the pattern they would take and would be able to intercede by exploring what was happening, discussing this openly with Myra. When the progress and adjustments they had made in learning to cope with the situation were reviewed with them, both expressed satisfaction with the changes that had occurred. They were told that they could return for further help if another crisis situation developed.

SUMMATION OF THE PARADIGM

Myra was an only child and rarely had to accept responsibility for others before her marriage. Because she had planned to wait 3 years before having a child, she had strong, mixed feelings about the responsibilities of motherhood before that time and felt unprepared. Her husband's adequacy in caring for the baby when she failed reinforced her mixed feelings. Loss of the social life shared with her husband, combined with the diversion of his attention from her to the baby, reinforced her strong feelings of rejection.

Because she was unable to recognize and accept her feelings of ambivalence and was also unable to tell her husband of her anger and frustration she turned them inward. Lack of previous experience in caring for infants made her unable to cope with the situation, increased her frustration and anger, and resulted in overt symptoms of depression and anxiety.

Late adulthood—theoretical concepts

Late adulthood is the final stage of development discussed in Erikson's theory of maturation (1950, 1959, 1963). If a person has successfully negotiated the preceding stages, he should be mature enough to accept responsibility for his life-style without regrets.

To the average person, reaching late adulthood implies that life patterns have been fairly well set and are no longer open to choices for change. Anxiety results if a man or woman has not demonstrated some capacity for success in either family or career roles. Symptoms of this are frequently noted in such forms as excessive use of alcohol, psychosomatic symptoms, feelings of persecution, and depression (English and Pearson, 1955).

Our culture seems unable to place any firm boundary lines on phases of the aging process. The general tendency is to view life as uphill from infancy and over the hill and decline after reaching the peak of middle years. With cultural emphasis on youthfulness it is not unusual for a person of 50 years to view his future with regret for things left unaccomplished. Hahn refers to this stage as "heads against the ceiling," a time when "the realization strikes home that the probability for appreciable advancement is remote. . . . The ceiling is encountered relatively early by some and at an amazing late time by others, but for all of us the ladder eventually ends at a ceiling." He further describes this as a period when "younger men and women are beginning to crowd into the competitive economic, political and social arenas."* With the rapid technological changes affecting business and professions, younger persons are often better prepared to supply the necessary knowledge and skills.

Family life changes as children grow up and become involved with school, careers, and marriage. For parents it is a time when specific tasks of parenthood are over, and they must return to the family unit of two, making reciprocal changes in role status in relation to their children and to the community. New values and goals must be developed in the marriage to replace those values no longer realistic in the present; failure to recognize this need can open the way to frustration and despair. The wife and mother now has freedom from parental responsibility, but if her entire life-style was centered around the parental role, she may lack interests, skills, and abilities with which to make the role change.

Menopausal changes occur in women at this time. Usually around the age of 45 years a relatively rapid decrease in activity of the sexual glands occurs over a period of 2 to 3 years. Sometimes this is accompanied by a syndrome of psychophysiological symptoms, such as hot flashes, dizziness, cold shivers, and anxiety attacks. According to English and Pearson (1955), it is thought that personality plays a larger part in the symptomatology than the cessation of glandular activity. Many women go through this phase without any stressful symptoms; others become panicky and afraid of a loss of sexual identity.

There appears to be no definite evidence that sexual gland activity in the male undergoes similar rapid decline and cessation; however, men can experience symp-

---

*From Hahn, M.E.: Psychoevaluation: adaption, distribution, adjustment, New York, 1963, McGraw-Hill Book Co., pp. 70, 92-93. Used with permission of McGraw-Hill Book Co.

toms similar to those of women at the same age period. English and Pearson (1955) consider these syndromes to be neuroses rather than a result of any changes in the sexual gland activity.

The unmarried person who may have had thoughts of eventual marriage and a family is now faced with the reality of advancing years. This is a particularly critical time for anyone who has relied strongly on physical attractiveness. He or she now faces the inevitability of physical decline. A person in this stage of life can continue to pursue career interests but may be confronted with limitations to further career advancements.

The following case study concerns a 40-year-old wife and mother whose planned changes in her family role after the marriage of her daughter seem to be threatened by the onset of early menopause.

Case study   *Late adulthood*

ASSESSMENT OF THE INDIVIDUAL AND THE PROBLEM

Mrs. C., a 40-year-old, youthful-appearing mother of three daughters (ages 17, 20, and 22 years) was referred to a crisis center by her physician because of severe anxiety and depression, as evidenced by recent anorexia, weight loss, insomnia, crying spells, and preoccupation, which had begun after a visit to her physician 3 weeks earlier. At that time she had been told that she was entering early menopause. Her youngest daughter was to be married in a month; the two older ones were already married and living out of the state.

She described herself to the therapist as having always been socially active both in community affairs and in her husband's business and social life. Mr. C. was employed as a senior salesman for a nationwide firm selling women's clothing. His work required frequent trips out of town and much business entertaining while at home. She seldom traveled with him (because of the children) but was deeply involved with planning and hostessing his in-town social engagements. She said that she enjoyed this and had always been confident of her ability to do it well. Part of her wife role was to wear the clothes of her husband's company as an unofficial model, and her husband had always expressed his pride in her attractiveness.

In recent weeks she had begun to feel inadequate in this role, and strong feelings of doubt regarding her ability had begun to plague her. At the same time she sensed that her husband was becoming indifferent to her efforts to keep herself and their home attractive to him. Her symptoms had overtly increased in the 2 days just past, until now she feared a complete loss of emotional control.

Mr. C. was 2 years older than she. He was socially adept, and her women friends frequently told her they thought he was "such a youthful, good-looking, and considerate person." She herself felt fortunate to have him for a husband. He was aggressive in business and could be sure of advancement. She said they had always been sexually compatible and shared interests and mutual esteem.

When asked about what had occurred in the past 2 days to increase her symptoms, she said that her husband had come home 2 nights ago and found her disheveled and crying and not ready to go to a scheduled business dinner for the second time in a week. He angrily told her that he did not know what to do and to "pull yourself together and find someone to help you because I've tried and I can't!" Then he left for the dinner alone. The next day he left town on a business trip after securing her promise to see a physician.

Mrs. C. said that she had seen several physicians during the past few months because of various physical complaints. None had found any organic cause, but all had advised her to get more rest—one even told her to find a hobby. The last physician, whom she saw 3 weeks ago, told her she was entering early menopause.

Mrs. C. had not told her husband of this because she feared his reaction in view of her own negative feelings; her initial reaction had been disbelief. This was followed by fear of "change of life," as she had heard of so many unfortunate things that could happen to a woman during this time. In common with all women, she did not want to become old and unattractive and was angry that it could be happening to her so soon! She thought that she would no longer be an asset to her husband in his work because his clothes were not designed for middle-aged women.

Mrs. C. had looked forward to traveling with her husband after their youngest daughter's marriage. They had planned such a future together enthusiastically, and she felt proud to have contributed to his success but was now afraid that he would not need her anymore and that all her plans were ruined.

Her expressed feelings of guilt and a fear of the loss of her feminine role were thought to be the crisis-precipitating events. She was not seen as a suicidal risk or as a threat to others, although she was depressed and expressed feelings of worthlessness. She was highly anxious but could maintain control over her actions.

PLANNING OF THERAPEUTIC INTERVENTION

Mrs. C. had withdrawn from her previous pattern of social and family activities. Her husband was frequently out of town, and the last of the daughters living at home had transferred many of her dependency needs to her fiance. Mrs. C. in the past 3 months had felt physically ill and had narrowed her social activities to infrequent luncheons "when I felt up to it." Her peer group was in the 35- to 40-year age level and were all actively involved in community affairs, family activities, and so on. Conversation with women friends still centered around problems of raising young children, and she believed that because her children were grown she no longer had much to offer to the conversation.

Her goals for a role change from busy parenthood to active participation with her husband in his business-social world were threatened, and she had no coping experiences in this particular situation. Previous methods of coping with stress were discussed. She related that she had always kept busy with their children and either forgot the problems or talked them out with close friends or her husband. She could not recall a close woman friend who had reached the menopausal stage and with whom she could discuss her feelings, and she was too fearful of the reaction she imagined her husband would have to discuss it with him. Her inability to communicate her feelings and the loss of busy work with her children eliminated any situational supports in her home environment, obviating the use of previously successful coping mechanisms. The goal of intervention established by the therapist was to assist Mrs. C. to an intellectual understanding of her crisis.

INTERVENTION

It was obvious to the therapist that Mrs. C. had little knowledge of the physiological and psychological changes that occur in menopause. She had no insight to her feelings of guilt and fear of the threatening loss of her feminine role. Unrecognized feelings about her relationship with her husband would be explored.

During the next 5 weeks, through the use of direct questioning and reflection of verbal and nonverbal clues with Mrs. C., it became possible for her to relate the present crisis and its effect to past separations from her husband (business trips) and her previous successful coping mechanisms.

Mrs. C. had married when she was 17 years old. She described herself as having been attractive and popular in school, busy at all sorts of school activities. Mr. C. had been what everyone considered quite a catch. He came from a prosperous family, had been a high school football captain and class president, and was sought after by many of her girlfriends. At the time of their marriage he was a freshman in college.

She always had a high regard for her physical attractiveness and her ability to fulfill the social role Mr. C. expected of her. Throughout the years when he traveled alone, she felt left out of a part of his life and had looked forward with great expectations to being able to be with him all of the time. Knowing that his business brought him in frequent contact with attractive women buyers and models, she regarded her own physical attractiveness as a prime requirement to "meet the competition." With Mr. C.'s frequent trips away from home she had magnified her role in the husband-wife relationship to be more on the physical-social level than in the shared role of parental responsibilities.

ANTICIPATORY PLANNING

Mrs. C. never questioned her physician after he informed her of his diagnosis of early onset of menopause, and obviously her knowledge was inadequate and based almost entirely on hearsay and myth rather than on fact. The physiological basis of

CASE STUDY: MRS. C

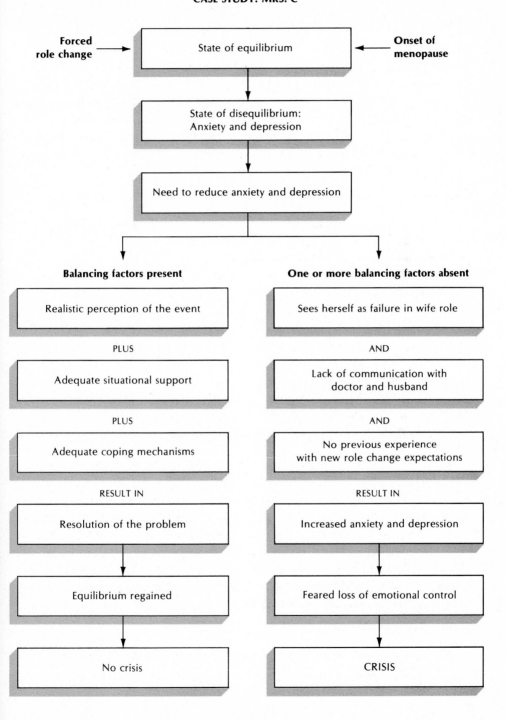

Forced role change → State of equilibrium ← Onset of menopause

State of disequilibrium:
Anxiety and depression

Need to reduce anxiety and depression

Balancing factors present

Realistic perception of the event

PLUS

Adequate situational support

PLUS

Adequate coping mechanisms

RESULT IN

Resolution of the problem

Equilibrium regained

No crisis

One or more balancing factors absent

Sees herself as failure in wife role

AND

Lack of communication with doctor and husband

AND

No previous experience with new role change expectations

RESULT IN

Increased anxiety and depression

Feared loss of emotional control

CRISIS

the process of aging was discussed, and much of her fear was allayed. This was an important phase of anticipatory planning.

She was given situational support in which to talk out her feelings of insecurity in her marriage and to view it in much more realistic terms. Relationships between the precipitating events and the crisis symptoms were explored.

By the third week Mrs. C. had made significant process toward reestablishing her coping skills. She no longer feared "getting old overnight" and was able to tell her husband that she was entering early menopause.

His response was, "What the hell! Is that why you have been acting so peculiar lately? You might have told me; the way you've been carrying on anyone would have thought you had just been told you had 6 months to live!" Although her first impulse was to interpret this as evidence of his indifference to her as a woman, she later saw it as positive proof of her own unrealistic fears. She returned to her medical doctor as advised for continuing care and planning for any physical problems that might arise in the future.

By the fifth week she expressed confidence in her ability to meet the goals that she and her husband had set for their future. Their daughter was married, and Mrs. C. was ready to leave town with her husband on a business trip. Before termination the adjustments she had made in coping with the crisis were reviewed and discussed with her.

SUMMATION OF THE PARADIGM

Mrs. C. had been unable to cope with the combined stresses of early menopausal symptoms and the need to change her family role. She avoided communicating her fears to anyone who might have given her situational support for fear they would confirm her own negative reactions. Increasing feelings of inadequacy, resulting in anxiety and depression, led to a crisis level of disequilibrium.

Initial intervention focused on the exploration of Mrs. C.'s knowledge of the physical and psychological changes that could occur in menopause. As she was encouraged to explore and ventilate her feelings about her relationship with her husband, her perception of the stressful situation became more realistic and her coping skills were reintroduced successfully.

Old age—theoretical concepts

Erikson's formulation of the stages of human development stops with late adulthood. Unfortunately, he has not extended his analysis to crisis stages encountered by the retrenching organism.

In human beings the aging process must not be viewed only in terms of chronological years but with regard for the complex interrelationships of biological, psychological, and sociological changes that occur during these years. There is no exact age of onset.

Generally, psychologists look on aging as a period of decline. The pace of physical decline is highly individual, occurring throughout life, yet it is most commonly attributed to the period loosely called old age. "Old age with respect to what?" is a most significant question. It could be one of many things—organic, sensory, or structural changes—and the significance of each is not fully understood.

Personality changes have been substantially investigated, but problems of interpretation have arisen because studies have been directed toward the segmentalized personality traits rather than the total organization or adaptiveness. Individual studies have found the aged to be "more set" in problem solving and to be "more stable" in their habits and tendencies than are younger subjects.

Abnormal behavior in the aged is difficult to diagnose because of the increase of organic damage with longevity. These abnormal patterns of experience and behavior develop along new lines with age and raise questions about the exact nature of endogenous psychosis and what part is played by reactive ill humor or somatically based psychosis. Abnormal mental attitudes may develop as reactions to loss of influence, destruction of or unfulfilled life goals, onset of human isolation, and threats to economic security.

Considerable research has been done in social attitudes and forces creating the role of the aged in our culture. Goffman's denotative grouping (1961) of total institutions defines those for the aged as being established to care for people thought to be helpless and insecure—the blind, orphaned, indigent, and aged. In essence this might define the negative attitudes of our society for the aged.

Our culture values mutual independence of the aged and their married children. Feelings of obligation on the part of adult children to support and care for their aging parents have declined with the establishment of social insurances of medical and other community forces. An exaggerated premium is placed on the physical and psychological attributes of youth. When a culture assigns a role to the individual, acceptance and performance of it depend greatly on her conception of the role as it relates to her own self-concept.

Sullivan (1953) refers to the "self" as the reflected appraisal of others that comes into being as a dynamism to preserve the feelings of security. As new evaluations are reflected, the individual is obliged to reconcile these new concepts of self with those preexisting. Increasing conflictual appraisals may result in increased tension and anxiety, leading to a state tantamount to the acceptance of, or resignation to, old-age status.

As in the first years of adolescence, these later years of life are characterized by physical, emotional, and social crises. The onset of physical infirmities may require that the aged person turn to her milieu for a measure of care and security. The presence or absence of environmental resources, as well as the degree to which help from others is required for survival, becomes of prime importance. The elderly who are economically secure, alert, and outgoing may be able to rise above social attitudes and be in the position of continuing to influence the lives of others, whereas those who are not in this position may be forced to play the roles designated by society's attitudes. Reisman's three ideal-typical outcomes of the aging process (1954) are as follows: (1) the autonomous people with creative resources who use them to advantage in old age, (2) those who are adjusted and remain so, and (3) those who are neither and so decay.

A study of centenarians by Dunbar and Dunbar, as quoted by Solomon (1954), found a high correlation between longevity and a particular type of ego structure, and most of the subjects had chosen independence from their children as a way of life. In many cases they contribute to the support of their dependents, many have an active sex life into the very late years, and few were found who retired to do nothing. They were not susceptible to feelings of uselessness and had maintained involvement in activities in which they took pride.

An apparent correlation between the degree of ego organization in early life and the degree maintained in the senescent years has been found. Those with strong ego organizations seem better able to withstand the increased stresses and conflicts of later years. According to Palmore (1973), it is highly probable that much of the functional mental illness among the aged is chiefly the result of stresses caused by loss of income, loss of role and status, bereavement, isolation through disability, and loss of cognitive functioning.

Fear of death is not unique to the aged; its proximity is undeniably closer to some. This is verified as groups of contemporaries become smaller because of attrition by death. The old *are* living longer. Various studies and observations have noted that feelings of anxiety about death are most commonly coped with by the mechanism of denial, but it is not unusual to hear the very aged speak of "welcoming death" or saying that they "have lived a full life and have no fear of death." The social taboos that our culture places on frank discussion about death may lead to suppression of fear, to increased anxiety, and to resulting disequilibrium.

The aged are also faced with the fear of invalidism or chronic debilitating illness that might lead to dependency on society for survival. This may lead to a regression to earlier childlike levels of ego organization as a means of adjusting. According to Slater (1963), the increased powerlessness and loss of authority status of the aged weakens the respect of youth. This may be followed by anger at the reversal in dependency roles, the ultimate destruction of the child role, and the anticipation of desertion by death. As a means of handling guilt that may arise as a result of ambivalence, young people project their feelings onto others. It is the aged who become malevolent, isolated, and alienated and who are denied participation in society for all the evils for which they are blamed.

Cumming and Henry (1961) have noted two critical events that take place during this period of life: the loss of a spouse and retirement. Both represent conclusions of central tasks of the adult life.

The loss of a spouse is particularly traumatic for the aging person. For both the widow and widower this represents the loss of a highly cathected person, one who has been a primary source of need satisfaction. There is a loss of emotional security and a feeling of intense loneliness at a time in life when only the most resourceful may be able to find means to redistribute the cathexis. The surviving spouse loses those aspects of social identity that were solely dependent on a marital partner role. Both the widow and the widower must develop social identities of their own, based on their own interests, economic status, and social skills as old social systems become closed to them and they are faced with finding and integrating into new ones.

Retirement is a highly critical time in a person's life. It is one thing if this occurs of one's own volition and planning; it becomes more complex when mandated by another. Losses include status identity based on identification with a productive and functional role in society. The retiree is also faced with the loss of a peer group.

Some people do not move easily into the role of pure sociability. Their focus of sociability has been directed toward their occupational peer groups, and loss of these groups through retirement leaves a void with few purely social skills to fill it.

Role reversal necessitated by a debilitating illness of a spouse is also a fertile area for the development of a crisis. Rarely is either spouse prepared socially, psychologically, or physically to assume all of the responsibilities of such a role change; the adjustments involved may be beyond the older individual's ability to cope and adapt.

It is evident that a continuation of maturational stages of development would be more difficult to define for the aged than for younger groups, since the processes of decline and growth occur concomitantly but not in equal balance. The process is highly individualized in all cases, and the variability of physiological, psychological, and sociological factors makes definite chronological relationships highly improbable.

When an elderly person seeks help, his symptomatology requires particularly close scrutiny before an interpretation for intervention is undertaken. The therapist must first be aware of his own tendencies to stereotype the client's appearance and symptoms as a normal aging syndrome. Determining which of the crisis symptoms may be the result of organicity is particularly important, since rapid onset of behavioral changes is not infrequently caused by cerebrovascular or other organic changes associated with longevity. A professional review of the current medical history of the individual must be a recognized part of the initial assessment phase.

Too often the individual, because of organic changes, cannot gain an intellectual understanding of the crisis or recognize his present feelings. It may also be that those who directed him to the therapist are themselves in crisis; if this is true, the therapist first may have to resolve the feelings of the referrer that have been projected toward the aged individual who seems to be in need of help.

In the aging process the ego organization needs to withstand increasing biopsychosocial threats to its integrity, and unfortunately the individual's coping abilities may fail to adapt to meet the threats. The ability to accept new value systems and adapt to necessary changes in the achieved maturational development of earlier years without loss of achieved integrity may indeed be a developmental task for the aged.

Case study   *Old age*

ASSESSMENT OF THE INDIVIDUAL AND THE PROBLEM

Sara was accompanied to the crisis center by her husband John, a former client who had come there for help when in crisis following the death of their only son about 10 years ago.

Sarah was 69 years of age, 3 years younger than John. She was neatly dressed, appeared to be slightly apprehensive, and walked with obvious difficulty, supported by a Canadian crutch and her husband's arm. After being assisted into a chair in the therapist's office, she quickly asked that John be allowed to remain with her during the interview. She stated that it "had really been John's idea that we both come here today. I'm sure that he can explain the problem better than I."

After a slight pause and several hesitations John began to speak. Sarah sat tensely forward on her chair, never taking her eyes from his face as he spoke.

According to John, their problem "probably first began" about 3 months ago when Sarah had fallen in the house and fractured her hip. After a month in the hospital she had been sent home in his care. The plan was for her to continue physiotherapy as an outpatient. Despite all of the therapy and exercises at home she was apparently not making the progress they had expected. "Look at her—she still can't walk alone! She still needs someone to help her about or she might fall again—and God knows what would happen to us then! It's been a worry for both of us."

As John continued to speak, it became quite obvious that he was avoiding any direct references to himself. He described Sarah as having recent symptoms of insomnia, anxiety, and depression and expressed the fear that she might be going into the same crisis symptoms that he had been treated for at the center 10 years ago. "It was sheer hell to feel the way I did then . . . she doesn't deserve to go through what I did then if she can be helped now."

As he spoke he was becoming obviously more agitated. He avoided eye contact with Sarah, kept moving about restlessly in his chair, was increasingly tense and tremulous, and chain smoked. His eyes frequently became tearful, and his voice broke on several occasions. In almost direct contrast to his behavior, Sarah had assumed a very supportive role, reaching out several times to pat his arm in a calming gesture and, finally, holding his hand tightly.

At the point when it seemed he might begin to cry openly, he abruptly stood up and said, "O.K., Sarah, I've told her all about the problem. Now I'm going to go take a walk for a while and let you do some of the talking, too." With that, he said he'd be back in about 20 minutes and left the office.

As soon as John had left, Sarah began to cry quietly. Then she gave several deep sighs and, for the first time, relaxed back into her chair. "Please," she asked the therapist, "can you help him again like you did the last time?" She stated that for the past week he had not slept more than an hour at a time during the night, paced constantly, cried easily and often for no apparent reason, and had reached the point where he now seemed too anxious and too preoccupied to make even the simplest of decisions.

According to Sarah, she and John had been married for 42 years. They had had only one son, who had died, unmarried, 10 years ago. While Sarah had never held a salaried job, she had always been very actively involved in both civic and church organizations in their community. After John's retirement from a federal service, she had withdrawn from several of these organizations in order to devote more time to activities that they could participate in together. They had developed many new social interests in common and maintained a fairly active social life. Sarah felt that the past 10 years had included some of the best times in their life together. They had always seemed to be planning something "for the future" and had acquired many new friends. Their home was completely paid for; they had planned wisely for financial security "in their old age"; and, until her accident, they had had few health problems to worry about.

Even after her hip fracture they had apparently been able to provide each other with the situational support needed to cope adequately with the many new changes arising in their daily lives. "After all," Sarah said, "it wasn't as though our world was going to come to an end because of this—only that it might have to slow down a bit until we could catch up again."

After a month in the hospital Sarah went home and arranged to continue therapy as an outpatient. Despite regular visits to physiotherapy and John's rigidly imposed schedule of exercising at home, her recovery had been much slower than they had anticipated. Last week her physician, also not satisfied with the rate of her progress, recommended that she seriously consider admission as a full-time inpatient to a well-known rehabilitation center in a nearby city. He was unable to guarantee how long she might have to remain, estimating only that it would be a minimum of 1 month.

She stated that at the time John seemed to be as much in agreement as she with the idea, although, she recollected, he had seemed a bit preoccupied on the drive home. He took her out to dinner that night to celebrate her improved chances for a full recovery.

That same night she was awakened several times by John getting out of bed and pacing about the house. When she mentioned it to him in the morning, he quickly apologized for disturbing her and blamed it on "too much coffee and food" the night before. She noticed, however, that he seemed very preoccupied that day, even to the point of having to be reminded by her when it was time for her exercises. Several times he asked if she felt confident that they were making the right decision, or if they should try to find another physician for her who might suggest "better treatments."

His tension and anxiety continued to increase over the next few days. He seemed unusually concerned with how she felt about the decision, and no amount of reassurance from her could convince him that she really wanted to go into the hospital for treatment. Several times yesterday she found him looking at her sadly with tears running down his face. His only explanation was that he felt "so sorry for you . . . having to go to a strange place . . . and I might not be there when you need me!" Last night he had not gone to bed at all but had sat chain smoking in the living room. She had not dared go to sleep for fear he would drop a cigarette and start a fire.

Several times during the past few days she had suggested he contact the crisis center to speak to his former therapist. At first he ignored her, then finally yesterday he had countered with the proposal that they go together. "I'm sure," he told her, "that you must be feeling just as anxious as I am about all of this." She said that she agreed to this because she could think of no other way to convince him to come alone. "Of course I'm upset about having to go back to a hospital," she told the therapist. "Anyone in my condition would like to have some sort of guarantee that they are going to improve—but my greatest concern is what this all has done to John." After discussing her feelings a bit longer with her, the therapist determined that Sarah appeared to be coping adequately with the recent events in her life and, although anxious and concerned about them, was indeed not in crisis.

Finding that John had returned from his walk, the therapist arranged to have Sarah wait outside and called him back into the office. He still appeared very tense, yet when confronted with his evident symptoms of depression and anxiety, he at first denied their severity. Then, after several evasive responses, he began to openly describe just how frightened and overwhelmed he had been feeling for the past week. "I just don't know what's going to happen to us next—I don't think I'll be able to handle much more. I was so sure she'd be back walking by this time. We did everything that the doctors told us to do—I worked so hard with her to keep up with the exercises and all of the appointments—and they haven't helped. Now she has to go back to the hospital. I feel that some of this is all my fault—maybe I didn't work hard enough with her—or maybe I was doing the exercises the wrong way. She hates being crippled like this. Sometimes I think she must hate me because she has to be so dependent on me for doing everything."

After Sarah had come home from the hospital 2 months ago, John had been kept very busy and involved in driving her to appointments, arranging the household schedules, and helping her exercise at home. He found many rewards in this role, feeling that he was contributing greatly toward her eventual recovery. However, as the weeks and months passed without too much apparent improvement in her condition, he was disturbed to find himself angry toward her, even at times blaming her for not trying harder. Lately he had been finding it increasingly difficult to hide these feelings from her and found himself wishing that he could just get away from the situation for awhile, to take a trip like they used to—even if it meant going off without her!

Now, because of her decision to go into the rehabilitation center for treatment, he was being given the opportunity to "get away from it all" for a while, to turn the responsibility for her daily exercises and care completely over to others, and he felt very guilty. Perhaps he had not really tried hard enough to help her walk; maybe he should have found ways to encourage her more. The more he ruminated on these thoughts, the more he convinced himself that her lack of progress was entirely his fault. Therefore it was his fault that she had to go back to a hospital, and it would be completely his fault if she were never able to return home again!

PLANNING THE INTERVENTION

The goals of intervention were to help John obtain a realistic perception of the situation, to assist him to ventilate his feelings about the effects of Sarah's disability on his life, and to provide him with situational support to help him cope with the pending loss of Sarah, albeit temporary at this point in time. Before the next session and with his consent, his personal physician was contacted to determine if there were any organic bases for his behavioral changes. The physician's report was negative.

INTERVENTION

During the next two sessions, through questioning and reflection, John was helped to ventilate his feelings about his fears that Sarah might never recover beyond her present level of functioning. With situational support supplied by the therapist, he was able to begin to openly discuss the anger that he had felt toward Sarah for "threatening the security of their future" by her accident. All of the careful planning they had made for their "old age" seemed to be falling apart more each day. "It wasn't just the financial security," he said, "we have enough insurance to take care of our illnesses. Our plans were all made for the *two* of us, *together*—not for just *one* of us, *alone*!" His fears of losing her had been displaced into anger against her for being the cause of his very unpleasant feelings.

It became quite apparent during the first session that John really did not have any clear idea as to the nature of Sarah's injury. To him, a broken bone was just that, regardless of which one. It broke; therefore it should heal! He had never sat down with her orthopedic surgeon to ask questions, leaving it to her to keep him informed. He was advised to make an immediate appointment with this physician in order to get direct information about Sarah's expected progress rather than to continue to rely on his own uneducated conclusions. By the next session he reported that he had followed through, kept the appointment, and was relieved to learn that while Sarah's progress was a bit slower than expected, the physician expected her to return to a fairly normal level of functioning. But, he was advised, it would take time, and he would be expected to help Sarah have patience. The recommendation that she enter the rehabilitation center in the next city was made in an effort to speed up her progress and was not to be construed by him as a sign that she might never recover.

As John's anxiety and depression decreased, he began to view the events leading up to his crisis in a more realistic manner. He realized that his anger was a normal response to his situation with Sarah but that she he *did* with that anger was not normal. Rather than openly discussing his feelings with Sarah as he would have at any other time in their lives, he found himself "protecting" her from them, yet blaming her for all of his misery. Since he lacked any other available situational support, his anxiety and depression had increased, even further distorting his perceptions of the event.

When the suggestion was made that Sarah enter a rehabilitation center for further therapy, John's anxiety level interfered with his ability to perceive this as anything other than the beginning of a final loss of Sarah from his life. As he later described it to the therapist, "I guess this is always in the back of a person's mind once they get around my age. When you're young you go to a hospital and the odds are good that you come home again—but when you get to be Sarah's and my age, the odds *aren't* so good that you come home again! And she was asking me to help her make the decision to go to that hospital—*me,* who was already mixed up in my feelings about having to take care of her like this the rest of my life!"

By the end of the third session John's symptoms had lessened greatly, and he was now able to help Sarah pack and move into the rehabilitation center without any increase in anxiety. He realized now that in overprotecting her from his true feelings, he had only created anxiety for her as well as a crisis for himself. He planned to visit her three times a week. They agreed that this would give her full time to concentrate on "being able to walk home," and he would begin to reestablish with their old friends so that he would not feel so lonely while she was away.

ANTICIPATORY PLANNING

Exploration with John about his feelings concerning the possibility that Sarah might not improve beyond her current level of functioning helped prepare him for this eventuality. He was able to begin to consider alternative modes of life for the two of them. For example, he decided that they should seriously consider selling their two-story home. "After all," he said, "if it isn't her broken hip, sure enough

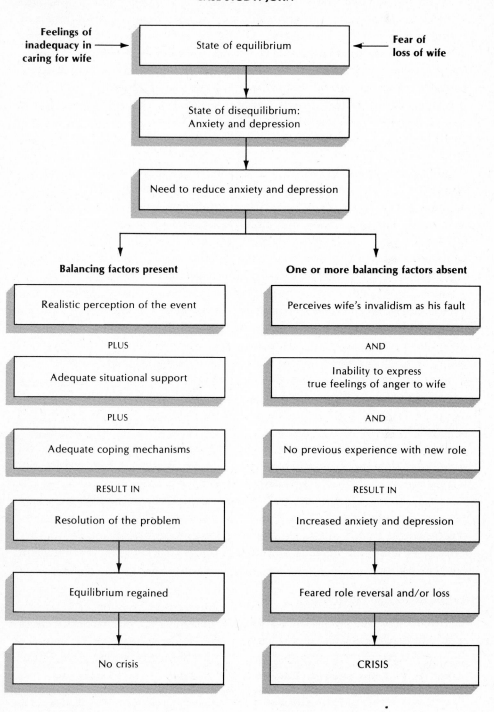

CASE STUDY: JOHN

Feelings of inadequacy in caring for wife → State of equilibrium ← Fear of loss of wife

State of disequilibrium: Anxiety and depression

Need to reduce anxiety and depression

Balancing factors present

Realistic perception of the event

PLUS

Adequate situational support

PLUS

Adequate coping mechanisms

RESULT IN

Resolution of the problem

Equilibrium regained

No crisis

One or more balancing factors absent

Perceives wife's invalidism as his fault

AND

Inability to express true feelings of anger to wife

AND

No previous experience with new role

RESULT IN

Increased anxiety and depression

Feared role reversal and/or loss

CRISIS

it's going to be my arthritis in the next few years that is going to make those stairs seem like Mount Whitney!" Furthermore, John found himself faced with the realities of what he would have to be able to do for himself if Sarah ever left him forever. While she was in the rehabilitation center, he knew that he would have to begin learning how to plan a life for himself. Although she might outlive him, he recognized that this time without her was a sample for him of what life "might be for him—and only a complete idiot would not recognize that I had better learn what to do and learn pretty damned fast!"

SUMMATION OF THE PARADIGM

Unprepared to assume his new role in caring for Sarah, John's increased anxiety distorted his perceptions of their stressful situation. When Sarah failed to make the progress that he had expected, he became frustrated and angry and saw himself as a failure in his new role. Unable to communicate these feelings appropriately, he displaced his anger on Sarah. When asked to help her decide about reentering a hospital, he felt threatened by a permanent role reversal and the eventuality of her loss. He lacked adequate coping mechanisms to deal with the increasing stresses of the situation; he became immobile and unable to make any decisions for their future.

Intervention focused on helping John to ventilate his feelings and to obtain a realistic perception of the event. As his anxiety and depression decreased, he became able to anticipate and plan for their future. The major focus of the last session was to help him recognize the accept that with increasing age there could be future threats to his biopsychosocial integrity and that he should learn to seek help as they arose and not try to assume all of the responsibility himself.

ADDENDUM

Two months later the therapist received a telephone call from John. Sarah had come home from the rehabilitation center about 2 weeks before. Her progress, unfortunately, was not what they had expected. However, according to John, she was at least able to stand there in the kitchen and make the "best damned dinner I have eaten in a month" and that was "good enough for me!" They had already put their home up for sale and were looking for a large mobile home into which they could move and begin traveling around the country to begin living the retirement they had planned.

References

Cameron, N.: Personality development and psychopathology, Boston, 1963, Houghton Mifflin Co.

Cumming, E., and Henry, W.E.: Growing old, New York, 1961, Basic Books, Inc., Publishers.

Dunbar, F., and Dunbar, F.: A study of centenarians. Quoted in Solomon, J.C.: A synthesis of

human behavior, New York, 1954, Grune & Stratton, Inc.

English, O.S., and Pearson, G.H.J.: Emotional problems of living, New York, 1955, W.W. Norton & Co., Inc.

Erikson, E.H.: Growth and crises of the health personality. In Senn, M.J.E., editor: Symposium on the healthy personality, New York, 1950, Josiah Macy, Jr., Foundation.

Erikson, E.H.: Identity and the life cycle. Psychological issues, vol. 1, No. 1, monograph I, New York, 1959, International Universities Press.

Erikson, E.H.: Childhood and society, ed. 2, New York, 1963, W.W. Norton & Co., Inc.

Goffman, E.: Asylums, New York, 1961, Doubleday & Co., Inc.

Hahn, M.E.: Psychoevaluation: adaptation, distribution, adjustment, New York, 1963, McGraw-Hill Book Co.

Palmore, E.B.: Social factors in mental illness of the aged. In Busse, E.W. and Pfeiffer, E., editors: Mental illness in later life, Washington, D.C., 1973, American Psychiatric Association.

Piaget, J.: The child's conception of the world, Totowa, N.J., 1963, Littlefield, Adams & Co.

Reisman, D.: Individualism reconsidered, New York, 1954, The Free Press.

Slater, P.: Cultural attitudes toward the aged, Geriatrics **18**:308, 1963.

Sullivan, H.S.: Conceptions of modern psychiatry, New York, 1953, W.W. Norton & Co., Inc.

Zachry, C.B.: Emotion and conduct in adolescence, New York, 1940, Appleton-Century-Crofts.

Additional readings

Aguilera, D.C.: Stressors in late adulthood, Fam. Community Health **2**(4):61, 1980.

Baumrind, D.: Reciprocal rights and responsibilities in parent-child relations, J. Soc. Issues **34**(2):179, 1978.

Bonnefil, M.C.: Crisis intervention with children and families, N. Directions Ment. Health Services **6**:23, 1980.

Breunlin, C., and Breunlin, D.C.: The family therapy approach to adolescent disturbances: a review of the literature, J. Adolescence **2**(2): 153, 1979.

Brown, H.F.: Crisis intervention in child abuse programs, Soc. Casework **7**:430, 1979.

Butler, R.N., and Lewis, M.I.: Aging and mental health: positive psychosocial and biomedical approaches, ed. 3, St. Louis, 1982, The C.V. Mosby Company.

Caley, B.: Outpatient services for the geriatric patient, Health Soc. Work **4**(1):201, 1979.

Cantor, M.: Neighbors and friends: an overlooked resource in the informal support system, Research on Aging **1**:434, 1979.

Cloudsley-Thomson, J.: Biological clocks, London, 1980, George Weidenfeld & Nicolson, Ltd.

Comfort, A.: The biology of senescence, New York, 1979, Elsevier.

Davis, R., editor: Aging prospects and issues, Los Angeles, 1981, University of Southern California Press.

Gelfind, D.E., and Fandetti, D.V.: Suburban and urban white ethnics: attitudes towards care of the aged, Gerontologist **20**(5):588, 1980.

Glick, P.C.: A demographer looks at the American family. In Savells, J., and Cross, L., editors: The changing family: making ways for tomorrow, New York, 1978, Holt, Rinehart & Winston.

Golant, S.M., editors: Location and environment of elderly population, New York, 1979, Halsted Press.

Goldman, G.D., and Milman, D.S., editors: Modern woman: her psychology and sexuality, Springfield, Ill., 1969, Charles C Thomas, Publisher.

Granetz, R., editor: Middle age, old age, New York, 1980, Harcourt Brace Jovanovich, Inc.

Grauer, H., and Frank, D.: Psychiatric aspects of geriatric crises intervention, Can. Psychiatr. Assoc. J. **23**:201, 1978.

Greenberg, J.: Old age: what is normal? Science News **115**:284, 1979.

Gross, S.J., and others: Crisis in the family: three approaches, New York, 1979, John Wiley & Sons, Inc.

Gwatkin, D., and Brandel, S.: Life expectancy and growth in the third world, Scientific American **246**:57, 1982.

Haley, J.: Leaving home, New York, 1980, McGraw-Hill Book Co.

Hefferin, E.A.: Life-cycle stressors: an overview of research, Fam. Community Health **2**(4):71, 1980.

Hellebrandt, F.A.: Aging among the advantaged: a new look at the stereotype of the elderly, Gerontologist **20**(4):404, 1980.

Herst, L.D.: Emergency psychiatry for the elderly, Psychiatr. Clin. North Am. **6**(2):271, 1983.

Hotchner, B.: Menopause and sexuality: gearing up or down? Top. Clin. Nurs. **1**:45, 1980.

Johnson, E.S., and Williamson, J.B.: Growing old: the social problems of aging, New York, 1980, Holt, Rinehart & Winston, Inc.

Kaluger, G., and Kaluger, M.F.: Human development: the span of life, ed. 3, St. Louis, 1984, Times Mirror/Mosby College Publishing.

Kent, S.: The evolution of longevity, Geriatrics **35**:98, 1980.

Kirschner, C.: The aging family in crisis: a problem in living, Soc. Casework **60**(4):209, 1979.

Kolbenschlag, M.: Kiss Sleeping Beauty goodbye: breaking the spell of feminine myths and models, New York, 1979, Doubleday & Co., Inc.

Kübler-Ross, E.: Questions and answers on death and dying, New York, 1974, Collier Books.

Lamy, P.P.: Consider all factors when treating the elderly, Long Term Care Health Serv. Admin. Q. **3**(3):194, 1979.

Malone, C.A.: Child psychiatry and family therapy: an overview, J. Am. Acad. Child Psychiatry **18**:4, Jan. 1979.

Miller, J.: Making old age measure up, Science News **120**:74, 1981.

Morely, W.E.: Crisis intervention with adults, N. Directions Ment. Health Serv. **6**:11, 1980.

Morgan, C.S.: Female and male attitudes towards life: implications for theories of mental health, Sex Roles: J. Res **6**:367, 1980.

Motto, J.A.: New approaches to crisis intervention, Suicide **9**:173, March 1979.

Murphy, L.B.: Coping, vulnerability, and resiliency in childhood. In Coehlo, G.V., and others: Coping and adaptation, New York, 1974, Basic Books, Inc.

Pelletier, K.: Longevity, New York, 1981, Delacorte Press.

Piaget, J., and Inhelder, B.: The psychology of the child, New York, 1969, Basic Books, Inc., Publishers.

Pruett, H.L.: Stressors in middle adulthood, Fam. Community Health **2**(4):53, 1980.

Reres, M.E.: Stressors in adolescence, Fam. Community Health **2**(4):31, 1980.

Ruffin, J., and Urquhart, P.: A comprehensive geratric mental health service in San Francisco, Int. J. Ment. Health **8**(3-4):101, 1980.

Schwenk, T.L., and Bittle, S.P.: Applicability of crisis intervention in family practice, J. Fam. Pract. **8**(6):1151, 1979.

Sexsmith, D.G.: Stressors in early adulthood, Fam. Community Health **2**(4):43, 1980.

Shanas, E.: The family as a social support system in old age, Gerontologist **19**(2):169, 1979.

Sheehy, Gail: Passages: predictable crises of adult life, New York, 1977, Bantam Books.

Sill, J.S.: Disengagement reconsidered: awareness of finitude, Gerontologist **20**(4):457, 1980.

Snow, D.L., and Gordon, J.B.: Social network analysis and intervention with the elderly, Gerontologist **20**(4):463, 1980.

Stern, D.: The first relationship—mother and infant, Cambridge, Mass., 1977, Harvard University Press.

Stevenson, J.S.: Issues and crises during middlescence, New York, 1977, Appleton-Century-Crofts.

Valente, S.M.: Stressors at school age, Fam. Community Health **2**(4):15, 1980.

Watson, W.H.: Stress and old age, New Brunswick, N.J., 1980, Transaction Books.

chapter 8

Burn-out syndrome

In this text *burn-out* refers to a progressive loss of idealism, energy, and purpose experienced by people in the helping professions as a result of the conditions of their work. These conditions may include insufficient training, client overload, too many hours, too little pay, inadequate funding, ungrateful clients, bureaucratic or political constraints, and the gap between aspiration and accomplishment.

The word burn-out came into professional literature in 1974 with the first of Freudenberger's articles on staff burn-out in alternative help-giving facilities, such as free clinics, that exist outside the established institutional structures of society and depend on dedicated volunteer help. It was then recognized that the concept applied equally well to the salaried or self-employed professional in an "establishment" position. Recently articles have been published on burn-out syndrome among teachers, police officers, attorneys, nurses, mental health workers, and day care staff (Ellison and Geng, 1978; Hendrickson, 1979; Maslach and Jackson, 1979; Maslach and Pines, 1977; Pines and Maslach, 1978; Shubin, 1978).

The most definitive work on burn-out syndrome is the text authored by Edelwich and Brodsky (1980). According to Edelwich and Brodsky, the four stages of disillusionment that occur are (1) enthusiasm, (2) stagnation, (3) frustration, and (4) apathy. Each of these stages of disillusionment is discussed briefly and a fifth stage, that of hopelessness, is included, as well as some intervention techniques.

Stages of disillusionment
Enthusiasm

Enthusiasm is the initial period of high hopes, high energy, and unrealistic expectations. During this period the person does not need anything in life but the job because the job promises to be everything. Overidentification with clients and excessive and inefficient expenditure of one's own energy are the major hazards of this stage.

People go into the human services to make a living but not to make money. Although the full extent of the inequities in salaries between publicly funded service positions and jobs in the private sector may become apparent only after a person has invested years of training and work in a helping profession, the person is generally aware that such professions do not pay especially well. The motivation is a desire to "help" people. Individuals become "helpers" because they really enjoy working with people and they want to make a difference in people's lives. Those who are genuinely involved far outnumber those who are cynical and self-seeking.

An important factor in bringing people into the human services is the example of others. People want to be like the people who have helped them. This is especially common in teaching and medicine, since every young person is exposed to teachers and physicians, some of whom are inspiring models.

In other human services fields the experience of being a client often engenders the desire to be a helper (Edelwich and Brodsky). The experience of being helped provides the strongest demonstration of the value of helping. At the same time, it creates expectations of what it would be like to assume the role of helper. People who have been counseled unsuccessfully do not become counselors. The people who become counselors are those who have been counseled successfully, and their experiences as cooperative clients who have benefited from the services offered them may give them unrealistic expectations. They may expect all clients to be as receptive and resourceful as they were and all counselors to be as competent and caring as those who counseled them.

Enthusiasm comes not only from high initial motivation but also from early successes and satisfactions on the job. The new counselor or social worker, needing a certain amount of structure and supervision, tends to be put to work in environments that are safer and more rewarding than those that they will face later. When the social worker has moved out into tougher, more demanding environments and has exhausted the capacity for self-reinforcement as well, she tends to look back on those halcyon days with a certain wistful nostalgia.

In the stage of enthusiasm it is commonly believed that the job is the person's whole life and that all gratifications are coming from the job. This unbalanced existence comes about by a kind of vicious cycle. On the one hand, an inflated conception of the job tends to obliterate personal needs and concerns. On the other hand, glorification of work may arise from deficiencies in an individual's personal life. The cycle of overcommitment is self-fulfilling because the longer the personal life is neglected, the more it deteriorates. The helper is thus left in a highly vulnerable position when the job ceases to furnish the rewards it once did (Edelwich and Brodsky).

Overidentification with clients is a major link in the chain that stretches from enthusiasm to burn-out, both because it leads the helper to act in ways that are detrimental to clients and because it makes the helper's emotional well-being depend on the client's living up to unrealistic expectations. Overidentification stems from an excess of energy and dedication, a lack of knowledge and experience in the field, and a confusion of personal needs with those of clients. It manifests itself as a lack of clarity in role definitions between client and helper. It leads well-meaning professionals and paraprofessionals to make themselves available to receive telephone calls at home at all hours of the night, a degree of accessibility that can have damaging effects on the helper's life.

The problem facing those who are dedicated to human services is to be realistic enough to cope with discouraging conditions without suffering a total loss of idealism and concern. This is also the lesson that needs to be conveyed to students and trainees. This is the area where intervention is the most crucial, especially when a person reflects that an initial lack of realism is what leaves him most vulnerable to eventual disillusionment.

Stagnation

According to Edelwich and Brodsky, stagnation refers to the process of becoming stalled after an initial burst of enthusiasm. It is the loss of the momentum of hope and desire that originally brought the person into the helping professions. No sharp distinction can be drawn between stagnation and frustration, or between any two of the four stages of burn-out. The progression through the four stages is not something that can be traced in precise chronological sequence in any given instance.

When accomplishments are reduced to a human scale, minor annoyances such as low pay and long hours begin to be noticed. The frustrations that occur at this point are not enough to question doing the job, but they are enough to question doing nothing but the job.

In stagnation a person is still doing the job, but the job can no longer make up for the fact that personal needs—to earn a decent living, to be respected on and off the job, to have satisfying family and social relationships, and to have some leisure time in which to enjoy them—are not being met. If those needs remain unmet, that person will not be able to keep on doing the job for very long.

Stagnation often begins with the discovery that it is not as easy as anticipated to see, let alone assess, the results of one's labors. Initially it is experienced not as a source of active discontent but as a kind of bewilderment that leaves a person wondering why the job is not quite what it appeared to be. At the heart of stagnation lies the feeling that one's career is at a dead end (Edelwich and Brodsky).

Frustration

In the stage of frustration, individuals who have set out to give others what they need find that they themselves are not getting what they want. They are not doing the job they set out to do. In essence, they are not really "helping." Besides the low pay, long hours, and low status, there is a more basic frustration in the helping professions. It is extremely difficult to change people—and it is even more difficult under negatively perceived working conditions.

The sensation of powerlessness is felt at many levels by people in the helping professions. Most obvious is the powerlessness felt by front-line workers who occupy the lowest positions in the decision-making hierarchy, for example, the therapist who has no way to compel his crisis patients to keep their appointments with him. Powerlessness is relative to a person's position. A frequent complaint of supervisors is that their subordinates credit them with more power than they actually have.

The feeling of powerlessness is universal: it goes beyond hierarchical status. Its broader implications are the inability to change the system and the inability to control patients, subordinates, superiors, or the agency. This is the frustration that leads directly to burn-out.

Notwithstanding the idealism that motivates people to enter the helping professions, the issues of power and control are central to the helping relationship. Some people complain that they do not have enough power, while others complain that they have too much power. The unresponsiveness of the system to the people working in it is seen as a lack of appreciation. Individuals who are not given responsibility, are not consulted about decisions, and are generally overlooked by the bureaucratic system will certainly believe they are not appreciated by their supervisor or by the organization as a whole.

Appreciation from clients is what enables the individual to go on despite lack of institutional support. A person can take the stress from the supervisor when he is appreciated and receives positive feedback from clients. When they, too, are unappreciative, it makes that person question the whole purpose in being there. Helping people is what it is all about.

The effects of frustration, and of stagnation as well, on the quality of services rendered to individuals is all too evident. Implicit and explicit in the accounts of overwork, inadequate funding, staff polarization, bureaucratic sluggishness, and other sources of discouragement and demoralization among staff members is the almost inevitable conclusion that the client is the one who suffers.

The importance of frustration for burn-out lies in what a person does with it. Reaction to frustration has a great deal to do with whether or not she will fall deeper into burn-out and, ultimately, whether or not she can stay in the field. A person can respond to frustration in three ways: (1) use it as a source of negative energy, (2) use it as a source of positive energy, or (3) just withdraw from the situation.

There is no doubt that frustration creates energy. When it is an energy of willful denial, a frenzy of activity aimed at evading the reality of frustration or doing away with the causes of frustration that are among the givens of the situation, then it is a self-destructive, negative energy. The energy of frustration can also be directed into a constructive effort. By taking responsibility, confronting issues, and taking actions that may bring about change, a person can release some of the emotional tension created by frustration. Frustration can be a major turning point in the progression through the stages. An individual who misses this turn is likely to descend into apathy.

Probably the most common response to frustration is not to express it at all, but to internalize it and withdraw from the threatening situation. The helper avoids clients because he has come to dislike or resent them, despairs of being able to do anything for them, or is physically exhausted. Some individuals walk away from their jobs and from their idealism and concern. Then they may get angry, assert themselves, and get back into the center of things. Others, unfortunately, drift into the fourth and last stage of burn-out—apathy (Edelwich and Brodsky).

Apathy

Apathy takes the form of a progressive emotional detachment in the face of frustration. The starting point is the enthusiasm, the idealism, and overidentification of the beginner. If one is to come down from the clouds and work effectively, some detachment is desirable and inevitable. But most individuals do not have ideal learning conditions and sympathetic guidance to help them reach an optimum level of detachment. Frustration comes as it will, sometimes brutally, and the detachment that develops in its wake is less a poised emotional distancing than a kind of numbness. In turning off to frustrating experiences, a person may well turn off to people's needs and to his own caring. Apathy can be felt as boredom. The once-idealistic helper can trace the erosion of the desire to help and the feeling of involvement with patients that he used to have. People who started out caring about others end up caring mainly about their own health, sanity, peace of mind, and survival.

The most severe, and saddest, form of apathy is that which is experienced when a person remains at a job for one reason only—because the job is needed to survive. The person has seen what is going on but has no inclination to try to change it. Certainly no risks will be taken when the individual can just go along, protecting the position while doing as little as possible. Security has become the prime concern.

Of all the stages of burn-out, apathy is the hardest to overcome and the one against which it is most difficult to intervene successfully. It is the most settled, the most deep-seated, the one that takes the longest to arrive at, and lasts the longest. It stems from a decision, reached over a period of time and reinforced by one's peers, to stop caring. In the absence of a major personal upheaval, vastly changed conditions on the job, or a concerted intervention, it can last forever.

Hopelessness

Edelwich and Brodsky did not discuss hopelessness as a stage in the process of disillusionment; it is, however, implicity evident in their stages of stagnation, frustration, and apathy. According to Horney (1967), hopelessness is the ultimate product of unresolved conflicts. It is looking forward to an event or an occurrence with the deeply held belief that the anticipated will not occur.

When hope is lost a person may be in the stage of stagnation, frustration, or apathy. Hopelessness may fluctuate throughout the stages, diminishing at times and then returning full force to make the individual feel like giving up the role of helper. When the helper is experiencing hopelessness he has a tendency to deny or to avoid revealing any personal thoughts or feelings that could be considered "un-professional" and to behave instead as if he were in control of the situation and do-ing well. Failing to share true feelings with others leads to the erroneous assump-tion that he is the only one having such problems. This error is further enhanced by the fact that the individual who believes he is alone in having these feelings will be especially careful not to reveal this response to others and will maintain the facade of professionalism.

Intervention

Intervention may be self-initiated or it may occur in response to an immediate frustration or threat. It may be fueled in part by a person's own strength and in part by support and guidance from peers, supervisors, family and friends, or who-ever else is important in her life. It may be a temporary stopgap or a real change.

Intervention can, and should, occur at any of the four stages of disillusionment. One of the major tasks of trainers and supervisors should be to help staff members experience the four stages with greater awareness and thus be less subject to violent swings of emotion. In reality though, intervention most often takes place at the stage of frustration, when it is almost too late. In the stage of enthusiasm people are having too good a time to see any need for intervention. Stagnation does not usual-ly provide the energy required to change course, though interventions in the areas of further education, skill development, and career advancement are sometimes ini-tiated at this stage. As for apathy, that stage is already a long way down into disillu-sionment, and the road back up is a long, hard one that some individuals negotiate successfully but many never attempt.

More often it is frustration that moves a person off center and impels change. Frustration is not so bad when it gets people angry enough to break out of a bad sit-uation instead of becoming apathetic.

Nothing is more important in handling burn-out than to know what responsi-bilities the individual does and does not have. The professional is not responsible for clients or for the institution but is responsible for herself. This does not mean that the professional does not become involved with patients or does not try to change the way the institution is run. It simply means that she is responsible for her own actions, not theirs, and remains responsible for her actions regardless of what they do or do not do.

When other systems in life are strengthened, the individual gains strength for coping with work as well. The things people do to strengthen their outside lives and create a larger world to live in vary from individual to individual. An important first step is to make a clear separation between work and other areas of life by limit-ing off-hours socializing with co-workers, or others in the same field, and controlling the tendency toward extracurricular preoccupation with job-related issues. The number of hours required at work is usually set, but the rest of the day is controlled by the individual. The professional can, however, refuse to give friends and relatives free professional assistance with their personal problems. The benefits of giving a home telephone number to clients in order to be available to them in an emergency must be weighed against the costs.

Probably the most important way of enlarging a person's world is through close personal and family relationships. Developing and maintaining these relationships requires, and in turn creates, time commitments and emotional commitments that keep the person from being devoured by the job. It may take a lot of work to negotiate with family and close friends the space needed for commitment to the job and the space all concerned need to be together and to be away from constant reminders of the job. But it is by making this effort that an identity independent of the job is created. There are, of course, many other reasons for wanting to have a fulfilling personal life. With regard to burn-out, however, the importance of close personal ties is clear and crucial. When one is loved and appreciated by the family, whether one is loved and appreciated by clients or supervisors is no longer a life-or-death matter. When deep and constant support of family and friends is enjoyed, a person's whole self is not put on the line every morning.

Other interventions could include the technique of planned, temporary social isolation. At a minimum, professionals need times when they can get away from those who are often the direct source of job stress—the recipients and, in some cases, the administrators. This can be accomplished through physical and psychological withdrawals and long vacations (Edelwich and Brodsky).

Another alternative is a "decompression routine" between leaving work and arriving home, a time in which they can engage in some solitary activity, preferably physical and noncognitive, in order to unwind and relax. By being alone for awhile, they are then more ready to be with people again, especially with those people who are close to them.

Some helping professionals deliberately use some of their off-duty hours to engage in activities with people who are normal, healthy, and well functioning. By having pleasant and successful interactions with these people, professionals can counteract the development of negative attitudes about clients and about their ability to work well with clients.

Case study   *Burn-out*

Alan was a 24-year-old trainee in crisis intervention at a community mental health center. Alan was a graduate in psychology from a very well known eastern university. At their first meeting he impressed one of his supervisors with his solid theoretical background and his great enthusiasm at being accepted as an intern at the mental health center. He was attractive, tall, had a physique like that of an athlete, and was very expressive. Because he was in that city for the first time the supervisor questioned him about his living arrangements. He stated that he was sharing a townhouse with two other interns and that they were having "a ball."

Because the center is very busy, after their orientation the interns were immediately booked to see clients. Alan spent his time in supervision discussing his clients with great enthusiasm and discussing his plans for intervention in each case. For the first 3 months everything went very well. He was apparently functioning well as an effective therapist. He was able to glow with pride when he had successes and was able to accept the fact that he could not "cure" everyone.

In the next 2 months Alan began to show some psychological changes. His enthusiasm was beginning to diminish and he appeared more concerned about his clients who were not responding to therapy—as *he* expected them to. When discussing this in his supervisory hour, he tried to pass over his concerns by saying, "I know I'm good—they won't do what I want because I'm too young." When questioned about what he did in his time off he smiled ruefully and said, "What time off? I am here 5 days a week and I volunteered to be a co-leader in four groups at another center every weekend." His supervisor asked why he believed he should "work" 7 days a week; he shrugged and said, "I feel it is a good learning experience—working as a co-leader." She continued to press the issue by saying, "Alan, when do you have fun? What about the girl you were dating and the sailing you used to do every weekend?" He said soberly, "Gone with the wind."

Alan appeared angry and bitter when the supervisor strongly suggested that he was jeopardizing his internship at the center by working on weekends and that he should terminate at the other center. He responded bitterly, "But they need me!" He was informed that he had no choice in the matter, that working with crisis clients was emotionally exhausting, and that everyone needs time for themselves to recoup from the stress of being on call every night for their clients if needed. He very reluctantly agreed to stop working weekends.

Over the next 2 months Alan began to withdraw from his peers and seemed tired, pale, and thin. He appeared for supervision each week but had little enthusiasm and was poorly prepared to discuss the clients he was seeing. When this was pointed out to him, he merely replied flatly, "I try to help them—but if they don't want it—so what." He denied that he was working weekends. He was informed that his performance at the center was poor and complaints had been received that he was not returning his clients' telephone calls. He responded by saying that "they are just neurotic and dependent." He was told that a meeting was scheduled with his other supervisors the next week and his presence would be required; he shrugged and agreed to be there.

Two days later, while in the main office where the switchboard is located, the supervisor was getting her mail when Alan walked in. The operator said, "Alan, I

CASE STUDY: ALAN

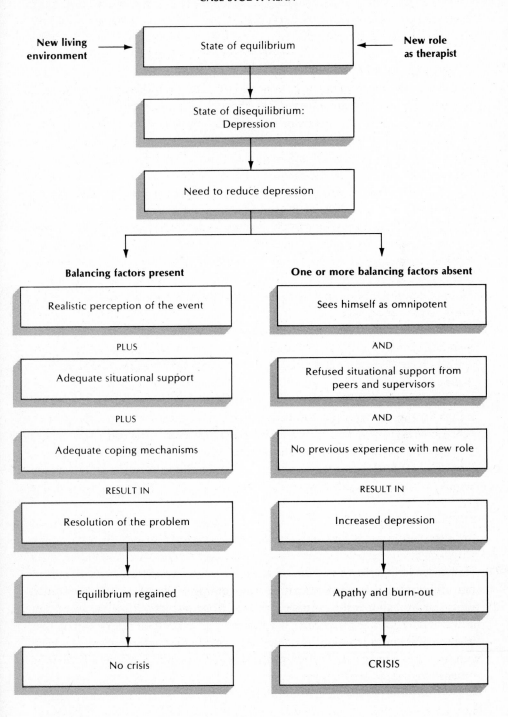

have a call for you—it's an emergency." Alan replied, "Just take a message." The supervisor turned to Alan and said firmly, "Alan, take that call at the other telephone." He sighed and agreed. He answered the telephone, listened for a few seconds, and then responded, "Oh my God! No!" and dropped the telephone. His supervisor picked it up and identified herself. On the line was a physician at a nearby emergency room; one of Alan's clients had successfully committed suicide. In his hand was his appointment card with Alan's name and the center's emergency telephone number. The supervisor took Alan by the arm (he was pale, trembling, and crying) and led him to her office. She let him cry and ventilate his feelings over losing a client and gave him coffee and facial tissues until he was able to control himself. She told him that she believed there should be an emergency meeting with him and his other supervisors. He agreed, the appropriate contacts were made, and a conference room was scheduled.

All of his supervisors gave Alan great emotional support as he told them his feelings after losing a client. As a group they all expressed to Alan how very much he needed a long vacation to recoup and to gain a different perspective on his role as a therapist. It was recommended that Alan return to his home in the East for a minimum of 3 months before resuming his internship at the center. He agreed that he would do as they asked.

Four months later Alan returned to continue his internship at the center with a surprise—a bride! He appeared relaxed, happy, and very sound. His wife, Kay, was delightful; they had gone to school together and they met again when he returned home.

The rest of Alan's internship went smoothly in every respect; he was more mature in his judgments, his enthusiasm was present, but, most importantly, he spent time off with his wife and they went sailing almost every weekend.

Alan apparently experienced burn-out, from enthusiasm to frustration, hopelessness, and then apathy. Fortunately, after an enforced vacation he was able to again function in a healthy manner as a therapist.

SUMMATION OF THE PARADIGM

Intervention focused on helping Alan to recognize that he had been overextending himself and had lost his sense of objectivity when working with his clients. He was living in a new environment and adjusting to a new role—that of a therapist. He became depressed when his clients did not respond as he believed they should; he truly believed he could "cure" everyone. He refused all situational support from his peers and supervisor. He had no previous experience or coping skills in his new role as a "helper," his depression increased, and he became apathetic, entering the fourth stage of burn-out and then crisis. With the assistance of his supervisors and with peer support he was finally able to accept the reality that a therapist can never become "all things to all people."

References

Edelwich, J., and Brodsky, S.: Burn-out: stages of disillusionment in the helping professions, New York, 1980, Human Sciences Press.

Ellison, K.W., and Geng, J.L.: The police officer as burned-out samaritan, FBI Law Enforcement Bulletin, March 1978.

Freudenberger, H.J.: Staff burn-out, J. Soc. Issues 30(1):159, 1974.

Hendrickson, B.: Teacher burn-out: how to recognize it; what to do about it, Learning 37, January 1979.

Horney, K.: Feminine psychology, New York, 1967, W.W. Norton and Co., Inc.

Larson, C., Gilbertson, D., and Powell, J.: Therapist burn-out: perspectives on a critical issue, Soc. Casework 59(9):563, 1978.

Maslach, C., and Jackson, S.E.: Burned-out cops and their families, Psychol. Today 12(12):59, 1979.

Maslach, C., and Pines, A.: The burn-out syndrome in the day care setting, Child Care Q. 6:100, 1977.

Pines, A., and Maslach, C.: Characteristics of staff burn-out in mental health settings, Hosp. Community Psychiatry 29:233, 1978.

Shubin, S.: Burn-out: the professional hazard you face in nursing, Nursing '78 8(7):22, July 1978.

Additional readings

Adler, G.: Helplessness in the helpers, Br. J. Med. Psychol. 45:315, 1972.

Berg, M.: Tune in, turn on, dropout? Imprint 27(4):11, 1980.

Daley, M.: Preventing worker burnout in child welfare, Child Welfare 58(7):443, 1979.

Depue, R.L.: Turning inward: the police officer counselor, F.B.I. Law Enforcement Bulletin 48:8, Feb. 1979.

Forbes, R.: Corporate stress, Garden City, N.Y., 1979, Doubleday Publishing Co.

Freudenberger, H., and Robbins, A.: The hazards of being a psychoanalyst, Psychoanalytic Rev. 66(2):275, 1979.

Freudenberger, H.J.: The staff burnout syndrome in alternative institutions, Psychotherapy: theory, research and practice 12(1):73, 1975.

Hall, R., and others: The professional burnout syndrome, Psychiatric Opinion 16(4):12, 1979.

Lamb, H.R.: Staff burn-out in work with long-term patients, Hosp. Community Psychiatry 30(6):396, 1979.

Maslach, C.: The client role in staff burn-out, J. Soc. Issues 34(4):111, 1978.

Spaniol, L., and Caputo, J.J.: Professional burn-out, Lexington, Mass., 1979, Human Services Association.

Storlie, F.: Burnout: the elaboration of a concept, Am. J. Nurs. 79(12):2108, 1979.

Valle, S.: Burn-out: occupational hazard for counselors, Alcohol Health Res. World 3(3):10, 1979.

Index